SLEEP MEDICINE: A GUIDE TO SLEEP AND ITS DISORDERS

Sleep Medicine: A Guide to Sleep and its Disorders

Second edition

JOHN M. SHNEERSON
MA, DM, FRCP, FCCP

Consultant Physician
Director of Respiratory Support and Sleep Centre
Papworth Hospital, Cambridge, UK

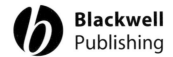
Blackwell Publishing

© 2005 John Shneerson
Published by Blackwell Publishing Ltd
Blackwell Publishing, Inc., 350 Main Street, Malden, Massachusetts 02148-5020, USA
Blackwell Publishing Ltd, 9600 Garsington Road, Oxford OX4 2DQ, UK
Blackwell Publishing Asia Pty Ltd, 550 Swanston Street, Carlton, Victoria 3053, Australia

The right of the Author to be identified as the Author of this Work has been asserted in
accordance with the Copyright, Designs and Patents Act 1988.

First edition published 2000
Second edition published 2005

Library of Congress Cataloging-in-Publication Data

Shneerson, John.
    Sleep medicine : a guide to sleep and its disorders / John M. Shneerson. — 2nd ed.
      p. ; cm.
    Rev. ed. of: Handbook of sleep medicine. 2000.
    Includes bibliographical references and index.
    ISBN 1-4051-2393-1 (alk. paper)
    1. Sleep disorders—Handbooks, manuals, etc.   2. Sleep—Physiological aspects—
  Handbooks, manuals, etc.   I. John M. Shneerson. Handbook of sleep medicine.
  II. Title.
    [DNLM: 1. Sleep Disorders.   2. Sleep—physiology.   WM 188 S558h 2005]
  RC547.S475 2005
  616.8′498—dc22

                                                                        2005006321

ISBN-13: 978-1-4051-2393-8
ISBN-10: 1-4051-2393-1

A catalogue record for this title is available from the British Library

Set in 9/11.5pt Sabon by Graphicraft Limited, Hong Kong
Printed and bound in India by Replika Press Pvt Ltd

Commissioning Editor: Maria Khan
Development Editor: Claire Bonnett
Production Controller: Kate Charman

For further information on Blackwell Publishing, visit our website:
http://www.blackwellpublishing.com

The publisher's policy is to use permanent paper from mills that operate a sustainable
forestry policy, and which has been manufactured from pulp processed using acid-free and
elementary chlorine-free practices. Furthermore, the publisher ensures that the text paper and
cover board used have met acceptable environmental accreditation standards.

Contents

Preface

Sleep disorders still often remain unrecognized and untreated despite the rapid advances in the understanding of their nature over the last few years. Sleep medicine as a specialty is only beginning to evolve and communication is often lacking between sleep specialists and other doctors who are developing an interest in sleep problems. I hope this book will bridge this gap by providing an up-to-date account of views on sleep and its disorders.

Sleep medicine crosses the conventional medical specialties and this has made it difficult for any one person to remain informed about the whole field. It has, however, opened up interesting interfaces between the specialties that have generated new ideas and treatments. The study of sleep disorders is one of the fastest developing areas of medicine with a rapidly growing scientific basis for clinical practice. The aim of this book is to provide an integrated view of clinical problems that fall within each of the medical sub-specialties and to illustrate how their assessment and treatment are based on an understanding of the abnormal processes occurring during sleep.

The initial chapter deals with the individual's need for sleep and the biological and social influences on this. This is followed by a detailed discussion of the physiology of sleep and its control. The assessment of sleep disorders and the increasingly important topic of drug-related sleep problems are covered. The remainder of the book concentrates on clinical presentations. The approach is primarily symptom-based, but there are two important chapters on respiratory complications and the final chapter deals with sleep problems in other medical disorders.

I hope that this book will be of interest to sleep specialists, respiratory physicians, neurologists, psychiatrists and general internal physicians involved with patients with sleep problems. The influence of age is emphasized and both paediatricians and those caring for the elderly will find topics of importance. The underlying mechanisms of sleep and its disorders should appeal to sleep researchers and those with a technical training. The integrated approach should prove helpful to nurses and other healthcare professionals involved in sleep problems.

I would like to thank Blackwell Publishing for their help with the preparation of this book, and especially Jill Dellar who has invariably coped without any fuss, met almost impossible deadlines and helped in many other ways with the preparation of the manuscript. Finally, my wife Anne has been a source of encouragement throughout and has been patient and understanding at every stage of the preparation of this book. Without her help it would not have been completed.

John M. Shneerson

1 Nature of Sleep and its Disorders

Characteristics of sleep

Sleep is recognizable by its contrast to wakefulness. It is a state of reduced awareness and responsiveness, both to internal and external stimuli. This reduced awareness is, however, selective [1]. It is an active process in which the significance of stimuli to the individual is interpreted and this determines whether arousal from sleep occurs. The crying of a child is, for instance, more likely to wake the parent than a different noise of the same intensity.

A second feature of sleep is motor inhibition (Table 1.1). The sleeping subject appears quiescent, but some movements occur, such as rapid eye movements. For each species there is a characteristic posture or type of movement that is adopted during sleep. Humans usually lie down, but many birds perch while asleep, horses may stand, vampire bats sleep upside down, dolphins and whales swim, and albatrosses can fly. In some of these animals, in contrast to humans, sleep is not accompanied by physical inactivity. Humans usually sleep with the eyes closed, but some animals, such as cattle, sleep with their eyes open.

Sleep is a cyclical or episodic phase which alternates with wakefulness. There is a wide variation in the duration of sleep between species, but humans, moles and pigs sleep for about 8 out of each 24 h. An important characteristic of sleep which differentiates it from most other states of altered consciousness is that it is promptly reversible. This is usually recognized by the sleeper, but brief episodes of sleep or wakefulness (microsleeps and microarousals) may emerge from the background state without any subsequent recall of the events.

The margin between sleep and wakefulness is seldom sharp. The transition between wakefulness and sleep often lasts several minutes, and the moment of falling asleep may be impossible to determine. The point at which sleep is attained, as judged by behavioural criteria, may differ from, for instance, the moment of sleep onset defined by electrophysiological standards. A period of drowsiness is often a transitional phase between wakefulness and sleep, but does not necessarily lead into sleep and may simply be a prolonged episode of subalertness followed by recovery of wakefulness. In a similar way the process of awakening can be sudden, particularly if there is a strong sensory stimulus; or gradual with a stage of partial recovery of wakefulness. Aspects of both sleep and wakefulness coexist in these transitional states, and awareness of the thoughts and images of dreams often persists into wakefulness after apparent arousal from sleep.

Structure of sleep (sleep architecture)

External influences and some internal stimuli have less influence on the brain during sleep than during wakefulness. To an extent the brain becomes de-afferentated, and partially deprived of sensory stimulation. This has in the past led to the concept of sleep as a passive phase, contrasting with the active state of wakefulness. This concept has been discarded in the light of physiological findings over the last 50 years. Most parts of the brain are active in sleep, although their functions and interrelationships differ from wakefulness.

Until the 1950s it was assumed that sleep was a homogeneous or unitary phenomenon which was the opposite of wakefulness. Electrophysiological studies in the 1950s, however, clearly demonstrated that there were two main states of sleep, non-rapid eye movement (NREM) and rapid eye movement (REM)

Table 1.1 Characteristics of sleep.

Episodic
Promptly reversible
Reduced awareness
Reduced responsiveness
Motor inhibition

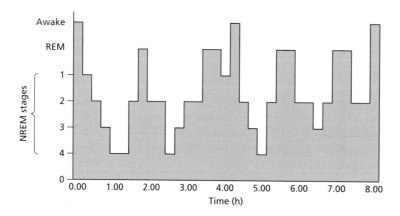

Fig. 1.1 Normal adult hypnogram.

sleep (Fig. 1.1) (Table 1.2). The fact that they usually occurred in sequence without an intervening episode of wakefulness probably delayed their recognition. Both NREM and REM sleep are themselves heterogeneous and at any one moment these two states and wakefulness may not be as distinct as has previously been thought. There is probably a continuous tendency to move in or out of one of these three states throughout the day and night. At any time, parts of the brain may be predominantly in, for instance, REM sleep whereas another part may be tending towards NREM sleep. The current methods of categorizing sleep into one or other state by conventional electrophysiological criteria give a false sense of rigidity to the constantly changing functional processes within the brain.

The exact onset of sleep is difficult to identify since precise criteria based on changes in subjective awareness, behavioural features or electrophysiological changes are hard to establish [2]. The lighter stages of NREM sleep appear first, and often alternate with brief episodes of wakefulness before the deeper NREM sleep stages are entered. NREM sleep, and

particularly its deeper stages, predominates early in the night, but REM sleep appears at around 90-min intervals. There are usually four to six of these sleep cycles each night and as the night progresses the REM episodes become longer, and NREM sleep both shorter and lighter. Brief arousals to wakefulness are a normal feature of sleep.

The drive to enter sleep increases with the duration since the last sleep episode (homeostatic drive). This is integrated with the circadian drive to sleep and wakefulness, which varies over each 24-h period. The circadian drive promotes sleep at night, and to a lesser extent between 2.00 and 4.00 PM, but at other times it facilitates wakefulness. Superimposed on these drives are reflex and psychological factors which adapt both sleep and wakefulness to changes in the environment of the subject.

Sleep in humans and other animals

A rest–activity pattern is detectable in almost all organisms and this may be related to the presence of clock genes which have been largely conserved throughout evolution. Whether or not these changes in activity are recognizable as sleep and wakefulness depends on the level of organization of the central nervous system of the organism. In invertebrates the heart rate is slower during 'behavioural sleep' than when they are more active, and there appears to be a homeostatic mechanism for rest and activity, such that if activity is prolonged the subsequent rest period is also longer.

All vertebrates have NREM-like sleep (Fig. 1.2), but stages 3 and 4 NREM sleep have not been detected in fish, amphibia or reptiles. REM sleep has not been definitely established in these groups either and, like stages 3 and 4 NREM sleep, its evolution appears to

Table 1.2 Nomenclature of sleep states and stages.

NREM	Quiet sleep (infants)
	Orthodox sleep
	Synchronized sleep
NREM stages 1 and 2	Light sleep
NREM stages 3 and 4	Deep sleep
	Slow-wave sleep
	Delta sleep
REM sleep	Active sleep (infants)
	Paradoxical sleep
	Desynchronized sleep

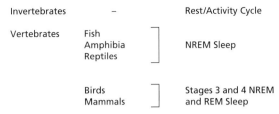

Fig. 1.2 Phylogeny of sleep.

be related to the extent of the development of the telencephalon. In birds, stages 3 and 4 NREM sleep may be present in only one hemisphere, leading to contralateral eye closure. The albatross, for instance, can fly with one hemisphere asleep. Birds who are sleeping on the edge of a flock often have unihemispheric sleep, with the eye facing outwards open in order to detect predators. REM sleep in birds is characteristically brief, often only 10–30 s, and the total duration of REM sleep is only about 25% that of mammals.

All mammals have both stages 3 and 4 NREM sleep and REM sleep. Monotremes, such as echidna and the platypus, appear to have REM sleep which is accompanied by slow waves on the electroencephalogram rather than the high-frequency waves seen in other mammals.

The duration of sleep varies widely among mammals and is not related to their evolutionary relationships as shown in the Linnaean classification, or the size of the cerebral cortex. Smaller mammals sleep for longer each day and they also have a higher metabolic rate. The metabolic rate within the brain is also increased, and the consequences of this may include increased glucose utilization and free radical generation.

In contrast, the duration of REM sleep in adult mammals is closely correlated with the degree of immaturity of the offspring at birth and is inversely related to birthweight. Mammalian neonates are more vulnerable than those of reptiles and birds which immediately lead an independent life. In mammals there is an urgent need to develop behavioural patterns, such as maternal bonding, which increase the chance of survival. The prolonged duration of REM sleep may have an important neurodevelopmental role soon after birth, but also persists throughout life.

In primates sleep is usually monophasic, although in most other mammals it is usually polyphasic, with episodes of sleep both during the day and at night. NREM sleep occurs in both the standing and lying positions, but REM sleep only appears when the animal is lying on the ground, probably because of the

motor inhibition which is characteristic of this state. In aquatic mammals, such as the dolphin, NREM sleep is unihemispheric. There is unihemispheric sleep rebound after sleep deprivation, emphasizing that sleep-related processes can be localized as well as generalized within the brain.

Sleep and wakefulness

Sleep and wakefulness are not totally distinct states. The constant flux in the activity of many parts of the brain may lead at any one time to either an overwhelming balance of activity in favour of one state or the other, or to features of both appearing simultaneously. The fluctuations between NREM and REM sleep are also much more dynamic and complex than is usually appreciated. The instability of these states underlies the appearance of a range of mixed or incomplete states of wakefulness, NREM and REM sleep (Table 1.3), and arousals.

The transitions between sleep and wakefulness may also be gradual, often lasting several minutes, rather than instantaneous. Consciousness and the awareness of activities, for example, can become separated from the performance of movements. The spinal cord can coordinate repetitive flexion and extension movements, such as those seen in walking, without higher control, and even complex activities can be organized by the basal ganglia and brainstem without the type of cerebral cortical involvement seen in wakefulness.

The characteristics of sleep are partially inherited and partially due to environmental factors. Most indices of the duration and type of sleep appear to be roughly equally genetically and environmentally determined, with a polygenic type of inheritance.

Mixed sleep–wake states

Mixed and transitional states are very variable, but can be categorized according to the state in which they arise.

Wakefulness

Sleep inertia is the drowsiness, often associated with physical incoordination and occasionally with confusion, that is present after waking from sleep. It may be the result of delayed activation of the prefrontal cortex at the transition from sleep to wakefulness. If it is severe it may cause a confusional arousal in which lack of awareness is combined with often complex motor behaviour.

Table 1.3 Mixed sleep–wake states.

Prior state	Effects of NREM sleep intrusion	Effects of REM sleep intrusion	Effects of wakefulness intrusion
Wakefulness: awareness, motor function	Unaware. Motor function retained (automatic behaviour)	Aware of dreaming. Loss of muscle tone (cataplexy and sleep paralysis)	—
NREM: unaware, no movements	—	—	Partially aware (sleep inertia and confusional arousal); motor function retained (automatic behaviour)
REM: unaware, REMs	—	—	Aware of lucid dreaming; motor function decreased (sleep paralysis) or increased (REM sleep behaviour disorder)

Sleep inertia often lasts for 30–120 min after waking in the morning. It almost always arises when waking occurs from NREM rather than REM sleep, particularly stages 3 and 4. It is commonest after oversleeping, after daytime naps if stages 3 and 4 NREM sleep are entered, which is usual if naps last for more than 30 min, and in idiopathic hypersomnia. Sleep inertia can be shortened by caffeine, suggesting that it may be related to an increased influence of adenosine after the onset of wakefulness.

Aspects of REM sleep can also intrude into wakefulness. The ability to recall dreams on awakening is a common example of this, and the hallucinations associated with delirium, such as delirium tremens, probably represent partial REM sleep intrusion into wakefulness. The loss of muscle tone with laughter (cataplexy) is an example of pathological REM sleep intrusion into wakefulness. Sleep-onset sleep paralysis may also be regarded as intrusion of a fragment of REM sleep into wakefulness.

NREM sleep
Intrusion of REM into NREM sleep does not cause any symptoms because sleep is maintained, but is very common. Muscle atonia, which is characteristic of REM sleep, is seen in NREM sleep, especially just before and after REM sleep episodes. The peripheral vasoconstriction of REM sleep also occurs up to 30 min before REM sleep episodes, and penile erections are common at times when a REM sleep episode would be anticipated, even if its electroencephalogram

features are not sufficient for it to be identified by conventional scoring systems. The narrative content of dreams in NREM sleep is also greatest when they arise close to a previous episode of REM sleep, suggesting that REM sleep mechanisms are responsible. All these features suggest that fragments of REM sleep are capable of intruding into what is conventionally classified as NREM sleep at times when there is pressure to enter REM sleep.

Intrusion of wakefulness is characteristic of 'disorders of arousal'. In these the transition from NREM sleep to wakefulness is incomplete or gradual and features of both states coexist temporarily. The commonest and mildest example is sleep inertia, in which sleep is followed by drowsiness or at least a sensation of feeling unrefreshed and of being no more alert after sleep than beforehand. This is often combined with temporary disorientation. The electroencephalogram shows some features of wakefulness and of stages 1 and 2 NREM sleep.

There is probably a spectrum of the degree of failure to arouse from NREM sleep which leads from sleep inertia through confusional arousals to activities such as sleep walking and sleep terrors.

REM sleep
Intrusion of wakefulness into REM sleep is responsible for sleep paralysis at the end of a period of sleep. Awareness of the environment is accompanied by the motor inhibition of REM sleep. Lucid dreaming, in which there is awareness of dreaming and the

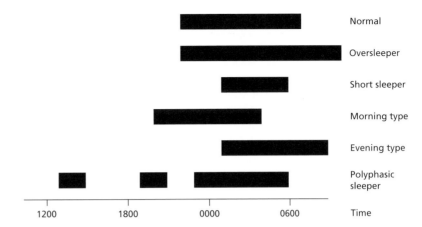

Fig. 1.3 Patterns of sleep.

ability to direct its content, reflects the combination of awareness typical of wakefulness, with continuing dream mentation. Retention of muscle 'tone' in the REM sleep behaviour disorder is dissociated from the continuing REM sleep dream mentation with the result that cerebral activities are physically enacted, unlike normal sleep in which they are suppressed by motor inhibition.

Duration of sleep

Normal sleep

About 60% of the adult population obtain 7–8 h sleep per night, with a mean of 7 h [3], but around 8% sleep for less than 5 h and 2% for more than 10 h (Fig. 1.3). The duration of sleep that is obtained often differs considerably from what is needed. For most adults the optimal duration of sleep appears to be 7–8 h per night, although many people function almost as well on 6–7 h [4]. Loss of NREM sleep, especially stages 3 and 4, probably causes more daytime sleepiness than loss of REM sleep. The duration of sleep should be sufficient to lead to a feeling of being refreshed on waking and remaining alert and able to function normally throughout the day [5]. The rate at which a sleep debt is built up following sleep deprivation is largely genetically determined, but there is little genetic difference in the way that it is relieved by brief naps.

Oversleeping

Epidemiological surveys have shown that long sleepers have a higher mortality than those who sleep for less than 8 h each day. Obtaining more sleep than is required, like eating more food than is needed, is of no benefit and can cause problems. Some subjects find it

difficult to oversleep, but others can readily do so. Towards the end of an extended sleep period the duration and depth of NREM sleep begin to increase as REM sleep takes the place of wakefulness in increasing the homeostatic drive to enter NREM sleep. Sleep inertia becomes more prominent and is often prolonged [6], and the subsequent night's sleep may become fragmented. Oversleeping should be distinguished from a prolonged sleep to compensate for a sleep debt due to sleep deprivation.

Short and long sleepers

Both short and long sleepers have approximately the same duration of stages 3 and 4 NREM sleep, but short sleepers have less stage 2 and have a shorter sleep latency. They probably have a higher homeostatic drive to enter sleep rather than living with a higher sleep debt. They often require a normal duration of sleep until adolescence, and thereafter, perhaps for social reasons, manage with less sleep than is usual.

Long sleepers have a longer duration of melatonin secretion at night and go to sleep closer to the peak of melatonin secretion. There may be a genetic basis, but the ability to extend sleep beyond physiological needs may be a psychophysiological trait. It is commoner in evening types and is usually associated with a normal sleep latency and sleep efficiency, whereas those who sleep for prolonged periods due to sleep deprivation have a short sleep latency and high sleep efficiency.

Timing of sleep

Regularity of sleep

A regular time of going to bed, going to sleep, waking up and getting up in the morning is an important factor in stabilizing and synchronizing the circadian rhythms. The most important of these is the regularity of the waking time. The exact times that are adopted vary according to, for instance, age, social constraints such as work patterns, and the individual tendency to be a long or short sleeper, or a 'lark' or 'morning type' or an 'owl' or 'evening type'. Regular sleep patterns ensure that the homeostatic drive to sleep is strong because they allow a sufficient interval after the previous main sleep episode. In the elderly especially, restricting the nocturnal sleep phase to 6–7 h is usually preferable to sleeping for longer and often improves insomnia.

Monophasic and polyphasic sleep patterns

Sleep in adults is usually taken as a single episode at night (monophasic pattern), but in 85% of mammals, particularly those with a small body mass, sleep is polyphasic. A single prolonged sleep episode may expose these animals to more danger. A monophasic pattern enables the sleep debt accumulated during the waking period to be fully discharged whereas a polyphasic routine pays back this sleep debt in smaller units.

There is evidence that hunter-gatherer communities adopt a polyphasic sleep pattern with at any one time around 25% of the population awake at night and 10% sleeping during the day. A problem with this sleep pattern is that there are repetitive episodes of sleep inertia if naps last for more than 20 min, and particularly if they are longer than 60 min. The polyphasic pattern does, however, reduce the exposure to danger, and can enable a broader division of labour in the society.

Although a monophasic pattern is usual in adults, children obtain polyphasic sleep, usually with around 3–5 h during the day at the age of 6 months and 2 h during the day at 2 years. Initially these sleep episodes are almost random, but once the circadian rhythms mature at 3–6 months, more sleep is obtained at night than during the day. The polyphasic pattern is often re-entered in the elderly who tend to nap during the daytime, but occasionally it is retained throughout life. Leonardo da Vinci, for instance, is said to have slept for 15 min every 4 h.

A polyphasic sleep pattern lessens the performance loss during sleep deprivation. The frequent naps repay the sleep debt exponentially. The deeper NREM sleep at the start of each nap is more time-effective than a more prolonged sleep episode with relatively more lighter NREM and REM sleep. Repayment of a sleep debt is facilitated if the naps coincide with an increased circadian or adaptive drive to fall asleep.

A biphasic sleep pattern is often adopted in Mediterranean countries, with a siesta taken in the mid-afternoon. It is common for nocturnal sleep to be postponed until after midnight. This pattern reflects the circadian tendency to promote sleep during the afternoon and at night, but in addition to this biological element there is probably also a cultural factor. The siesta also avoids taking physical activity during the hottest part of the day.

The influence of the REM sleep ultradian 90-min cycle on the timing of sleep is uncertain. A 90-min cycling in reaction time performance and in the tendency to daydream has been found, but it is uncertain whether or not this predisposes to enter sleep at these times.

Sleep chronotypes

Most people have a tendency to be more alert early in the morning soon after waking (morning types, larks) or late at night prior to falling asleep (evening types, owls). The tendency to be in one or other category can be assessed using the Horne Ostberg questionnaire [7] (Appendix 1).

These patterns merge into the advanced and delayed sleep phase syndromes respectively (page 110). There is a tendency during adolescence to become an evening type and from early adult life onwards to progressively becoming a morning type by old age. There is some evidence that morning and evening types tend to marry each other more frequently than by chance. The biological basis of this may be that it increases the duration during the day when one or other parent is awake and able to protect the children.

Morning types tend to have a shorter latency before entering stages 3 and 4 NREM sleep, are unable to sleep late in the morning and often complain of poor sleep quality with more frequent awakenings, especially late in the night, and early morning waking. They have an earlier peak melatonin secretion and core body temperature nadir. They may have a shorter circadian periodicity. There is a longer delay between the temperature nadir and waking, so that in effect waking occurs later in the circadian phase, facilitating alertness soon afterwards. They have a high sleep efficiency and are intolerant of working night shifts and can only sleep longer by going to bed earlier.

Evening types tend to have a larger amplitude of circadian rhythms such as temperature. Their sleep is more closely entrained by light. They have a later melatonin peak and temperature nadir and may have a long circadian periodicity [8]. They wake closer to the temperature minimum than morning types. They nap less easily during the day, but for longer than the morning types, and feel more refreshed afterwards. They obtain more sleep by waking later in the morning rather than going to bed earlier, and if this is impossible because of, for instance, work commitments a sleep debt is built up which is usually discharged at weekends by sleeping longer. Alertness in the morning can be promoted by taking nicotine or caffeine. Evening types have more irregular sleeping times, and adapt better to time zone changes and to nocturnal shift work than morning types. In adolescence, however, they are often more sleepy on school days, with resulting attention problems, under-achievement at school, and more injuries, and they take more caffeine.

Naps

Daytime naps are normal in young children and common in the elderly and are taken especially at between 2.00 and 4.00 PM when the circadian rhythms favour sleep. They are often taken to compensate for sleep deprivation at night, but may be a manifestation of excessive daytime sleepiness from other causes.

The structure of sleep during a nap depends on the duration since the last sleep episode and its position in the circadian rhythm. Stages 3 and 4 NREM are more likely if the nap occurs after a prolonged period of wakefulness, which is usually later in the day. These stages of sleep are also more likely if a nap lasts for more than around 60 min, but are unlikely if it is less than 20 min. REM sleep may be entered if a nap coincides with the ultradian REM sleep cycle which probably persists in a mild form throughout wakefulness as well as sleep. This is otherwise unusual in normal subjects. Frequent dreaming during daytime naps suggests the diagnosis of narcolepsy.

'Sleep attacks' have been thought to be characteristic of narcolepsy and Parkinson's disease, perhaps triggered by dopaminergic agents, but they can occur with any cause of severe daytime sleepiness. They may be slightly more likely in REM rather than NREM sleep disorders or deprivation, and can be confused with transient loss of consciousness due to cardiac dysrhythmias or epilepsy.

Long naps may be followed by sleep inertia, and brief 'power' naps are often more refreshing. This may be not only because they may contain stages 3 and 4 NREM sleep, but also because the act of entering sleep from wakefulness itself leads to feeling refreshed. This implies that features of stages 3 and

4 NREM sleep may not be the best indicator of whether or not sleep is refreshing.

In narcolepsy naps of 5–30 min or even less are refreshing. Longer naps are required in obstructive sleep apnoeas and even prolonged naps of up to 2 h may be unrefreshing in idiopathic hypersomnia. Shift workers often have unavoidably modified nocturnal sleep routines and require naps at other times during the day in order to compensate for this.

Sleep hygiene

The quantity, quality and timing of sleep are affected by many everyday activities and attitudes (Table 1.4). The importance of these in assisting or interfering with sleep is generally underestimated. In developed societies sleep is being increasingly squeezed into the time left over after family, social, work and recreational activities with the result that insomnia, excessive daytime sleepiness and other sleep symptoms are becoming increasingly common.

The aim of sleep hygiene is to translate an understanding of the nature and the control of sleep into practical advice about how to promote this through changes in lifestyle and the environment.

Sleep hygiene is useful in a wide range of sleep disorders and combines advice about homeostatic, adaptive and circadian aspects of sleep control, how to avoid sleep deprivation, and how to respond to awakenings from sleep if these occur. Some aspects of sleep hygiene fall into more than one of these categories, but in general it entails the following.

1 Altering the sleep environment so that the bed is comfortable and the bedroom warm, dark and quiet.

2 Improving sleep–wake patterns. Increasing the physical activity during the day; preparation for sleep (for instance by mentally winding down and taking a hot bath); regular meals and sleep and wake times, and avoiding daytime and evening naps may all be of help.

3 Changing drug intake. Avoiding caffeinated drinks in the evening and discontinuing other stimulants, such as glucocorticoids, and altering the timing of diuretics in order to minimize nocturia may all be of benefit.

Sleep and age

The pattern of sleep varies considerably with age [9], partly because of intrinsic changes in the sleep–wake cycles and sleep structure (Figs 1.4 and 1.5), but also because of the presence of age-related medical

Table 1.4 Sleep hygiene.

Good practice	Time	Bad practice
Wake up at same time	Awakening	
Take exercise	Daytime	Take more than 6 caffeinated drinks per day
		Take a nap in the day
Set aside time to deal with tomorrow's stresses	Early evening	
Set aside time to unwind		
Establish regular patterns, e.g. hot bath	Late evening	Take exercise within 3 h of desired sleep time
Relaxation routines		Take caffeine in the evening
Take a light snack and a milky drink		Go to sleep hungry
Go to bed when drowsy		Have a heavy meal within 3 h of desired sleep time
		Drink excess fluid in the evenings
		Drink alcohol late in the evenings
		Continue to work within 1.5 h of desired sleep time
		Watch exciting videos or TV late in the evening
Ensure your bed is comfortable	In bed	Use bedroom for watching TV or as an office
Ensure bedroom is quiet, dark and neither too hot nor too cold		Read stimulating books in bed before sleeping
Put the light out soon after going to bed		Try too hard to fall asleep
Ignore intrusive ideas and thoughts		Lie in bed feeling angry if you are unable to sleep

disorders. The most important stages in the development of sleep patterns are as follows.

Prenatal phase

A rhythmic cycling of motor activity is detectable at around 20 weeks gestation and at 28–32 weeks a regular sleep–wake cycle is detectable with alternating periods of body movements, rapid eye movements and irregular respiratory movements ('active sleep', probably equivalent to REM sleep), interrupted by brief episodes of inactivity ('quiet sleep', probably equivalent to NREM sleep) [10]. By 24 weeks gestation the EEG recordings show intermittent high amplitude signals alternating with periods in which the EEG is 'flat', and which gradually become more prolonged. From 32 weeks onwards, active and quiet sleep become more easily distinguishable and resemble REM and NREM sleep respectively. Any circadian influence on rest and activity prenatally is due to maternal rather than fetal rhythms.

Early postnatal phase

At birth the fetus moves from an environment of continuous darkness into one with intermittent light exposure, and the nature of other external stimuli such as feeding and social contact also changes vastly. Normal full-term infants show almost randomly timed phases of wakefulness, active sleep, and quiet sleep on behavioural criteria, although about 3% of their time is spent in an indeterminate state [11]. Around 16 h per day is spent asleep, which is entered through REM sleep. Premature infants at 30 weeks appear to be in REM sleep for 80% of their sleeping time, at 36 weeks for 60%, and at 40 weeks for 50%.

3–12 months

At this age, as in the early postnatal phase, the interpretation of the electrophysiological tracings is difficult. The total sleep time gradually falls. Quiet sleep predominates by around 3 months. Conversely, active sleep, which may at this age be equivalent to REM sleep or possibly an immature form of wakefulness, occupies around 50% of the total sleep time in normal infants at birth and is responsible for only around 40% at 3 months and 30% at 6–12 months. The latency before entering REM sleep gradually increases during the first year.

By 3 months K-complexes and sleep spindles are detectable on the EEG and the latter increase in number by 6 months, although until the age of 2 years there is often interhemispheric asynchrony of spindles. High-voltage, low-frequency theta (4–8 Hz) or delta (0.5–4 Hz) waves are detectable, particularly over the occipital area from 1 month of age. By 6–12 months

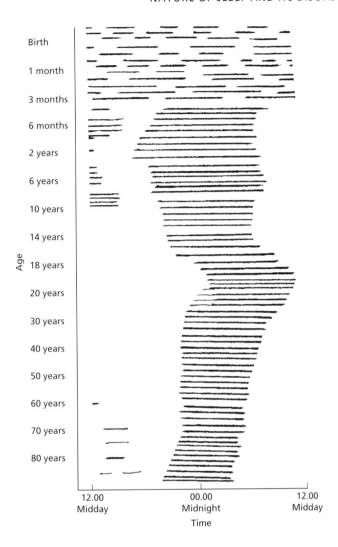

Fig. 1.4 Changes in sleep patterns with age. Horizontal lines indicate sleep episodes at different ages.

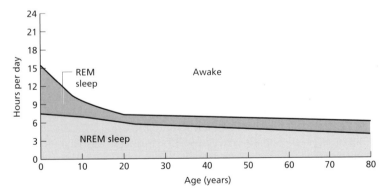

Fig. 1.5 Changes in duration of NREM and REM sleep with age. NREM, non-rapid eye movement; REM, rapid eye movement.

the four stages of NREM sleep are distinguishable electrophysiologically. By 6 months 30% of sleeping time is REM sleep and the total sleep time is 14–15 h per night. REM density remains high.

The sleep pattern until around 3 months is thought to be related to feeding which probably increases the tendency to sleep afterwards. Both sleeping and feeding occur at 3- to 4-h intervals, but by 3–6 months a circadian rhythm in the child's sleep patterns, body temperature, and melatonin secretion becomes detectable. This is initially free-running but gradually comes under the control of external stimuli, including light exposure. By 6 months it is common to sleep throughout the night and signs of a predominantly biphasic pattern with an afternoon sleep appear.

Cycles of REM sleep develop by around 3 months. These are initially approximately of 45 min duration, but gradually lengthen to around 60 min by 1 year of age. Intermittent retention of muscle tone during REM sleep is responsible for smiling, grimacing facial movements, brief vocalizations, irregular respiratory movements and twitching of the limbs and whole body.

1 year to puberty

By the age of 1 year children spend around 11 h asleep at night and up to $2\frac{1}{2}$ h asleep during one or two naps in the daytime. Thirty per cent of their sleep is REM sleep. The morning nap is usually discontinued at the age of 2–3 years, but the afternoon nap is often retained until around 4–5 years.

The total sleep time at 2 years is around 13 h, at 4 years 12 h, at 5 years around 11 h and at the age of 10 years around 10 h. The REM sleep cycles lengthen, but the first REM sleep episode is shorter than those later in the night. Body movements become much less common in REM sleep at this age, and by the age of 5 years REM sleep occupies only around 25% of the sleeping time.

The sleep latency is shorter than in later life at 5–10 min with few arousals by the age of 8. The sleep efficiency is around 95% and the percentage of stages 3 and 4 NREM sleep is greater at around 5 years than at any other age. There is a strong monophasic sleep cycle centred on the night time, possibly related to the high melatonin levels at this age.

Environmental factors often have a significant impact on sleep in childhood. Some physical disorders such as middle ear infections are more painful at night, but may not be recognized, and nocturnal asthma or gastro-oesophageal reflux may also severely disrupt sleep. Bedtime fears and rituals may delay the initiation of sleep, and family situations can cause hyper-arousal of the child shortly before the intended sleep time. Irregular sleeping times and peer group pressures may also lead to sleep problems.

Puberty

At this stage most children sleep for around 9 h, of which around 40% is stages 3 and 4 NREM sleep and 25% REM sleep. A biphasic sleep pattern begins to emerge with occasional complaints of daytime sleepiness, usually in the afternoon.

Adolescence

Most adolescents begin to go to sleep later and wake up later in the morning. The total sleep time increases slightly, perhaps related to the metabolic changes during the growth spurt. A delayed sleep phase syndrome is common, but whether this is due to an endogenous change in the circadian sleep rhythm or to social factors such as opportunities for late evening and night entertainment or work is uncertain. The sleep latency is usually longer than in childhood and REM sleep comprises 25% of total sleep time. The sleep cycle lengthens to the adult duration of 90 min.

Sleep restriction due to school and social pressures is common, and irregular sleep–wake patterns often develop [12]. Excessive caffeine or alcohol intake and recreational drugs may contribute to these patterns. Unrecognized depression and anxiety are also common.

Young and middle-aged adults

At the age of 20 years the sleep efficiency is still usually around 95%, but it then falls progressively. By 35 years the duration of stage 4 NREM sleep is only around 6% of the total sleep time which is only half of what it is at 20. Wakefulness at night is twice as prolonged and the duration of stage 1 NREM sleep is increased slightly at around 5% of total sleep time. The percentage of REM sleep remains constant at around 22–25% throughout early and middle adult life, but REM density gradually falls. Changes in the circadian rhythms prevent subjects over the age of around 45 from adapting as fast and as completely to changes in sleep patterns, e.g. shift work. Other environmental factors such as a reduction in exposure to light due to indoor employment, restriction of sleep time and medical and psychological disorders influence sleep patterns.

Old age

The total sleep time during the night is reduced, but if daytime naps are frequent or prolonged, the total amount of sleep during each 24 h may be similar to that of younger subjects. The sleep efficiency falls to 70–80% with an increase in the number of awakenings and a reduction in stages 3 and 4 NREM sleep [13]. This is around 18% at age 20 years, but may be only around 10% at the age of 60 and by 75 there may be no stage 4 NREM sleep, especially in males. The amplitude of the delta waves falls by about 75% relative to childhood, probably as a result of loss of cortical synchronization due to degeneration of the sleep regulating processes and to cerebral atrophy which causes fewer cortical neurones to be sampled by the surface electroencephalogram (EEG). The duration of stages 1 and 2 NREM sleep is increased (up to 15% stage 1), sleep spindles become fewer, poorly formed, of small amplitude and their frequency may fall from 16 to 12–14 Hz. The elderly often take naps during the day and this may be associated with a poor prognosis.

The sleep pattern deteriorates in men at a younger age than in women, and men have more arousals from sleep than women between the ages of 60 and 80. At these ages there is no detectable gender difference in the duration of REM sleep and its overall percentage remains almost constant at around 20% even into old age, although it may then fall slightly. REM sleep latency shortens to 70–80 min, but the first episode of REM sleep is often prolonged, possibly related to changes in the circadian rhythm. This results in REM sleep episodes of similar duration throughout the night rather than the pattern of lengthening REM sleep cycles seen in younger subjects.

These changes in the sleep patterns of the elderly are influenced by the following factors.

Changes in circadian rhythms

There is no change in the endogenous length of the circadian cycle, which remains around 24.2 h, but the circadian rhythm reduces in amplitude and often alters its timing. The peak blood melatonin level, which is controlled by exposure to light, falls in the elderly and the amplitude of the temperature rhythm is attenuated. The sleep onset and time of wakening and temperature nadir become almost 1 h earlier per decade after the age of 60 years. This is a form of the advanced sleep phase syndrome and is a continuation of the phase change from the delayed sleep phase syndrome of adolescence through the normal sleep phase of middle adult life. There may also be internal desynchronization of circadian rhythms, particularly of sleep, temperature and hormone secretion.

Reduction in homeostatic sleep drive

The sleep–wake controlling mechanisms disintegrate with less delta wave activity, and there are more frequent arousals which may be either spontaneous or due to a lower threshold to, for instance, light and noise. The duration of arousals remains similar to that of young adults at a mean of around 15 s [14]. The elderly wake closer to the peak of melatonin secretion and the temperature nadir than younger adults. The

increased vulnerability of the elderly to these stimuli reduces the continuity of sleep and together with changes in the circadian rhythm leads to a polyphasic sleep pattern with frequent daytime naps. By the age of 70, 25% of men nap during the day and by 80 the figure rises to 45%.

Changes in environment

It is common for entraining factors of the circadian rhythms to be attenuated in old age. The exposure to light falls because the elderly remain indoors for longer, and often have cataracts and macular degeneration which reduce the amount of light stimulating the retina. Institutionalization in nursing homes, reduction in activity, either due to lack of opportunity or physical restrictions, social isolation and boredom all adversely affect the control of sleep. Conversely, some habits such as physical and social activity [15], regular meal times, bedtime and wake-up time tend to consolidate sleep–wake patterns. Exposure to bright light in the morning may exacerbate the advanced sleep phase syndrome. Light exposure at night, even if it is brief, may reduce melatonin secretion and worsen insomnia.

Sleep and gender

There are only minor differences in sleep requirements between males and females. The duration of sleep appears to be slightly longer in females and their circadian rhythm period length may be a few minutes shorter. The changes in sleep structure seen in the elderly are delayed in women compared to men and the dreams of women have a different content to those of men (page 187).

Sleeping in women is considerably modified by the following.

Menstrual cycle

In the follicular pre-ovulation phase oestrogen secretion is increased and this inhibits REM sleep. In the luteal (post-ovulation) phase increased progesterone production promotes sleep, particularly NREM sleep. There is no clear-cut difference in the quality of sleep at night or daytime sleepiness between these two phases, but both premenstrual insomnia and excessive daytime sleepiness may occur. Premenstrual parasomnias, particularly sleep talking and sleep walking, are also recognized.

Little is known about the effects of the oral contraceptive pill on sleep, but progesterone containing preparations can cause excessive sleepiness.

Pregnancy

In pregnancy there is an increase in both oestrogens, which inhibit REM sleep, and progesterones, which promote NREM sleep. Other hormonal changes, such as an increase in cortisol secretion, also modify the sleep patterns. Increase in prolactin during pregnancy increases the duration of REM sleep. Oxytocin is increased at night and may lead to excessive sleepiness.

The duration of sleep is often increased during the first trimester, falls to normal in the second and is reduced in the third [16]. The complaint of excessive daytime sleepiness is most common in the first trimester and is associated with an increase in the total sleep time at night, but with reduced sleep efficiency. During the third trimester the duration of stages 3 and 4 NREM sleep is particularly reduced and daytime naps are frequently taken. Insomnia is commonly due to backache, nocturia, abdominal distension, fetal movements and heartburn.

Several specific sleep disorders arise in pregnancy [17].

Upper airway obstruction

The increase in oestrogen secretion causes hyperaemia, mucosal oedema and hypersecretion in the upper airway, particularly in the third trimester, with an increase in upper airway resistance. Snoring is more common and obstructive sleep apnoeas may develop. Weight gain during pregnancy may also contribute.

There is an association between an increase in upper airway resistance during sleep and pregnancy hypertension and pre-eclampsia. Each arousal from upper airway obstruction increases the blood pressure temporarily and increases catecholamine secretion. The fetal outcome in pre-eclampsia is worse if obstructive sleep apnoeas are present, and the blood pressure can be reduced slightly by the application of nasal continuous positive airway pressure (CPAP) treatment.

Changes in respiratory drive

Increased progesterone secretion increases the ventilatory drive. It acts on chemoreceptors on the ventrolateral surface of the medulla to reduce the arterial $P\text{CO}_2$. This leads to central sleep apnoeas. There is a reduction in functional residual capacity and residual volume and an increase in ventilation–perfusion mismatching and elevation of the diaphragm due to the increased intra-abdominal pressure. The metabolic rate is also increased. These changes may lead to respiratory failure in neuromuscular and skeletal disorders, particularly during sleep [18].

Restless legs and periodic limb movements in sleep

Between 15 and 20% of women develop the restless legs syndrome during pregnancy. This is mainly related to iron deficiency, but folic acid deficiency may also be relevant. The restless legs syndrome occurs particularly in the third trimester especially if there are twins or triplets. Discomfort in the legs, insomnia and excessive daytime sleepiness may all develop, but usually resolve within 10 days of delivery of the fetus. Reduction in caffeine intake during pregnancy and iron supplementation are often effective.

Narcolepsy

This may first appear during pregnancy or be worsened by pregnancy.

Sleep walking and sleep talking

These are less common in pregnancy, probably because of a decreased tendency to arouse from stages 3 and 4 NREM sleep as a result of increased progesterone secretion.

Labour

In the 24 h before labour there is an increase in oestrogen secretion and a reduction in progesterone. Immediately after delivery there is a rapid reduction in secretion of both these hormones and a reduction in NREM and REM sleep. Maternal factors related to caring for the new-born child and the need for feeding also contribute. This is followed by a period of hypervigilance for the child at night and a reduction in total sleep time and sleep efficiency for at least 1 month after delivery. Postnatal depression may also cause insomnia.

Lactation

During lactation oestrogen and progesterone levels fall, but prolactin is secreted, particularly during stages 3 and 4 NREM sleep. Mothers who breast-feed have more prolonged stages 3 and 4 NREM sleep and less stages 1 and 2 NREM sleep than those who bottle-feed. REM sleep duration is increased in breast-feeding due to surges in prolactin secretion.

Menopause

At the menopause the reduction of oestrogen and progesterone produced by the failing ovaries leads to increased gonadotrophin secretion. Insomnia is common and may be related to nocturnal hot flushes (flashes). The flushes begin with a sudden sensation of heat, particularly in the upper part of the body, associated with sweating. They usually last only a few minutes and vary considerably in intensity. They are most frequent after 6.00 PM, probably because of a circadian influence, and are due to abnormalities in temperature control in the preoptic hypothalamus, probably as a result of either oestrogen withdrawal or fluctuations in noradrenergic or 5HT activity within the brain. They can be relieved by oestrogen replacement treatment.

The blood pressure may rise and the risk of developing obstructive sleep apnoeas is increased fivefold after the menopause. This is partly due to a change in the distribution of body fat so that more is laid down in the upper part of the body, as in males. Hormone replacement treatment is slightly protective against obstructive sleep apnoeas after the menopause, but the risk of these occurring is still twice that of a pre-menopausal woman.

Sleep and obesity

The control of sleep is closely linked to feeding behaviour and energy expenditure. These determine the body weight and in particular the body fat and lean body mass. Body weight and body mass index (weight in kg/height in m squared) are only indirect indicators of obesity because they do not assess body composition. Other measures, such as the waist to hip ratio and collar circumference, give an indication of the distribution of body fat and in particular whether it has a central rather than a peripheral location. Central fat deposition is more common in males and post-menopausal females, and peripheral fat is more common in pre-menopausal females.

Control of sleep and obesity

The control of feeding and of exertion involves environmental, social and psychological factors, as well as complex neurological and humoral control systems. The ventromedial nucleus of the hypothalamus acts as a satiety centre, and inhibits the more lateral feeding centre, which is otherwise tonically active.

Several humoral factors are relevant to the physiological control and abnormalities of sleep.

Leptin

Leptin is a protein secreted by adipocytes in white fat, which is mainly subcutaneous. Its blood level therefore is an indirect marker of the quantity of energy stored as fat. Its release is increased by insulin, glucocorticoids and sympathetic activity. It inhibits the synthesis of neuropeptide Y, thereby increasing sympathetic activity and energy expenditure. It also interacts with melanocortin and agouti-related peptide (Agrp) in the arcuate nucleus in the hypothalamus. Leptin also stimulates melanocyte stimulating hormone (MSH) and cocaine and amphetamine regulated transcript (CART), which inhibit appetite. Leptin is a respiratory stimulant, as well as increasing physical activity and energy expenditure and inhibiting appetite.

A genetic failure to produce leptin can lead to obesity of early onset, but in obesity there is usually an increased leptin level due to leptin resistance. Leptin is also increased in obstructive sleep apnoeas due to increased sympathetic activity, but is reduced in narcolepsy, where there is also a loss of the physiological nocturnal increase in leptin secretion.

Chemicals arising from the gut

Ghrelin
This is a growth hormone-like peptide, which is released from the stomach in response to gastric distension. Blood levels therefore rise during meals and fall afterwards. Ghrelin not only stimulates growth hormone secretion through its action in the hypothalamus, but also increases appetite and feeding, leading to obesity.

Cholecystokinin (CCK)
This is secreted by the small intestine in response to distension following food intake. It reduces appetite and food intake.

Oxyntomodulin
The secretion of this is related to the meal size. It acts on the arcuate nucleus to reduce appetite and increase energy expenditure.

Neuropeptide Y
This is produced in the small intestine and not only delays gastric emptying, which reduces appetite, but also is present in the neurones of the arcuate nucleus that project to the paraventricular nuclei. It decreases food intake.

Glucagon-like peptide 1 (GLPl)
This is produced by the gastro-intestinal tract and also in the brain. It induces a feeling of satiety.

Insulin

Insulin is secreted by the pancreas in response to a rise in blood sugar after meals. It promotes NREM sleep.

Neurotransmitters

Orexins (hypocretins)

Orexin modifies feeding behaviour to increase food intake. It also inhibits sleep and limits the duration of REM sleep.

Cannabinoids

These increase appetite.

Endorphins

These lead to satiety.

Pituitary hormones

Growth hormone and cortisol regulate anabolism and catabolism respectively, and both control and are controlled by the state of sleep. Thyroid function also influences obesity and is itself controlled both by circadian rhythms and by sleep.

Obesity and sleep disorders

Obesity is related to the following sleep conditions.

Sleep deprivation and fragmentation

Sleep deprivation and fragmentation lead to insulin resistance and other hormonal and autonomic changes (page 135) with the result that appetite is increased and obesity and the 'metabolic syndrome' often develop.

Obstructive sleep apnoeas

Obstructive sleep apnoeas are caused by obesity and may also contribute to it through inducing the metabolic syndrome with insulin resistance, diabetes mellitus, an increase in lipids and hypertension. The serum leptin is raised due to increased sympathetic activity both during the day and at night, but falls once effective CPAP treatment is started.

Narcolepsy

An increase in appetite, particularly for carbohydrates, is common at the onset of symptoms, but later in the natural history food intake appears to be reduced, although some subjects retain a craving for carbohydrate food during the night. Carbohydrates in general appear to have an increased tendency to promote sleep in narcolepsy.

The serum leptin level is reduced, probably because of a reduction in sympathetic activity, and there is also loss of the nocturnal increase in leptin.

Kleine–Levin syndrome

The episodes of hypersomnia are commonly associated with a voracious non-selective appetite.

Sleep eating and drinking

This commonly causes obesity.

Treatment of obesity

Behavioural treatments

These include cognitive behavioural therapy which aims to alter attitudes about comfort eating, and anxiety about lack of food availability and the moral duty to finish meals. There is, however, a high relapse rate after this type of therapy.

Drug treatment

Drugs which increase the metabolic rate

These include thyroxine, amphetamines, fenfluramine and dexfenfluramine. These have all been used in the past, but reduce the lean body mass as well as adipose tissue, and have other adverse side-effects.

Orlistat

This inhibits lipase action within the gut and reduces fat absorption. It may cause diarrhoea with malabsorption, but is effective in leading to weight loss. It increases insulin sensitivity and also reduces low-density lipoproteins.

Sibutramine

This is a 5HT and noradrenaline re-uptake inhibitor. It is as effective as orlistat in leading to weight loss, but may cause hypertension and tachycardia.

Bariatric surgery

Liposuction of large quantities of fat reduces body weight to a corresponding degree, but does not have any significant metabolic effects or lead to changes in feeding behaviour. In contrast, surgery directed to the gastro-intestinal tract does not cause any immediate weight loss, but alters feeding behaviour and may assist the subject to obtain more control over what is eaten. Bariatric surgery is of two types.

Restrictive

This reduces the capacity of the stomach and small intestine through techniques such as resection of part of the stomach and banding of the stomach. Newer techniques allow the gastric banding to be adjusted according to the effect that it has on food intake. Both of these methods reduce ghrelin production and thereby reduce appetite.

Malabsorptive

This includes techniques such as bilio-pancreatic diversion and proximal gastric bypass. These have complex hormonal effects. Proximal gastric bypass, for instance, appears to significantly increase neuro-peptide Y.

These surgical methods may lead to dramatic weight loss, particularly in the grossly obese, together with secondary benefits, such as improvement in hypertension, serum lipids and insulin resistance. They are usually reserved for subjects whose body mass index is greater than 40.

Sleep and the partner

Sleep disorders may affect the bed partner, family, friends, carers and even neighbours in addition to the patient. The partner may become concerned because of the implications of the sleep disorder, especially when the patient stops breathing, as in obstructive and central sleep apnoeas and Cheyne–Stokes respiration, appears to choke and makes sudden vigorous movements, as with epilepsy and REM sleep behaviour disorder, and if there is a possibility of injury while sleep walking. Snoring and abnormal movements during sleep due to, for instance, the restless legs and periodic limb movements may fragment the partner's sleep and cause a significant degree of excessive daytime sleepiness. Severe insomnia at night or sleep reversal can also put considerable strain on the family and carers, particularly if the patient also becomes confused at night and wanders from the bedroom.

These problems may lead to feelings of frustration, annoyance or anger which are often directed by the partner or family at the subject with the sleep disorder, who comes to feel guilty about causing the problem. Occasionally the partner may be aggressive or violent to the patient while he or she is asleep.

Partners often take hypnotics or alcohol, or both, in order to obtain adequate sleep. The patient and partner often decide to sleep in separate beds or separate bedrooms, at least for part of the night, or on some nights, and the sleep disorder is quite commonly considered as a factor leading to either separation or divorce.

The sleep disorder may also affect the partner less directly by impairing the daytime function of the patient. Excessive daytime sleepiness due to, for instance, obstructive sleep apnoeas or narcolepsy restricts or even prevents family and social activities. Patients often fall asleep readily in the evenings and are unable to interact with other members of the household. The excessive sleepiness may cause difficulties at work, with job insecurity, failure to be promoted and loss of earnings for the family. Other symptoms such as cataplexy may prevent the patient from being left alone in the home or make it unsafe for the individual to care for children without another person being present. This can cause considerable difficulties and tensions.

The partner may also have to adjust to the treatment required for the sleep disorder. This may be intrusive, as with nasal continuous positive airway pressure (CPAP) systems for sleep apnoeas. Prescribed drugs may have side-effects which indirectly affect the partner's sleep.

The presence of a bed partner can also modify the patient's sleep and sleep complaints. The partner's snoring, movements during sleep or nocturia can cause frequent awakenings leading to sleep fragmentation [19]. This may exacerbate the patient's underlying disorder, such as sleep walking, or worsen symptoms of conditions that lead to excessive daytime sleepiness, such as sleep apnoeas or periodic limb movements. Sleeping in separate beds or bedrooms may help one or both partners to sleep.

Young children often wake their parents or carers during the night and the insomnia that this causes can become a long-term problem. Similarly, pets in the home, such as cats and dogs, often prefer to sleep in the bedroom or in or on the bed and can disturb the individual's sleep. This may be due to movements, purring or barking, but their presence may also lead to nocturnal asthma through an allergic mechanism, or by disturbing the dust in the bed and increasing its inhalation.

Effective treatment of the patient's sleep disorder has the advantage, compared with treatment of most other medical conditions, of often being directly of benefit to both the patient and the partner [20]. Relief of obstructive sleep apnoeas, for instance, improves the patient's daytime sleepiness and reduces the disturbance to the partner's sleep as well. Treatment of REM sleep behaviour disorder not only reduces the risk of injury to the patient, but also to the partner. The partner's description of the changes in the patient's sleep disorder with treatment is often important in evaluating its effectiveness, as it is in the initial assessment of the type and severity of the patient's sleep problem.

Location of sleep

Most people fall asleep more readily and sleep more soundly in familiar surroundings, except those with psychophysiological insomnia. This is exemplified by the 'first night' effect in the sleep laboratory, which is characterized by increased sleep latency, reduced stages 3 and 4 NREM sleep and in many subjects an increase in heart rate and blood pressure due to raised sympathetic activity induced by the uncertainty and unfamiliarity of the surroundings. There are, however, features that are specific to certain locations of sleep.

Intensive care units

Sleep is almost invariably disturbed in intensive care units. There is a reduction in total sleep time at night, and a lack of consolidation of sleep, with a reduction in stages 3 and 4 NREM and REM sleep. Naps are frequently taken during the day and the circadian rhythms are readily disturbed. The main causes of these changes are as follows.

Continual sensory stimulation

In most intensive care units there is little daylight, but there is considerable artificial illumination at night. The environment is noisy, not just because of the communication between members of staff and patients, but also because of alarms and other mechanical and electrical sounds [21]. Frequent observations and procedures have to be carried out on patients, which disturb their sleep, and the ambient temperature is usually high.

Medical conditions

Hunger, thirst, pain and other symptoms, including nausea and diarrhoea, frequently disturb sleep. In sepsis there is a reduction in REM sleep with little definition of individual sleep states, which may even resemble status dissociatus.

Treatment effects

Drugs prescribed as sedatives and analgesics often considerably modify the sleep pattern. Even treatments such as mechanical ventilation can affect sleep, for instance by reducing arterial $P\text{CO}_2$, leading to central apnoeas, and if irregular ventilator triggering leads to arousals from sleep [22]. There is also a reduction in stages 3 and 4 NREM and REM sleep in response to surgery.

Psychological aspects

Anxiety about the cause, course and effects of the illness is almost universal in critical care units. Separation from the patient's family and friends may contribute to insomnia, and confusion may result from sedative drugs or the effects of the illness itself.

The sleep restriction that develops may lead to hallucinations and delirium, which, combined with the underlying illness and medication, may cause amnesia for the episode. The post-traumatic stress disorder, with nightmares and flashbacks of the events, may also arise.

Residential and nursing homes and institutions

Disrupted sleep at night is often the cause of elderly people requiring long-term residential and nursing home care, but the environment that these institutions provide frequently exacerbates the sleep disruption. Lack of exercise, naps during the day, being put to bed early in the evening, noise and light exposure at night, with little exposure to light during the day, and wakening at night, for instance to reposition the subject, may all contribute to sleepiness during the day, insomnia at night and to waking feeling agitated, particularly if dementia is also a problem. Exposure to light during the day decreases the sleep latency, causes fewer nocturnal awakenings and increases daytime activity and alertness. Unrecognized sleep disorders such as obstructive sleep apnoeas may also contribute to sleep-related symptoms.

Cholinesterase inhibitors which are commonly prescribed for dementia also cause insomnia as well as intense dreams through their REM sleep promoting action. Conversely, antipsychotic drugs, often prescribed at least partly for their sedative effect at night, will increase daytime sleepiness. This is also the problem with most hypnotics except those with a short duration of action. Daytime sleepiness increases the risk of accidents and falls, but insomnia and getting out of bed at night also contribute to this.

Sleep and space travel

It is common for there to be a prolonged episode of wakefulness before take-off on space travel. There may be as long as 30 h of continuous wakefulness before sleep is first obtained during the trip. It is usual for around 6 h sleep in total to be taken each 24 h, but this is not consolidated into a single sleep episode.

The earth is encircled every 90 min so that during this interval the external illumination is the equivalent of a normal day and night. Masks are therefore usually worn when attempting to sleep.

Sleep hygiene is difficult, particularly since there is little opportunity for physical exercise. Hypnotic use is common among astronauts. The weightlessness during space travel requires the sleeper to be attached to a point in the cabin to prevent drifting around. It also causes backache because of lengthening of the spinal column by 2–4 cm due to reduced pressure on the intervertebral discs.

The environment in space reduces the gravitational effect on the structures in the upper airway. This reduces the upper airway resistance during sleep. Snoring and sleep-disordered breathing are less likely and there are fewer respiratory arousals during sleep as a result. There is also a reduction in respiratory frequency and heart rate before sleep and in the latter during stages 3 and 4 NREM sleep.

Hyberbaric environments

Hyberbaric environments are usually encountered in workers on the sea-bed. Several people are usually present in a confined space and reduction of stages 3 and 4 NREM sleep, an increase in stages 1 and 2 and slight reduction of REM sleep are common. Sleep fragmentation is a problem and there is increased dream recall.

The extent of excessive daytime sleepiness is approximately proportional to the barometric pressure, especially at depths greater than 200–300 m. The increased gas density leads to a sensation of nasal blockage which causes awakenings from sleep. Snoring and obstructive sleep apnoeas are more common than at sea level. There is also an initial polyuria which interrupts sleep and is due to haemodynamic changes.

Awareness of sleep disorders

Sleep occupies approximately 8 h of each 24-h cycle, but much less attention has been paid to the medical problems during this phase of life than to those that occur during wakefulness.

There are several reasons for this. Patients are often reticent about events which occur during sleep. They regard this as a personal and private time and are more reluctant to talk about problems occurring during sleep than about those occurring during wakefulness. They may be unaware of the existence of a sleep disorder causing their abnormal movements at night, or of obstructive sleep apnoeas, which may only be reported if the partner becomes alarmed. Sleep-related symptoms are often attributed to problems occurring in everyday life. 'Tiredness', for example, may be thought to be due to age or overwork, rather than to a sleep disorder.

The consequences of sleep deprivation and sleep disorders are almost certainly increasing in developed societies without a corresponding increase in the awareness of these problems by the general population. More public education about the need for sleep and the main components of good sleep hygiene is required. The effects of shift work should be more widely recognized. Awareness of these issues should become an important influence on those who make decisions regarding practices at work, in educational establishments, and in relation to social activities. If government policy reflected the importance of sleep problems in everyday life, better provision for, for instance, the sleepy driver would be made on motorways, which pose the greatest risk for sleep-related accidents.

In addition to this under-reporting of sleep problems, medical and other healthcare professionals are generally less aware of sleep disorders and how to assess and manage them than of conditions arising during wakefulness. Medical consultations take place while the patient is awake so that direct observation of a sleep disorder by the doctor is unusual. A survey of British medical schools has shown that only a few minutes are spent on the study of sleep disorders during the whole of the undergraduate and postgraduate training [23]. An American survey has indicated that the mean number of questions asked in response to the complaint of insomnia is only 2.5. This probably reflects the lack of awareness of the possible causes and effects of this symptom, and how to formulate a management plan for it.

It is important that doctors and other healthcare workers become aware of the impact of sleep disorders and that these become a regular part of their training programme. Clear checklists or protocols might be helpful for general practitioners to assist in identifying significant sleep disorders and providing treatment. The provision of specialist sleep centres should reflect the need for them by society, and within each centre a multidisciplinary approach should be developed.

Costs of sleep disorders

There are several aspects of the costs of sleep disorders to society.
1 Development of other diseases which could have been avoided if the sleep disorder had been recognized and treated earlier. An example is the occurrence of strokes or myocardial infarctions associated with untreated obstructive sleep apnoeas.

Table 1.5 Classification of important sleep disorders.

Disordered function	EDS	Insomnia	Behavioural abnormalities	Respiratory disorders
Homeostatic drive and NREM sleep	IH	Idiopathic insomnia	Disorders of arousal	—
Ultradian drive and REM sleep	Narcolepsy	Narcolepsy	REM sleep behaviour disorder	—
Adaptive drive	Poor sleep hygiene	Poor sleep hygiene	—	—
Circadian rhythms	DSPS, ASPS	Depression, DSPS, ASPS	—	—
Dissociation of sleep states	Sleep inertia	—	Confusional arousal	—
Arousals	OSA	Hyperarousal states	PLMS	—
Autonomic function	—	—	Sleep terrors	Asthma
Behaviour in sleep	PLMS	PLMS	Epilepsy	OSA, CSA

ASPS, advanced sleep phase syndrome; COPD, chronic obstructive pulmonary disease; CSA, central sleep apnoea; DSPS, delayed sleep phase syndrome; EDS, excessive daytime sleepiness; IH, idiopathic hypersomnia; NREM, non-REM; OSA, obstructive sleep apnoeas; PLMS, periodic limb movements in sleep; REM, rapid eye movement.

2 Reduction in the quality of life [24]. Excessive daytime sleepiness leads to irritability and difficulties in interpersonal relationships, which not only impair social activity, but also reduce productivity at work. Studies of those with obstructive sleep apnoeas before and after using continuous positive airway pressure treatment have shown a considerable reduction in quality of life which improves with treatment. The same has been demonstrated for those with narcolepsy before and after receiving treatment with modafinil.

3 Financial consequences of sleep-related accidents. Excessive daytime sleepiness impairs efficiency at work and leads to accidents which may have considerable financial consequences. The duration of sick leave is increased in those with excessive daytime sleepiness and insomnia.

These costs could largely be avoided with better awareness of sleep disorders and availability of advice and treatment for them. The cost of providing care for sleep disorders and education about good sleep hygiene practice has to be offset against these potential savings. Sleep laboratories are expensive, and investigations such as polysomnography are costly and require trained staff.

These resources should be used in a cost-effective manner in order to provide the best value for money. The simplest effective test should be used rather than proceeding directly to polysomnography unless the additional information that this provides is required. Most drugs used to treat sleep disorders are cheap, particularly benzodiazepines and other hypnotics and antidepressants, but some drugs and equipment such as continuous positive airway pressure systems and light therapy are more expensive. The cost of ongoing medical or paramedical supervision of the patient also has to be balanced against the benefit that it provides.

Classification of sleep disorders

The pathophysiology and main symptoms of sleep disorders form the basis of the approach to these conditions in this book (Table 1.5). The complaints of insomnia and excessive daytime sleepiness are covered in Chapters 6 and 7. The circadian rhythm disorders are separately identified since they form a physiological entity (Chapter 5). Abnormal experiences and events taking place during sleep are covered in Chapters 8 and 9; and the respiratory disorders of sleep, which are a subgroup of these, are discussed in Chapters 10 and 11. The links between the pathophysiology, clinical features and treatment of these sleep disorders are emphasized throughout these chapters.

This approach has many similarities to, but also some differences from, the widely used 1997 third revision of the International Classification of Sleep Disorders (ICSD) produced by the American Sleep Disorders Association (ASDA) in association with other national and international sleep societies [25] (Table 1.6). This groups insomnia and excessive daytime sleepiness as dyssomnias and distinguishes them from disorders occurring during sleep (parasomnias). It also has two other categories which are less satisfactory. First, a group of medical and psychiatric disorders which includes epilepsy and mood disorders, all of which interact with the sleep mechanisms in a similar fashion to the disorders in the dyssomnia and

Table 1.6 ASDA classification of sleep disorders 1997.

1 Dyssomnias

A Intrinsic sleep disorders
1 Psychophysiologic insomnia — 307.42–0
2 Sleep state misperception — 307.49–1
3 Idiopathic insomnia — 780.52–7
4 Narcolepsy — 347
5 Recurrent hypersomnia — 780.54–2
6 Idiopathic hypersomnia — 780.54–7
7 Post-traumatic hypersomnia — 780.54–8
8 Obstructive sleep apnoea syndrome — 780.53–0
9 Central sleep apnoea syndrome — 780.51–0
10 Central alveolar hypoventilation syndrome — 780.51–1
11 Periodic limb movement disorder — 780.52–4
12 Restless legs syndrome — 780.52–5
13 Intrinsic sleep disorder NOS — 780.52–9

B Extrinsic sleep disorders
1 Inadequate sleep hygiene — 307.41–1
2 Environmental sleep disorder — 780.52–6
3 Altitude insomnia — 289.0
4 Adjustment sleep disorder — 307.41–0
5 Insufficient sleep syndrome — 307.49–4
6 Limit-setting sleep disorder — 307.42–4
7 Sleep-onset association disorder — 307.42–5
8 Food allergy insomnia — 780.52–2
9 Nocturnal eating (drinking) syndrome — 780.52–8
10 Hypnotic-dependent sleep disorder — 780.52–0
11 Stimulant-dependent sleep disorder — 780.52–1
12 Alcohol-dependent sleep disorder — 780.52–3
13 Toxin-induced sleep disorder — 780.54–6
14 Extrinsic sleep disorder NOS — 780.52–9

C Circadian-rhythm sleep disorders
1 Time zone change (jet lag) syndrome — 307.45–0
2 Shift work sleep disorder — 307.45–1
3 Irregular sleep–wake pattern — 307.45–3
4 Delayed sleep–phase syndrome — 780.55–0
5 Advanced sleep–phase syndrome — 780.55–1
6 Non-24-hour sleep–wake disorder — 780.55–2
7 Circadian rhythm sleep disorder NOS — 780.55–9

2 Parasomnias

A Arousal disorders
1 Confusional arousals — 307.46–2
2 Sleepwalking — 307.46–0
3 Sleep terrors — 307.46–1

B Sleep–wake transition disorders
1 Rhythmic movement disorder — 307.3
2 Sleep starts — 307.47–2
3 Sleep talking — 307.47–3
4 Nocturnal leg cramps — 729.82

C Parasomnias usually associated with REM sleep
1 Nightmares — 307.47–0
2 Sleep paralysis — 780.56–2
3 Impaired sleep-related penile erections — 780.56–3
4 Sleep-related painful erections — 780.56–4
5 REM sleep-related sinus arrest — 780.56–8
6 REM sleep behavior disorder — 780.59–0

D Other parasomnias
1 Sleep bruxism — 306.8
2 Sleep enuresis — 788.36–0
3 Sleep-related abnormal swallowing syndrome — 780.56–6
4 Nocturnal paroxysmal dystonia — 780.59–1
5 Sudden unexplained nocturnal death syndrome — 780.59–3
6 Primary snoring — 786.09–1
7 Infant sleep apnea — 770.80
8 Congenital central hypoventilation syndrome — 770.81
9 Sudden infant death syndrome — 798.0
10 Benign neonatal sleep myoclonus — 780.59–5
11 Other parasomnia NOS — 780.59–9

3 Sleep disorders associated with mental, neurologic, or other medical disorders

A Associated with mental disorders — 290–319
1 Psychoses — 290–299
2 Mood disorders — 296–301, 311
3 Anxiety disorders — 300, 308, 309
4 Panic disorders — 300
5 Alcoholism — 303, 305

B Associated with neurologic disorders — 320–389
1 Cerebral degenerative disorders — 330–337
2 Dementia — 331
3 Parkinsonism — 332
4 Fatal familial insomnia — 337.9
5 Sleep-related epilepsy — 345
6 Electrical status epilepticus of sleep — 345.8
7 Sleep-related headaches — 346

C Associated with other medical disorders
1 Sleeping sickness — 086
2 Nocturnal cardiac ischemia — 411–414
3 Chronic obstructive pulmonary disease — 490–496
4 Sleep-related asthma — 493
5 Sleep-related gastroesophageal reflux — 530.81
6 Peptic ulcer disease — 531–534
7 Fibromyalgia — 729.1

4 Proposed sleep disorders
1 Short sleeper — 307.49–0
2 Long sleeper — 307.49–2
3 Subwakefulness syndrome — 307.47–1
4 Fragmentary myoclonus — 780.59–7
5 Sleep hyperhidrosis — 780.8
6 Menstrual-associated sleep disorder — 780.54–3
7 Pregnancy-associated sleep disorder — 780.59–6
8 Terrifying hypnagogic hallucinations — 307.47–4
9 Sleep-related neurogenic tachypnea — 780.53–2
10 Sleep-related laryngospasm — 780.59–4
11 Sleep choking syndrome — 307.42–1

Table 1.7 American Academy of Sleep Medicine Classification of sleep disorders 2005. Permission for single-use of the information contained in this table was obtained from the American Academy of Sleep Medicine, April 2005.

1 **Insomnia**
  Adjustment Insomnia (Acute Insomnia)
  Psychophysiological Insomnia
  Paradoxical Insomnia
  Idiopathic Insomnia
  Insomnia Due to Mental Disorder
  Inadequate Sleep Hygiene
  Behavioral Insomnia of Childhood
  Insomnia Due to Drug or Substance
  Insomnia Due to Medical Condition
  Insomnia Not Due to Substance or Known Physiological
    Condition
  Unspecified (Nonorganic Insomnia, NOS)
  Physiological (Organic) Insomnia, Unspecified

2 **Sleep Related Breathing Disorders**
  Central Sleep Apnea Syndromes
    Primary Central Sleep Apnea
    Central Sleep Apnea Due to Cheyne Stokes Breathing Pattern
    Central Sleep Apnea Due to High-Altitude Periodic Breathing
    Central Sleep Apnea Due to Medical Condition Not Cheyne
      Stokes
    Central Sleep Apnea Due to Drug or Substance
    Primary Sleep Apnea of Infancy (Formerly Primary Sleep
      Apnea of Newborn)
  Obstructive Sleep Apnea Syndromes
    Obstructive Sleep Apnea, Adult
    Obstructive Sleep Apnoea, Pediatric
  Sleep Related Hypoventilation/Hypoxemic Syndromes
    Sleep Related Nonobstructive Alveolar Hypoventilation,
      Idiopathic
    Congenital Central Alveolar Hypoventilation Syndrome
  *Sleep Related Hypoventilation/Hypoxemia Due to Medical
  Condition*
    Sleep Related Hypoventilation/Hypoxemia Due to
      Pulmonary Parenchymal or Vascular Pathology
    Sleep Related Hypoventilation/Hypoxemia Due to Lower
      Airways Obstruction
    Sleep Related Hypoventilation/Hypoxemia Due to
      Neuromuscular and Chest Wall Disorders
  Other Sleep Related Breathing Disorder
    Sleep Apnea/Sleep Related Breathing Disorder, Unspecified

3 **Hypersomnias of Central Origin**
  **Not Due to a Circadian Rhythm Sleep Disorder, Sleep Related
  Breathing Disorder, or Other Cause of Disturbed Nocturnal
  Sleep**
  Narcolepsy With Cataplexy
  Narcolepsy Without Cataplexy
  Narcolepsy Due to Medical Condition
  Narcolepsy, Unspecified
  Recurrent Hypersomnia
    Kleine-Levin Syndrome
    Menstrual-Related Hypersomnia
  Idiopathic Hypersomnia With Long Sleep Time
  Idiopathic Hypersomnia Without Long Sleep Time
  Behaviorally Induced Insufficient Sleep Syndrome
  Hypersomnia Due to Medical Condition
  Hypersomnia Due to Drug or Substance
  *Hypersomnia Not Due to Substance or Known Physiological
  Condition (Nonorganic Hypersomnia, NOS)*
  *Physiological (Organic) Hypersomnia, Unspecified (Organic
    Hypersomina, NOS)*

4 **Circadian Rhythm Sleep Disorders**
  *Circadian Rhythm Sleep Disorder, Delayed Sleep Phase Type
    (Delayed Sleep Phase Disorder)*
  *Circadian Rhythm Sleep Disorder, Advanced Sleep Phase Type
    (Advanced Sleep Phase Disorder)*
  *Circadian Rhythm Sleep Disorder, Irregular Sleep-Wake Type
    (Irregular Sleep-Wake Rhythm)*
  *Circadian Rhythm Sleep Disorder, Free-Running Type
    (Nonentrained Type)*
  *Circadian Rhythm Sleep Disorder, Jet Lag Type (Jet Lag
    Disorder)*
  *Circadian Rhythm Sleep Disorder, Shift Work Type (Shift Work
    Disorder)*
  Circadian Rhythm Sleep Disorder Due to Medical Condition
  *Other Circadian Rhythm Sleep Disorder (Circadian Rhythm
    Disorder, NOS)*
  *Other Circadian Rhythm Sleep Disorder Due to Drug or
    Substance*

5 **Parasomnias**
  Disorders of Arousal (From NREM Sleep)
    Confusional Arousals
    Sleepwalking
    Sleep Terrors
  Parasomnias Usually Associated With REM Sleep
    REM Sleep behavior Disorder (*Including Overlap Disorder
      and Status Dissociatus*)
    Recurrent Isolated Sleep Paralysis
    Nightmare Disorder
  Other Parasomnias
    Sleep Related Dissociative Disorders
    Sleep Enuresis
    Sleep Related Groaning (Catathrenia)
    Exploding Head Syndrome
    Sleep Related Hallucinations
    Sleep Related Eating Disorders
    Parasomnia, Unspecified
    Parasomnia Due to Drug or Substance
    Parasomnia Due to Medical Condition

6 **Sleep Related Movement Disorders**
  Restless Legs Syndrome
  Periodic Limb Movement Disorder
  Sleep Related Leg Cramps
  Sleep Related Bruxism
  Sleep Related Rhythmic Movement Disorder
  Sleep Related Movement Disorder, Unspecified
  Sleep Related Movement Disorder Due to Drug or Substance
  Sleep Related Movement Disorder Due to Medical Condition

7 **Isolated Symptoms, Apparently Normal Variants and
  Unresolved Issues**
  Long Sleeper
  Short Sleeper
  Snoring
  Sleep Talking
  Sleep Starts (Hypnic Jerks)
  Benign Sleep Myoclonus of Infancy
  *Hypnagogic Foot Tremor and Alternating Leg Muscle
    Activation During Sleep*
  Propriospinal Myoclonus at Sleep Onset
  Excessive Fragmentary Myoclonus

8 **Other Sleep Disorders**
  Other Physiological (Organic) Sleep Disorder
  *Other Sleep Disorder Not Due to Substance or Known
    Physiological Condition*
  Environmental Sleep Disorder

parasomnia categories. The second group of 'proposed sleep disorders' is heterogeneous and emphasizes the descriptive aspects and includes partly developed concepts such as the 'sleep choking syndrome'.

The 2005 version recognises eight categories of sleep disorder (26) (Table 1.7) with insomnia and hypersomnias separated, but motor disorders during sleep included in the parasomnia, sleep related movement disorders and isolated symptoms sections. The term 'parasomnia' has not been used in this book because of the wide range and heterogeneous nature of sleep conditions that it has come to represent, but the important influence of drugs is recognised by a separate chapter devoted to their effects. The AASM 2005 classification includes drug related sleep disorders in several different categories, but excludes disorders such as sleep related epilepsy and several medical and psychiatric disorders causing sleep related symptoms.

References

1 Velluti RA. Interactions between sleep and sensory physiology. *J Sleep Res* 1997; 6: 61–77.

2 Terzano MG, Parrino L. Origin and significance of the cyclic alternating pattern (CAP). *Sleep Med Rev* 2000; 4(1): 101–23.

3 Groeger JA, Zijlstra FRH, Dijk D-J. Sleep quantity, sleep difficulties and their perceived consequences in a representative sample of some 2000 British adults. *J Sleep Res* 2004; 13: 359–71.

4 Ferrara M, Gennaro L de. How much sleep do we need? *Sleep Med Rev* 2001; 5(2): 155–79.

5 Horne J. Is there a sleep debt? *Sleep* 2004; 27: 1047–9.

6 Jewett ME, Wyatt JK, Ritz-de Cecco AD, Khalsa SB, Dijk D-J, Czeisler CA. Time course of sleep inertia dissipation in human performance and alertness. *J Sleep Res* 1999; 8: 1–8.

7 Horne JA, Ostberg O. A self-assessment questionnaire to determine morningness–eveningness in human circadian rhythms. *Int J Chronobiology* 1976; 4: 97–110.

8 Taillard J, Philip P, Coste O, Sagaspe P, Bioulac B. The circadian and homeostatic modulation of sleep pressure during wakefulness differs between morning and evening chronotypes. *J Sleep Res* 2003; 12: 275–82.

9 Ohayon MM, Carskadon MA, Guilleminault C, Vitiello MV. Meta-analysis of quantitative sleep parameters from childhood to old age in healthy individuals: developing normative sleep values across the human lifespan. *Sleep* 2004; 27: 1255–73.

10 Mirmiran M, Maas YGH, Ariagno RL. Development of fetal and neonatal sleep and circadian rhythms. *Sleep Med Rev* 2003; 7(4): 321–34.

11 Weerd AW de, Bossche RAS van den. The development of sleep during the first months of life. *Sleep Med Rev* 2003; 7(2): 179–91.

12 Wolfson AR, Carskadon MA. Understanding adolescents' sleep patterns and school performance: a critical appraisal. *Sleep Med Rev* 2003; 7(6): 491–506.

13 Hume KI, Van F, Watson A. A field study of age and gender differences in habitual adult sleep. *J Sleep Res* 1998; 7: 85–94.

14 Boselli M, Parrino L, Smerieri A, Terzano MG. Effect of age on EEG arousals in normal sleep. *Sleep* 1998; 21(4): 351–7.

15 Benloucif S, Orbeta L, Ortiz R, Janssen I, Finkel SI, Bleiberg J, Zee PC. Morning or evening activity improves neuropsychological performance and subjective sleep quality in older adults. *Sleep* 2004; 27(8): 1542–51.

16 Pien GW, Schwab RJ. Sleep disorders during pregnancy. *Sleep* 2004; 27: 1405–17.

17 Santiago JR, Nolledo MS, Kinzler W, Santiago TV. Sleep and sleep disorders in pregnancy. *Ann Intern Med* 2001; 134(5): 396–408.

18 Shneerson JM. Pregnancy in neuromuscular and skeletal disorders. *Monaldi Arch Chest Dis* 1994; 48: 227–30.

19 Strawbridge WJ, Shema SJ, Roberts RE. Impact of spouses' sleep problems on partners. *Sleep* 2004; 27(3): 527–31.

20 McArdle N, Kingshott R, Engleman HM, Mackay TW, Douglas NJ. Partners of patients with sleep apnoea/hypopnoea syndrome: effect of CPAP treatment on sleep quality and quality of life. *Thorax* 2001; 56: 513–18.

21 Freedman NS, Gazendam J, Levan L, Pack AI, Schwab RJ. Abnormal sleep/wake cycles and the effect of environmental noise on sleep disrupton in the intensive care unit. *Am J Respir Crit Care Med* 2001; 163: 451–7.

22 Parthasarathy S, Tobin MJ. Effect of ventilator mode on sleep quality in critically ill patients. *Am J Respir Crit Care Med* 2002; 166: 1423–9.

23 Stores G, Crawford C. Medical student education in sleep and its disorders. *J R Coll Phys* 1998; 32: 149–53.

24 Reimer MA, Flemons WW. Quality of life in sleep disorders. *Sleep Med Rev* 2003; 7(4): 335–49.

25 International Classification of Sleep Disorders. (Revised). Diagnostic and Coding Manual. Rochester: American Sleep Disorders Association, 1997.

26 American Academy of Sleep Medicine. International classification of sleep disorders, 2nd ed.: Diagnostic and Coding Manual. Westchester, Illinois: American Academy of Sleep Medicine, 2005.

2 Physiological Basis of Sleep and Wakefulness

Introduction

Knowledge about the physiological basis of sleep has increased rapidly over the last few years. It is now recognized to be a highly complex and heterogeneous state, which is intimately connected with the state of wakefulness. There is a dynamic balance between the processes controlling both these states, which is complex and has important implications for many sleep disorders.

Functions of sleep

The functions of sleep are still uncertain, but NREM and REM sleep almost certainly have different functions. Sleep is in many ways a vulnerable state, because of the reduced awareness and responsiveness to the environment, but it has been highly conserved during evolution suggesting that it has a survival advantage. The proposed functions for sleep fall into the following categories.

Biochemical

Several anabolic hormones, such as growth hormone, are secreted primarily during sleep, whereas catabolic hormones, such as cortisol, are produced mainly during wakefulness. The metabolic rate slows during NREM sleep, in which energy is conserved, the body temperature falls, and protein synthesis and other anabolic processes are accentuated.

Wakefulness may also have important biochemical effects on neurones which are compensated for by sleep. During wakefulness neuronal glucose utilization is more rapid, and intracellular stores of glycogen within astrocytes are consumed. This process is reversed during sleep so that glucose can be available for neuronal activity and to enable normal metabolic functioning during the next episode of wakefulness. Replenishment of other metabolites or removal of oxygen free radicals during NREM sleep may also be important.

Physiological

Sleep has been considered to be a restorative or a recovery phase, or to prepare the organism physiologically for the next phase of wakefulness. Cell division is most rapid during NREM sleep, at which time protein synthesis is increased. Sleep also has important effects on the immune system and is itself influenced by, for instance, cytokines which are an integral component of immunity. Energy is conserved during sleep, but this is only between 100 and 200 calories per night and is probably of little significance.

Neurological

Synchronization of cortical activity during NREM sleep may in some way coordinate cortical networks. The prefrontal cortex is inactive during NREM sleep as well as REM sleep, and this may also have some benefit.

REM sleep may have a neurodevelopmental role. It is most prolonged in mammals whose offspring are least mature at birth, and in neonates and young children. The ability to form new neurones (neurogenesis) slows early in life and new behaviour patterns are mainly due to the development of neural networks. During REM sleep the cerebral cortex is open to sensory inputs and makes loose associations which are not possible during wakefulness. The basal ganglia are also active so that behavioural patterns that are essential for survival can be developed without them being manifested by motor activity. The REM sleep processing and integration of newly acquired information into existing neural templates enables future responses to also reflect the previous experience of the individual and the inherited potential [1]. These are given an emotional charge through the activity of the limbic system.

Psychological

Both NREM and REM sleep appear to be involved in consolidation of memory, but they almost certainly have different influences on this. Acquisition of new information during sleep is extremely limited, but consolidation or maintenance of memory from experiences during the previous day is considerable [2]. Learning of visually acquired information is improved during the first night of sleep, and sleep deprivation on this night impairs recall of information. Retention is best if stages 3 and 4 NREM sleep in the first 2 h of the night are followed by REM sleep in the last 25% of the night. The sequence of NREM and REM sleep appears to be important.

Learning of motor sequences improves during the first night of sleep and appears to be dependent particularly on stage 2 NREM sleep later in the night, during which individual components of the learnt sequence can be integrated, particularly the most complex parts.

Recall of cognitive procedures is better if there is a sequence of NREM and then REM sleep, but declarative memory appears not to require REM sleep [3]. Probabilistic learning, in which associations are made according to the likelihood of events being related, improves after sleep on the first night after the experience. Declarative memory during sleep may be related to spindle activity in stage 2 NREM sleep [4].

Dreams are a manifestation of the underlying cerebral activity and reflect the loose mental associations of REM sleep which enable new neuronal networks to be formed, probably promoting creative mental activity and improving problem-solving ability. At sleep onset explicit images of the day's events are often recalled if the subject is awoken during stage 1 NREM sleep, but as the REM sleep episodes progress during the night these become incorporated into associative networks and are less readily recognizable. This creative activity of REM sleep complements its function in memory consolidation.

Social

In non-developed societies it is usual for some members of a group to be awake while others are sleeping in order to afford protection for the group. The rapid reversibility of sleep to the waking state in response to significant stimuli also gives protection against adverse environmental events.

Non-rapid eye movement (NREM) sleep

Neurophysiology

The thalamocortical pathways synchronize cortical activity, particularly during the deeper stages of NREM sleep. The cortex is in effect removed from the influence of ascending sensory input by the thalamic 'gate' and also by reduction in the activity of the ascending reticular activating system. This disconnection contrasts with wakefulness and REM sleep (Table 2.1).

The synchronization of the cortical activity is not homogeneous. Early in NREM sleep it is most marked in the prefrontal area, suggesting that this region, which is particularly active during wakefulness, develops a greater homeostatic drive to enter NREM sleep. This regional difference is particularly marked after sleep deprivation.

Thalamic activity in NREM sleep stabilizes this state and inhibits arousals. Arousal stimuli may however lead to a reduction in delta activity and an increase in alpha and beta rhythms. The threshold for painful stimuli causing arousal increases from stage 1 through to stage 4 NREM sleep. Impulses ascending in the spinoreticular tract can be inhibited in the nucleus

Table 2.1 Comparison of NREM and REM sleep.

Characteristic	NREM sleep	REM sleep
Cerebral cortex	Prefrontal cortex inactive Limbic cortex inactive Deafferented	Prefrontal cortex inactive Limbic cortex active Active information processing Dreams
Somatic reflexes	Reduced	Intense inhibition
Movements	Constant for each stage (1–4) Reduced	Rapid eye movements
Autonomic function	Constant for each stage (1–4) Parasympathetic dominance	Fluctuates Overall parasympathetic dominance
Metabolic	Reduced metabolic rate Anabolic	Slightly reduced metabolic rate

reticularis gigantocellularis so that afferent stimuli are prevented from causing arousals.

Functional neuro-imaging

Functional neuro-imaging has revealed global shifts in cerebral function between wakefulness and NREM sleep, particularly stages 3 and 4. In this state there is reduced activity in the brainstem, particularly the pons and cerebellum, in the basal forebrain and limbic cortex, such as the anterior cingulate gyrus, and especially in the dorsolateral prefrontal and inferior parietal cortex. There is little change in activity relative to wakefulness in the basal ganglia and primary sensory and motor cortex.

On waking from NREM sleep there is an increase in brainstem activity, followed by increasing activity in the cerebral cortex. The prefrontal cortex is the last to be activated after waking, and this sequence may explain the features of sleep inertia. Activity patterns midway between normal wakefulness and NREM sleep are seen during wakefulness following sleep deprivation. Wakefulness in the evening is associated with increasing brainstem and hypothalamic metabolic activity, possibly due to increased input from the circadian rhythm generators to maintain wakefulness.

Electroencephalogram (EEG) activity

The depth of NREM sleep can be quantified by electroencephalogram (EEG) fluctuations. Four stages of NREM sleep are recognized on conventional EEG criteria (page 61). These are categorized by the frequency and amplitude of the EEG, the presence of sleep spindles and K-complexes, and electro-oculogram (EOG) and electromyogram (EMG) findings.

Mental activity

Subjects woken during NREM sleep frequently report awareness of fragmented, thought-like processes, particularly in the lighter stages and later in the night. These contain less action than the dreams that occur during REM sleep. The simpler dream mentation in NREM sleep is probably due to the functional disconnection of the cortex from sensory input by the thalamus. This may represent a process of reorganization of neural networks in an analogous, but different, manner to that which occurs in REM sleep.

Motor activity

The separation of the cerebral cortex from brainstem functioning during NREM sleep frees the somatic reflexes from higher control. Reflex activity is depressed, with the result, for instance, that tendon reflexes are

reduced, and in 50% of subjects there is an upgoing plantar (Babinski) reflex during NREM sleep.

Autonomic function

There is a relative increase in parasympathetic to sympathetic activity. The parasympathetic activity is also increased due to circadian factors at night. In contrast, the sympathetic system is more influenced by the sleep–wake state than circadian rhythms. The parasympathetic activity increases from stage 1 through to stage 4 of NREM sleep, and, in contrast to REM sleep, within each stage the balance of parasympathetic to sympathetic activity remains stable.

Metabolic rate

The metabolic rate is reduced in NREM sleep by 5–10%.

Temperature control

The core body temperature normally falls as NREM sleep is entered at the start of the night, and the control of sleep is closely related to thermoregulation. The reduced metabolic rate and vasodilatation of NREM sleep tend to reduce body temperature.

Respiratory function

The minute ventilation falls (1.23) and the arterial P_{CO_2} rises by 2–3 mmHg. The stage of NREM sleep oscillates frequently at sleep onset and the threshold for carbon dioxide to act as a respiratory stimulus fluctuates correspondingly. This may lead either to frequent central sleep apnoeas or to Cheyne–Stokes respiration. During the apnoeic phases the P_{CO_2} rises progressively at a rate determined by the metabolic rate, and when it exceeds the apnoeic threshold, respiration restarts, often with a phase of hyperventilation until the P_{CO_2} again falls below the threshold and the next apnoea begins.

The threshold for arousal from NREM sleep rises progressively from stage 1 to stage 4, but remains lower than in REM sleep [5] (Table 2.2).

The reduction in cerebral cortical influence on the respiratory centres and the reduction in somatic reflexes have important effects on respiration in NREM sleep. The respiratory drive is reduced, although it remains greater than in REM sleep. Within each NREM sleep stage the respiratory pattern is regular, but it varies between stages as the threshold for responding to P_{CO_2} (apnoeic threshold) alters. The threshold for the ventilatory response to P_{CO_2} increases from wakefulness to stage 1 NREM sleep and progressively into the deeper stages of NREM sleep with the effect that a

Table 2.2 Effects of REM and NREM sleep on respiration.

	REM sleep	*REM and NREM sleep*	*NREM sleep*
Physiological changes from wakefulness	↓↓ Drive ↓↓ Upper airway dimensions ↓↓ Chest wall muscles ↓ Functional residual capacity		↓ Drive ↓ Upper airway dimensions ↓ Chest wall muscles
Reversible pathological changes		Alkalosis Sedatives and alcohol Obesity Hypokalaemia Malnutrition Hyperinflation	
Irreversible pathological changes	Diaphragm weakness	Upper airway abnormalities Reduced chest wall muscle strength Impaired chest wall mechanics	Reduced reflex drive

NREM, non-rapid eye movement; REM, rapid eye movement.

$P\text{CO}_2$ which stimulates respiration during wakefulness may lead to apnoeas during sleep.

The activity of the chest wall muscles is globally reduced, unlike REM sleep in which the diaphragm is selectively spared, so that the ratio of rib cage to abdominal movement is greater in NREM than in REM sleep (Fig. 2.1). The reduction in respiratory activity almost parallels the reduced ventilatory requirements needed to cope with the lower metabolic rate during NREM sleep.

The action of the upper airway muscles during sleep is complex. The dilators and constrictors are reciprocally inhibited and the dilators and the diaphragm are activated together. There is a sequence of activation from the alae nasi to the diaphragm so that the upper airway is stabilized a few milliseconds before the negative pressure is developed by chest wall muscle contraction. Negative pressure itself is sensed by receptors in the upper airway and this leads to further activation of the dilator muscles.

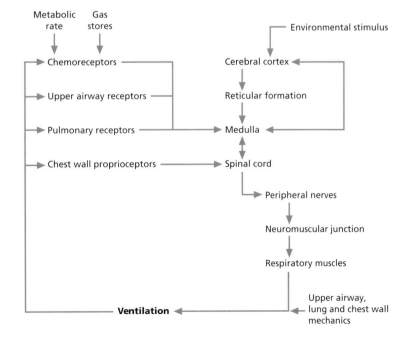

Fig. 2.1 Control of ventilation.

This response is less during NREM sleep than in wakefulness.

The upper airway resistance increases in NREM sleep compared to wakefulness, but to a lesser degree than during REM sleep. It increases the work of breathing and predisposes to obstructive sleep apnoeas.

Cardiovascular function

Even before the onset of NREM sleep the heart rate falls in parallel with the reduction in body temperature and is related to the fall in metabolic rate. Vasodilatation is due to reduced sympathetic activity and possibly accumulation of adenosine.

The cardiovascular system is more stable during NREM sleep than during REM sleep. The heart rate falls shortly after sleep onset, and there is then little further change between stages 2, 3 and 4 NREM sleep, although it continues to fall during the night because of a circadian rhythm.

The blood pressure is not under circadian control, but is more sleep-state dependent. It falls by 5–15% shortly after sleep onset due mainly to a reduction in cardiac output, but also to peripheral vasodilatation. There is little difference between either the systolic or diastolic blood pressures in stages 2, 3 and 4 NREM sleep. This fall in blood pressure is absent if there is increased sympathetic activity, as in hypertension or obstructive sleep apnoeas, and in chronic renal failure and Cushing's syndrome.

NREM sleep has been thought to be cardio-protective in that the coronary blood flow remains fairly constant during sleep, but there is a reduced perfusion pressure which may lead to ischaemia if there is coronary artery disease.

The cerebral blood flow is coupled to the metabolic rate of the central nervous system [6], and this auto-regulation is both regional within the brain and independent of the autonomic nervous system. The cerebral blood flow falls by 10–20% in NREM sleep compared to wakefulness, and is less than during REM sleep. It is reduced particularly in the prefrontal cortex.

Cerebral blood flow increases if hypercapnia develops because this causes cerebral vasodilatation and an increase in cardiac output. It also increases during wakefulness in the presence of hypoxia, but this response is absent in stages 3 and 4 NREM sleep. As a result there is a potential for reduction in oxygen delivery to the brain in hypoxic situations such as during obstructive and central sleep apnoeas. This may influence medullary function, and thereby modify upper airway and chest wall muscle control.

Cutaneous blood flow is increased due to vasodilatation, but there is probably little change in distribution of visceral blood flow during NREM sleep.

Gastrointestinal function

Less saliva is produced during sleep than during wakefulness, possibly partly related to a reduction in oromotor activity, but the volume is similar in NREM and REM sleep. The sensation of a dry mouth is common during sleep, particularly in the presence of snoring and sleep apnoeas. The swallowing frequency is similar to that during wakefulness in stage 1 NREM sleep, but in the deeper stages is less frequent. Swallowing may occur without causing any electroencephalogram features of arousal.

Gastro-oesophageal reflux commonly occurs during sleep, and clearance of acid from the oesophagus is slowed, probably because of a reduction in swallowing and oesophageal peristaltic activity. There are rhythmic gastric contractions approximately every 20 s in NREM sleep. The interval between peristaltic contractions in the small intestine and colon is increased in NREM sleep compared to wakefulness and there is an increase in colonic activity after waking [7]. Changes in the stability of the anal sphincter have been found during sleep.

Genito-urinary function

There is considerable diurnal variation in renal function. Water and sodium are retained at night and of the 1–2 l of urine that is normally excreted in the 24 h, around 80% is produced during the day.

Endocrine function

This changes considerably during NREM sleep compared to wakefulness (page 39).

Immunological function

The changes in immune function in sleep are less well documented than the autonomic changes, but the blood eosinophil and cortisol levels, and natural killer (NK) cell activity fluctuate with a circadian pattern. There is a relationship between melatonin, cytokines and interferon, all of which have immunological actions and influence sleep. The T-lymphocyte level rises in sleep, but the peripheral blood monocyte concentration falls, largely because the cells are sequestered in the spleen. In addition, changes in autonomic activity regulate the local immune responses through, for instance, alterations in regional blood flow. Peripheral release of cytokines may also affect sleep through

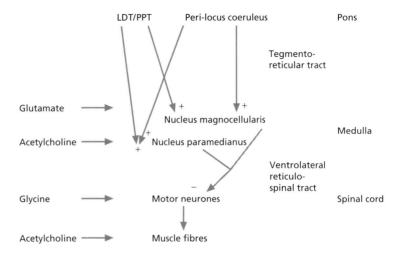

Fig. 2.2 Muscle atonia in REM sleep.

stimulation of vagal afferents which reach the brainstem, as well as through direct transfer across the blood–brain barrier.

Rapid eye movement (REM) sleep

Neurophysiology

Cortical activity

There are regional differences in cortical activity in REM sleep. The dorsolateral prefrontal cortex is particularly inactive. Unlike NREM sleep in which the thalamic 'gate' partially disconnects the cortex from the brainstem, the cortex still reacts to sensory information but in a different way than during wakefulness. The exception is that there is little activity in the spinoreticular tract which mediates pain, and painful sensations are very unusual in dreams.

There is evidence for interhemispheric disconnection compared to wakefulness, but similar to that which is seen after sectioning of the corpus callosum. Transcranial magnetic stimulation has revealed this disconnection particularly in the frontal and central areas of the cortex compared with the parietal and occipital regions [8]. It may be responsible for some of the lack of insight during dreams, time distortion and failure of some subjects to report dreams.

Muscle atonia

The pontine reticular formation ventral to the locus coeruleus (peri-locus coeruleus), including the LDT/PPT nuclei (page 41), projects to the nucleus magnocellularis and nucleus paramedianus in the medial medullary reticular formation via the lateral tegmento-

reticular tract (Fig. 2.2). Glutamate, which acts on receptors of the NMDA type, and acetylcholine are released and excite neurones in these nuclei. They project via the ventrolateral reticulospinal tract to the alpha motor neurones. The medial medullary centres are also activated by the locus coeruleus and the red nucleus which thereby reduce muscle tone. The motor neurones in the cranial nerve nuclei and spinal cord are inhibited by release of glycine, and this leads to the intense muscle atonia which is characteristic of REM sleep.

The continuous activity of the cerebral cortex is transmitted to the basal ganglia which remain active in REM sleep, but the complex behaviour patterns that they formulate are not enacted because of the intense inhibition of skeletal muscle tone.

Phasic activities

Many of the manifestations of REM sleep occur irregularly and apparently spontaneously due to intrinsic activity of the brainstem mechanisms responsible for REM sleep. These phasic activities include:

1 Rapid eye movements. These are controlled by the pontine and midbrain cranial nerve nuclei.

2 Ponto-geniculo-occipital (PGO) waves. These can be detected in animals by electrodes on the surface of the brain, but are not detectable by scalp electrodes in humans. They arise in the cholinergic peribrachial area of the pontine reticular formation and impulses project to the lateral geniculate nucleus of the thalamus, a visual relay station, and to the occipital visual cortex.

PGO waves are characterized by electroencephalogram spikes usually in bursts of 3–5 Hz which occur synchronously with rapid eye movements and probably represent higher neurological activity related to these and to other phasic REM events. They may have a role in visual dream imagery.

3 Actions of other cranial nerve nuclei and brainstem centres involved with cardiovascular and respiratory function. The changes in heart rate and respiratory frequency appear chaotic and probably represent the output from multiple partially independent lower brainstem 'pacemakers'.

Functional neuro-imaging

In REM sleep the pons and areas corresponding to the ascending reticular activating system are active. The dorsolateral prefrontal cortex is completely inactive as in stages 3 and 4 NREM sleep, but in contrast several areas of the limbic system are highly active. These include the anterior cingulate gyrus amygdala, lateral hypothalamus, the orbitomedial prefrontal cortex and the parahippocampal gyrus. Inactivity in the dorsolateral prefrontal cortex, which is involved in executive and planning functions, probably underlies the illogicality, but retention of social awareness, which is characteristic of dream mentation.

The overall metabolic rate of the brain in REM sleep is the same as in wakefulness, but greater than in NREM sleep.

Electroencephalogram (EEG) activity

The EEG reflects the intense cerebral cortical activity that distinguishes REM from NREM sleep, and its similarity to the EEG of wakefulness led to the term 'paradoxical' sleep for REM sleep. The depth of REM sleep is hard to quantify except perhaps through the REM density and the duration of REM sleep. The characteristic electrophysiological features of REM sleep are a combination of a wide range of 'desynchronized' EEG frequencies, loss of EMG activity and the presence of rapid eye movements.

Mental activity

REM sleep is characterized by loose mental associations, and the cortical processes responsible for these and for dreams are activated primarily by intrinsic activity within the pontine centres rather than by external or internal stimuli as in wakefulness. Mental activity in REM sleep is reflected in dreams which are characteristically full of activity, narrative and incidents, especially those occurring later in the night. They differ from the more thought-like content of NREM sleep, and often, but not invariably, coincide with phases when rapid eye movements are present.

Motor activity

The intense inhibition of alpha motor neurones in REM sleep prevents dreams and other cortical processes from being enacted. Tone is only retained in certain essential muscles, such as those of the middle ear, diaphragm and the posterior crico-arytenoids and to a lesser extent the parasternal intercostal muscles. Occasional jerking of the limbs during REM sleep represents a brief failure of inhibition of muscle tone and the rapid eye movements characteristic of REM sleep are a similar phasic phenomenon. These occur particularly during dreams, but also at other times during REM sleep, and may be accompanied by bursts of small movements of the facial, limb and trunk muscles.

Autonomic function

Autonomic activity is extremely variable in REM sleep. In general, sympathetic activity is reduced and parasympathetic activity increased. The rapid fluctuations in their balance may coincide with changes in activity in the pontine reticular formation or possibly in the cerebral cortex. The limbic cortex, in particular, is able to influence the hypothalamus, which translates cortical activity into autonomic function.

Metabolic rate

The metabolic rate during REM sleep is similar to that during wakefulness while resting.

Temperature control

Homeostatic temperature control is grossly impaired in REM sleep.

Respiratory function

The minute ventilation is reduced compared to NREM sleep and wakefulness [9], and the arterial $P\text{CO}_2$ rises by 2–5 mmHg. Arousal in response to stimulation from mechanoreceptors in the lungs, airways and chest wall, cough receptors and chemoreceptors occurs at a higher threshold in REM sleep than in NREM sleep.

The ventilatory responses to hypercapnia and hypoxia are reduced to a greater extent in REM than in NREM sleep and the combination of a reduction in reflex responsiveness and irregular cerebral cortical activity leads to an erratic and unpredictable pattern of respiratory activity. This appears to be due to multiple semi-independently functioning respiratory pacemakers in the pontine reticular formation [10].

Central apnoeas are more frequent and prolonged during REM sleep if other factors such as sleep deprivation, chronic hypercapnia, alkalosis, sedative drugs or alcohol are present. The respiratory frequency is not related to perceived physical activity during dreams, but is greater than in NREM sleep. The tidal volume and frequency both vary considerably in REM sleep. The intervals between respirations may be sufficiently prolonged to be classified as central sleep apnoeas according to the conventional criterion of a lack of airflow for 10 s or more.

The intense supraspinal inhibition of motor activity in REM sleep contributes to the reduction in reflex responsiveness and is manifested by a reduction in tone in the postural muscles, including all the respiratory muscles except the posterior crico-arytenoid muscles which abduct the vocal cords and maintain glottic patency, the diaphragm and to a lesser extent the parasternal intercostal muscles. Respiration becomes virtually dependent on diaphragmatic function and, if this is impaired, 'central' sleep apnoeas and hypoventilation appear.

Selective sparing of diaphragm activity in REM sleep leads to abdominal expansion increasing relative to the rib cage expansion. Loss of activity in the other chest wall muscles alters the compliance of the chest wall so that the functional residual capacity falls. This not only reflexly reduces the upper airway dimensions, but worsens ventilation and perfusion matching, reduces lung compliance and reduces the volume of the stores of oxygen in the lungs.

In REM sleep there is little tone in the upper airway dilator muscles and their reactivity to reflexes generated by negative pressure in the upper airway is reduced. The upper airway resistance rises, increasing the work of breathing, and may lead to closure of the airway and obstructive sleep apnoeas.

Cardiovascular function

Homeostatic control of cardiovascular function in response to, for instance, changes in blood volume or temperature is poor in REM sleep. There is considerable variability of heart rate and blood pressure according to fluctuations in the sympathetic–parasympathetic balance. This is primarily the result of erratic activity in the brainstem reticular formation. Overall, blood pressure is similar to that in wakefulness and the heart rate is greater than in NREM sleep. Cardiac output fluctuates according to the heart rate and blood pressure changes.

The coronary artery blood flow varies according to changes in blood pressure and heart rate. In general it is slightly greater than in NREM sleep, but the myocardial work is also increased.

Cerebral blood flow is similar to that in wakefulness, but greater than in NREM sleep, especially in the pons, thalamus and occipitotemporal cortex. As in NREM sleep it is coupled to central nervous system metabolic activity, and increases with hypercapnia. The intracranial pressure rises particularly in REM sleep possibly due to increases in cerebral blood flow.

Renal blood flow is slightly reduced in REM sleep due to an increase in sympathetic activity, and this also underlies the reduction in skeletal muscle blood flow.

Gastrointestinal function
This is described on page 26.

Genito-urinary function
Sleep-related erections (nocturnal penile tumescence) develop rapidly during REM sleep, and may persist into NREM sleep. Their frequency is not affected by sexual abstinence or activity. There is little change in their frequency with age, even in the elderly, and they may occur in prepubertal children.

Endocrine function
This is considerably different during REM sleep compared to NREM sleep or wakefulness (page 39).

Immunological function
This is different during sleep compared to wakefulness (pages 26, 37), but there are no known specific effects of REM sleep.

Control of sleep and wakefulness

Whether an individual is awake or asleep depends on the balance of forces promoting and inhibiting each of these two states [11]. At times the balance can be almost equal and the subject may begin to fall asleep if he or she had previously been awake, or to lighten from sleep if previously asleep. The mechanisms determining whether sleep or wakefulness predominates are incompletely understood, but three processes interact with each other and with circadian rhythms (Fig. 2.3).

NREM sleep homeostatic (intrinsic) drive (process S)
This drive to enter sleep increases, probably exponentially, with the duration since the end of the previous episode of NREM sleep. It builds up during wakefulness and probably in REM sleep as well. The duration of NREM sleep in each sleep cycle is inversely related to the duration of REM sleep in the previous cycle.

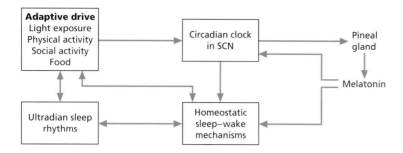

Fig. 2.3 Mechanisms of sleep–wake control. SCN, suprachiasmatic nuclei.

This drive declines once NREM sleep has been initiated, again probably exponentially. Its time constant is short at around 150 min so that after a few days of partial sleep deprivation a steady level of sleep drive is attained.

The homeostatic drive reinforces the cyclical nature of sleep and wakefulness and is analogous to other physiological needs such as hunger or thirst. The increased need to sleep according to the length of time awake is similar to the increase in hunger as the duration of abstinence from food increases.

An increase in homeostatic drive increases the duration and depth of NREM sleep at the expense of REM sleep. There is an increased duration and depth of NREM sleep (NREM sleep rebound) on the first night after sleep deprivation, but once the NREM sleep debt has been repaid after one or two nights, REM sleep duration increases.

REM sleep ultradian rhythm

REM sleep is almost never normally entered from wakefulness except in infants. It is preceded by NREM sleep, usually stages 1 and 2. It can therefore be regarded as a type of arousal from NREM sleep [12]. There are two drives which appear to determine whether or not REM sleep occurs.

Homeostatic drive

This increases with the duration since the previous REM sleep episode in a similar manner to the NREM sleep homeostatic drive, and decreases during REM sleep [13]. It increases throughout episodes of NREM sleep, but wakefulness appears to be a substitute for REM sleep in this respect and the REM sleep homeostatic drive only increases slightly in wakefulness. As a result there is little pressure to enter REM sleep at the onset of sleep, but this builds up increasingly during the night after episodes of NREM sleep. During wakefulness, although there may have been a considerable interval since the last episode of

REM sleep, the tendency to manifest features of REM sleep is limited to a 90-min cycle of transient feelings of drowsiness or a tendency to daydream.

Circadian rhythm

The tendency to enter REM sleep peaks at around 9.00 AM independently of the duration of previous REM or NREM sleep. This appears to be under circadian control and may be related to the increase in catabolic hormone secretion, such as cortisol, and the reduction in production of anabolic hormones.

As a result of these two drives, REM sleep appears at approximately 90-min intervals during the night. This ultradian rhythm may simply be a reflection of the two separate drives to enter REM sleep and their balance with NREM sleep and wakefulness. No specific anatomical location for this drive has been found. The increased duration of REM sleep later in the night is probably due to the combination of an increase in homeostatic and circadian drives to enter REM sleep and the reduced homeostatic NREM sleep drive towards the end of the night.

Adaptive drive

This includes a variety of mechanisms that influence sleep but which are independent of the time spent awake and of circadian and ultradian rhythms. They modify the sleep–wake cycle according to changes in the environment which are significant for the individual. They are important but complex and ill-understood components of the sleep–wake control system. They have three main elements.

Behavioural factors

These include motivation, attention and other psychological responses to the environment. The voluntary choice of, for instance, deciding whether to take exercise or to move to a more stimulating situation influences the probability of remaining awake or falling asleep. The degree of conscious or subconscious awareness of the significance of different sensory inputs influences whether arousal from sleep occurs. Once aroused, the conscious brain is able to recognize the source of the stimulus and to respond accordingly. The conscious decision either to try to fall asleep or to stay awake and knowledge of the clock time then influence whether or not the individual stays awake or falls asleep.

Social activity usually induces alertness but, through its association with physical activity and exposure to light, may have complex effects on sleep. Sleep is more likely after social interactions, and the resulting synchronization of sleep and wake patterns within a group or community may have a biological survival advantage.

Psychological factors

Mental stimulation before falling asleep makes doing so difficult, particularly if there are worries or anxieties which cannot be resolved. The ability to relax both mentally and physically affects whether or not sleep can be entered. Watching a television or video can be mentally stimulating because of the changing pictures, sounds and often exciting action, but equally they can induce sleep through boredom, immobility and low ambient light levels.

The degree to which the bedroom is mentally associated with sleep and how much it is, for instance, used as an office or a kitchen, affects the mental associations between going to bed and initiating sleep. Most people also find it more difficult to sleep in an unfamiliar environment, such as a hotel or sleep laboratory.

Reflex factors

The level or lack of sensory stimulation influences the sleep–wake state, and can be broken down into the following elements.

Light exposure

Light exposure has complex and important effects on sleep and wakefulness [14, 15]. The seasonal changes in the duration of daily light exposure lead to cyclical alterations in the duration of rest and activity. The duration of melatonin secretion and of sleep is longer in winter than in summer in non-tropical latitudes. At high latitudes with prolonged nights the long nocturnal sleep phase in winter may break into two episodes with an intervening stage of quiet wakefulness. Seasonal changes in light duration also influence

mood and behaviour, as exemplified by the seasonal affective disorder.

During sleep, 5–10% of ambient light reaches the retina even through closed eyelids. This has an alerting effect during NREM sleep, increasing the electroencephalogram frequency and causing arousals from sleep, with the result that there may be a later rebound increase in NREM sleep. The effects on REM sleep are less clear, but this can be promoted by brief episodes of darkness.

During wakefulness, light exposure has several important physiological effects that are independent of vision and visual pathways to the brain. These include an increase in the level of alertness, which is particularly marked with bright light and at night. Light exposure also significantly improves motor performance, for instance in shift workers, and elevates mood. Acute light exposure also increases the heart rate and core body temperature.

A separate non-visual effect is the influence of light on the timing of the circadian rhythms. Exposure to light resets these each day so that they are coordinated with environmental time. These effects are mediated by the influence of light on the suprachiasmatic nuclei and its suppression of melatonin secretion (Fig. 2.4).

The effects of light on the circadian rhythms depend on the following:

Intensity. There is probably an exponential or logarithmic relationship between the intensity of the light exposure and its effect in modifying circadian rhythms. Exposure to 25 lux for around 20 min will entrain the circadian rhythm in around 75% of subjects, and while the maximum effect can be seen with around 1000 lux, around 50% of this is obtained with only 100 lux, which is less than the light level in most domestic situations during the day (Table 2.3).

Duration. Brief light pulses can influence the circadian rhythms, but continuous exposure for 10–20 min has a significantly greater impact.

Wavelength. The individual wavelengths of light influence the circadian rhythms to different extents. The most effective in resetting them are between 445 and 475 nm, particularly around 460 nm, which is close to the wavelength to which melanopsin in the retinal ganglion cells is most sensitive.

Timing. The sleep phase can be shifted by up to 1–2 hours per day by light exposure according to its

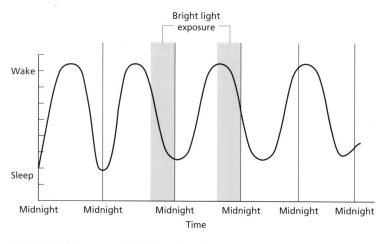

Fig. 2.4 Delay in sleep phase following exposure to bright light on the second and third evenings.

Table 2.3 Light exposure in different situations.

Situation	Light exposure (lux)
Starlight	0.01
Full moonlight	1
Television	1–15
Dim indoor light	100
Bright indoor light	300–500
Cloudy outdoors	1000
Sunlight outdoors	10 000

1 lux = illumination from a candle at 1 m from the surface; 1-foot candle = 10.76 lux.

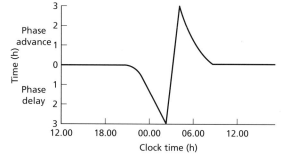

Fig. 2.5 Phase response curve to light. Bright light exposure in the evening leads to a sleep phase delay, but after 3.00–5.00 AM advances the next sleep phase.

timing. The phase response curve of sleep to light is complex (Fig. 2.5). The circadian rhythms are insensitive to light exposure during the day. There is little sleep phase delaying effect before around 9.00 PM or phase advance after around 10.00 AM. Light exposure at night, when there is normally little light and when melatonin is secreted, can have a major effect on the circadian rhythms. A rapid shift in the response to light occurs around the nadir of temperature and at the time of peak melatonin secretion, usually 3.00–5.00 AM. Light exposure before this phase-shift transition point delays the next sleep phase, but afterwards leads to a sleep phase advance. The magnitude of both of these effects is greatest close to the temperature nadir.

Noise

A noisy sleep environment can impair sleep but the threshold for arousal varies according to the age of the subject and the stage of sleep.

Arousal is also more likely if the noise is of significance to the sleeper, such as the crying of a child to the mother. Children sleep through more noise than adults, and older subjects are readily aroused from sleep by noise unless they are deaf. The threshold for arousal increases from stage 1 through to stage 4 NREM sleep. Arousal is therefore more likely later in the night after the initial episodes of stages 3 and 4 NREM sleep have been completed.

International standards for nocturnal environmental noise have been drawn up. In general they recommend a mean nocturnal noise level within the sleeping area of less than 40 dB and the avoidance of peak levels greater than 60 dB. Noise greater than 40 dB frequently causes difficulty in initiating sleep and greater than 50 dB often causes awakenings during the night. These thresholds, however, vary considerably between individuals, between nights and within each night, and with other environmental factors, such as room temperature. In young adults, for example, the threshold for arousal from stage 4 NREM sleep is around 100 dB, but this falls to 70 dB at age 70 years.

Adaptation to environmental noise occurs rapidly, and people living, for instance, close to railways, motorways and even airports may sleep soundly. Measures to isolate sleepers from noise can be successful and include earplugs and double glazing.

Pain and discomfort
Both internal and environmental stimuli can cause arousals from sleep despite the pain threshold being increased during sleep. Chronic disorders such as rheumatoid arthritis and multiple sclerosis commonly cause arousals of this type, and while a hard bed may help to reduce backache, it also leads to more frequent changes of position during sleep which are associated with brief awakenings.

Temperature
A constant environmental temperature of around 18°C (65°F) is ideal for inducing and maintaining sleep and for the optimal balance of NREM and REM sleep. Both high and low environmental temperatures lead to fragmentation of sleep. Rapid eye movement sleep is particularly sensitive to temperature changes and is significantly shortened in cold environments. REM sleep is facilitated by a rise, and NREM sleep by a fall, in core body temperature.

Physical exercise
Exercise promotes wakefulness not only at the time of the activity, but for around 3 h afterwards. This alerting effect is present both in normal subjects and also in, for instance, those with narcolepsy.

Exercise early in the day may cause a phase advance, reducing the sleep latency on the next night. It increases the total sleep time and the duration of stages 3 and 4 NREM sleep, and may reduce the duration of REM sleep. Exercise within around 3 h of the desired time of sleep onset may delay this and reduce melatonin secretion.

Food intake
Hunger is associated with wakefulness. This has a survival advantage in that wakefulness is retained until sufficient food has been eaten. After eating, humans tend to relax and readily fall asleep. This is due to complex reflex and humoral factors (page 13).

Carbohydrates and milky drinks which contain tryptophan, a precursor of 5HT, and melatonin, have a greater sleep-promoting effect than other foods. Tryptophan is also present in bananas, peanuts and figs. Lettuce contains lactucarium, an opioid which may promote sleep. Dietary unsaturated fatty acids such as oleamide bind to GABA receptors and can promote sleep and reduce motor activity. Conversely a low serum cholesterol level has been associated with violence. High protein foods which are rich in tyrosine may promote noradrenaline synthesis and lead to wakefulness.

Large meals taken before sleep can cause gastro-oesophageal reflux leading to heartburn and awakenings. Large volumes of liquid should be avoided before sleep since they may lead to nocturia, especially if there is renal impairment or prostatic hypertrophy.

Very severe malnutrition can induce excessive daytime sleepiness and inactivity, but, in general, weight loss, whether it is due to anorexia nervosa, mania or thyrotoxicosis, leads to insomnia and hyperactivity. Weight loss in depression is associated with insomnia, but if weight is gained, as in seasonal affective disorder, sleepiness is common. There may be a link in otherwise normal subjects between weight loss, hyperactivity and insomnia, and between weight gain, inactivity and excessive daytime sleepiness. The chemical basis of these associations is uncertain, but weight gain may also lead to excessive daytime sleepiness through causing obstructive sleep apnoeas.

Sexual activity
Sexual intercourse usually promotes the onset of sleep, in contrast to other types of physical activity.

Circadian rhythms

Circadian rhythm periodicity
Circadian rhythms have a periodicity of around a day, which is longer than ultradian rhythms of, for instance, REM sleep and shorter than infradian rhythms such as the menstrual cycle. The intrinsic circadian rhythm ranges between 23.5 and 24.5 h with a mean of around 24.2 h in humans. Approximately 25% of subjects have a rhythm which is less than 24 h and 75% a rhythm longer than this.

The circadian rhythms are generated by an internal pacemaker, oscillator or biological clock whose activity is modified by external factors (time givers, cues or zeitgebers). These reset or entrain the internal clock and gear it to the external environment. In certain situations the clock can become dissociated from the time givers, in which case it becomes 'free running' and desynchronized from the environment.

Suprachiasmatic nuclei (SCN)
The suprachiasmatic nuclei (SCN) in the supra-optic region of the anterior hypothalamus are the centres responsible for the most important circadian rhythms.

These two tiny bilateral nuclei about 3 cm behind the eyes each have a volume of only 0.1 ml and each contains around 10 000 neurones.

Each SCN has 'a core' of neurones which secrete either vaso-intestinal peptide or gastrin-releasing peptide. They respond particularly to light stimuli via the retino-hypothalamic tract and have melatonin receptors. The 'shell' of arginine vasopressin- and calretinin-releasing neurones responds to non-photic stimuli. This region probably controls the circadian elements of motor activity and feeding behaviour. Gamma-aminobutyric acid (GABA)-secreting neurones are present in both the core and the shell.

Each of the cells in the SCN is capable of spontaneous depolarization. The coordination of these is the source of circadian rhythmicity, but within the SCN there are subpopulations of cells with different cycle times [16]. These are usually entrained by diffuse chemical, rather than synaptic, mechanisms to a single rhythm but under certain circumstances they can become dissociated from each other.

The SCN is active during the day, both in diurnal and nocturnal animals. In humans it promotes wakefulness and influences the structures which control the onset and maintenance of sleep, but is not solely responsible for this.

SCN clock genetics

The characteristics of this rhythm generator are largely genetically determined. At least 12 genes have been identified on chromosome 5 which, through inhibiting or promoting protein transcription, form a complex negative feedback system which has the properties of an oscillator or clock. Examples of the genes are period 1–3, clock, BMAL, cryptochrome 1 and 2, and casein kinase. They are all DNA transcription activators and repressors with complex interactions which result in fluctuating levels of messenger RNA during the day and night. The clock genes have other functions such as encoding proteins related to cardiovascular function and haem synthesis.

Input to SCN

Impulses reach the SCN from retinal receptors which lie particularly in the lower and nasal quadrant of the retina. The receptors are the retinal ganglion cells and their light-sensitive pigment is melanopsin which is particularly sensitive to radiation with a wavelength of around 460 nm. These cells are glutamatergic and comprise around 4% of the fibres in the optic nerve in most species.

The retinal ganglion cells are distinct from the rods and cones which lead to the sensation of vision, and whose fibres run in the optic nerves, synapse in the lateral geniculate nuclei and connect to the primary visual sensory cortex in the occipital lobes. Impulses from retinal ganglion cells travel in the retino-hypothalamic tract, which also runs within the optic nerve, to monosynaptically reach the SCN independent of any visual sensation. Other impulses from the retinal ganglion cells reach the pretectum, superior colliculus and sub-paraventricular zone. These probably mediate the pupillary light reflex and the effects of light exposure on NREM and REM sleep, but do not lead to any visual sensations.

The cholinergic pedunculopontine and laterodorsal tegmental (LDT/PPT) nuclei and basal forebrain neurones also project to the SCN, as do the ascending reticular activating system and other areas of the brainstem (Fig. 2.6). These probably mediate the effects of physical exercise on advancing or delaying the sleep phase. This is also influenced by melatonin which inhibits the activity of the SCN and promotes sleep.

Output from SCN

Fibres leave the SCN to reach the ventrolateral preoptic area (VLPO) of the anterior hypothalamus multisynaptically. They initially relay in the sub-paraventricular zone before synapsing predominantly in the dorsomedial nucleus of the hypothalamus and then in the VLPO. At each of these locations integration of the circadian rhythms with other influences controlling not only sleep but temperature and endocrine function takes place.

Fibres also travel from the SCN to the hypothalamus, to control pituitary function, to the thalamus, the medial preoptic nucleus and multisynaptically to the pineal gland. The latter take a tortuous course descending through the periventricular hypothalamus into the intermediolateral cell column of the thoracic spinal cord from which preganglionic sympathetic neurones project to the superior cervical ganglion and then postganglionic sympathetic fibres travel along the internal carotid artery to reach the pineal gland.

Pineal gland

The pineal gland contains a circadian pacemaker in some vertebrates, such as perching birds (passerines). In humans this function is taken over by the SCN in the anterior hypothalamus, which controls the cycle of pineal melatonin secretion.

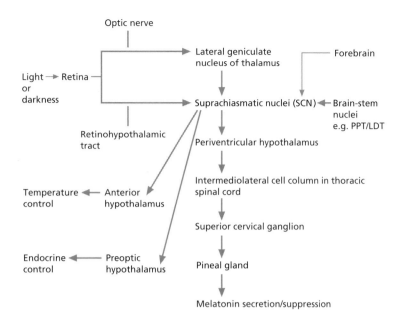

Fig. 2.6 Pathways linking retina, suprachiasmatic nuclei (SCN) and pineal gland. LDT, laterodorsal tegmental nuclei; PPT, pedunculopontine nuclei.

The human pineal gland contains glial cells and pinealocytes which have similarities to the photo-receptors of amphibia, but in humans they are only indirectly, not directly, light sensitive. The pinealo-cytes secrete several hormones and related chemicals such as GABA and 5HT, but their most important hormone is melatonin.

Melatonin

Melatonin production
Melatonin (N-5-methoxy-N-acetyl-tryptamine) is synthesized from tryptophan after it has been converted to 5HT [17]. Its synthesis can be increased by oral tryptophan or vitamin B6, a coenzyme in tryptophan metabolism. Little melatonin is stored in the pineal gland, but it is synthesized and secreted in pulses in response to noradrenaline release at synapses within the pineal gland. Its release is increased by selective serotonin re-uptake inhibitor (SSRI) antidepressants and antipsychotic drugs, but is inhibited by caffeine, beta blockers, benzodiazepines and non-steroidal anti-inflammatory drugs. It is also produced in the retina and gastro-intestinal tract.

Endogenous control
Without any exposure to light the endogenous rhythm of the SCN leads to a circadian rhythm of melatonin secretion of around 24.2 h by the pineal gland. Melatonin is a marker of the circadian clock function,

but it also acts as a hormone of darkness to reinforce the synchronization of sleep with the light–dark cycle of the environment. The pineal gland in effect acts as a transducer, converting a photo-period signal into a chemical signal.

Age and melatonin
Under the age of 3 months little melatonin is secreted and there is no variation with light exposure. A nocturnal secretion pattern then emerges and the peak nocturnal concentration rises to around 1400 pmol/l at around the age of 3 years. This then declines, especially during puberty, to a level which is maintained until around 40 years of age before it falls further. The peak nocturnal level in adults is 250–500 pmol/l and a total of 30 μg is usually secreted in each circadian cycle, although melatonin is often undetectable (less than 40 pmol/l) during the day.

Light exposure and melatonin
Melatonin secretion is particularly suppressed with wavelengths of around 460 nm.

Light exposure can either phase advance or delay melatonin secretion, according to its timing. Light exposure in the evening delays melatonin secretion, and darkness in the morning prolongs it and helps maintain sleep. This mechanism underlies the phase response curve of the circadian sleep rhythm to light.

Reduction of melatonin secretion at night is seen with low-frequency (50–60 Hz) electromagnetic

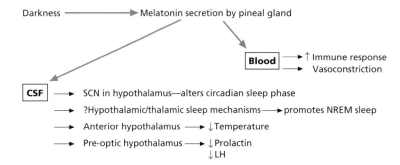

Fig. 2.7 Effects of melatonin secretion. CSF, cerebrospinal fluid; LH, luteinizing hormone; NREM, non-rapid eye movement; SCN, suprachiasmatic nuclei.

radiation from, for instance, electric cables, pylons and mobile (cellular) telephones. Exposure to light early in the morning induces an earlier onset of melatonin secretion the next evening. A brief light stimulus at night inhibits melatonin secretion temporarily. Complete suppression requires more than 1000 lux for more than 2 h, but as little as 100 lux may halve melatonin secretion.

Timing of melatonin secretion

Melatonin secretion increases shortly before sleep, usually around 9.00–10.00 PM. The peak nocturnal level in adults is reached between 3.00 and 5.00 AM, which is around the transition point of the phase response curve to light. This is usually around 4 h before waking in young subjects and 3 h in the elderly but varies with the Chronotype.

Pharmacology of melatonin

Melatonin is lipid soluble and is released both into the cerebrospinal fluid and into the blood so that it becomes widely distributed within the brain and the rest of the body, to which it acts as an indirect chemical messenger of the SCN. The concentration in the periventricular areas of the brain, which are exposed to the cerebrospinal fluid, may be very much higher than the blood levels.

Melatonin has a half-life of 30–45 min in the blood and is mainly inactivated in the liver by conversion to 6-hydroxymelatonin. It is then conjugated with sulphuric or glucuronic acid. These metabolites are excreted in the urine, particularly 6-sulphatoxymelatonin whose concentration runs in parallel, but with a delay of around 1 h behind the serum melatonin concentration.

Effects of melatonin

These are three melatonin receptors. MT1 is present in the SCN and the pars tuberalis of the pituitary gland, and inhibits the wake promoting effect of the SCN and influences endocrine funtion. MT2 is present in the SCN and the retina and can entrain the SCN. The role of the MT3 receptor is uncertain. Melatonin binds to calmodulin within the cells, but the details of its biochemical effects are unclear.

Its main actions are as follows.

Effects on SCN

Melatonin appears to have two effects on the SCN which are mediated either by a direct effect on the circadian rhythm generating cells or by activation of GABA-ergic neurones within the SCN which inhibit its activity (Fig. 2.7). First, it entrains the SCN, modifying the timing of its circadian rhythms and reducing body temperature, predisposing towards NREM rather than REM sleep and influencing the timing of sleep. This action is greatest in the evening when the circadian drive to wakefulness is strongest. It causes a phase advance of the sleep pattern with opening of the 'gate' for sleep through loss of the normal 'wakefulness maintenance zone' shortly before the usual sleep time.

Secondly, melatonin may synchronize other circadian rhythms, such as temperature and cortisol secretion, either through an action on the SCN or directly on the centres controlling these rhythms. The sleep and temperature rhythms, for instance, can be dissociated either because of incoordination of sub-populations of cells in the SCN which control the two rhythms, or through divergences in the mechanisms controlling them outside the SCN.

Hypnotic effect

Melatonin has a soporific effect which is greatest during the day. This may be through inhibiting the wake promoting effect of the SCN or by a direct action on other sleep mechanisms, perhaps in the thalamus or hypothalamus. Its effect is probably mediated by activation of inhibitory GABA-ergic neurones, possibly through the action of cytokines. It does not appear to alter the proportions of NREM and REM sleep, but if given during the day usually leads to stages 1 and 2 NREM sleep.

Inhibition of reproductive function
Melatonin reduces prolactin and luteinizing hormone levels and delays puberty. The fall in its serum concentration at puberty may enable sexual development to take place. A high peak melatonin level at night is associated with infertility in both males and females.

The steadily changing seasonal duration of exposure to light alters the duration for which melatonin is secreted each night. This may influence reproductive activity, although humans are less sensitive to this photoperiod signal than many animals which have well-defined seasonal reproductive cycles.

Effects on immune function
Resection of the pineal gland is followed by immunosuppression and changes in the thymus, probably due to loss of melatonin secretion. Melatonin's effects on immune function are:

1 augmentation of natural killer (NK) cell activity in killing tumour and virus infected cells;
2 binding to T-lymphocytes, especially CD4+, and augmenting T-helper cell activity increasing their production of interferon gamma and interleukin-1 (IL-1), and release of IL-2;
3 increasing antibody responses, probably by augmenting T-helper cell function;
4 preventing apoptosis of T-lymphocytes;
5 antagonizing corticosteroid-induced immunosuppression, probably through its effects on cytokine availability.

Vasodilation. The heat loss through the skin due to peripheral vasodilation when melatonin is secreted in the evening lowers the body temperature and facilitates sleep onset.

Mild anticonvulsant action

Coordination of circadian rhythms
The clock in the SCN, through its neurological connections, has a circadian influence not only on sleep, but also on temperature control, hormone secretion and other functions. The multisynaptic processing of the SCN output allows circadian rhythm and other controlling influences to be coordinated through integration with other inputs at each stage. Removal of the SCN causes a loss of most of these rhythms, but does not prevent sleep from taking place or temperature from being controlled.

In normal circumstances these functions have a constant relationship, but they can become desynchronized. This may occur even if the SCN is working normally, if there are unusual environmental situations, such as time zone changes, which can disturb their coordination. The potential for this internal desynchronization varies between the various circadian rhythms. Loss of function of the SCN increases the duration of sleep, indicating that the SCN has a wakefulness maintaining effect and tends to counteract the homeostatic drive to sleep.

Individual circadian rhythms
The most important SCN-related circadian rhythms concern cell growth and proliferation, autonomic and immune function, sleep, temperature and endocrine secretion.

Cell growth and proliferation
The genetic control of clock function and circadian rhythms through protein production is closely linked with a diurnal variation in cell growth and proliferation in many tissues. The clock genes for instance control the production of a rate limiting enzyme in haem synthesis. Regeneration of liver cells varies diurnally, and division of the squamous cells of the skin is most rapid at night.

Several tissues such as the liver and kidneys have local pacemakers which are capable of sustaining a circadian rhythm for several days independently of the SCN. These local pacemakers represent an inherent circadian rhythm which may be present in all cells of the body, and which feed back to the main circadian rhythm controller in the SCN, and are also controlled through changes in autonomic innervationand melatonin. Circadian cell growth and proliferation cycles may be relevant to the development of malignancy.

Autonomic and immune function
Several autonomic functions, including bronchoconstriction, heart rate and renal function, have a circadian rhythm, and several aspects of immune function have a similar pattern. Parasympathetic activity has a circadian rhythm with a peak at 4.00 AM and a nadir in the late afternoon, whereas sympathetic activity is more related to the sleep–wake state.

Motor and feeding behaviour
Motor activity and feeding behaviour have a circadian pattern which is closely related to the sleep–wake rhythms, but is also controlled by, for instance, orexins and leptin.

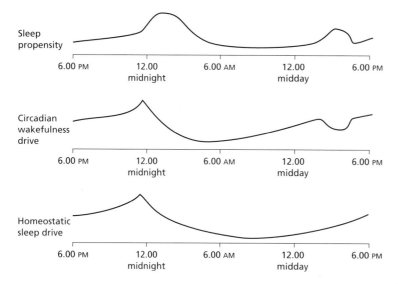

Fig. 2.8 The influence of circadian rhythms and homeostatic sleep drive on sleep–wake states. The sleep propensity is the sum of the circadian and homeostatic drives.

Sleep rhythms

The diurnal cycling of sleep–wake rhythms maintains sleep and wakefulness in line with environmental time, but by itself is insufficient to initiate sleep (Fig. 2.8). Loss of function of the SCN increases the duration of sleep, indicating that it has a wakefulness maintaining effect and tends to counteract the homeostatic drive to sleep. In effect it raises the threshold of the other sleep drives for initiating sleep. It does not selectively promote either NREM or REM sleep.

The SCN promotes wakefulness during the day, except between 2.00 and 4.00 PM, and particularly in the evenings shortly before the usual time of sleep onset which is when the homeostatic drive to sleep is greatest. The circadian rhythm opposes this and leads to the 'wakefulness maintenance zone' or 'forbidden zone'. At this time just prior to the usual time of sleep it is difficult to fall asleep. The end point of this zone occurs when the homeostatic drive, together with an input from the adaptive drive, overcomes this circadian influence. The onset of secretion of melatonin by the pineal gland also inhibits the SCN activity.

The circadian drive to wakefulness is at its least before the habitual wake-up time of the subject in the morning. This helps to consolidate sleep at the end of the night when the homeostatic drive to sleep is waning. At the time of waking the circadian drive to wakefulness increases sharply and its wakefulness effect overcomes any residual homeostatic drive to sleep.

Temperature cycle

The sleep and temperature cycles are usually closely coupled [18], although in free-running experiments the sleep cycle usually becomes around 1 h longer than the temperature cycle. The temperature of the blood is sensed in the paraventricular nucleus which is close to, but separate from, the VLPO and other sleep-regulating sensors in the preoptic area of the anterior hypothalamus. Activity in these centres suppresses arousals and increases NREM sleep as well as reducing the core body temperature. Melatonin secretion facilitates sleep and also lowers the core body temperature. The peak melatonin level is seen at the nadir of the core body temperature at 3.00–5.00 AM.

The paraventricular nucleus reacts to a rise in temperature by increasing heat loss through cutaneous vasodilatation and sweating. If the temperature falls, the posterior hypothalamus causes heat conservation by cutaneous vasoconstriction and increased heat production through skeletal muscle activity, including shivering, and piloerection.

The amplitude of the circadian temperature cycle is 0.5–0.75°C, although this is reduced in the elderly. The temperature rises to a peak of 37°C at 3.00–5.00 PM and falls only slowly until around 9.00 PM. The drop in core temperature which precedes sleep is associated with an elevation of skin temperature due to cutaneous vasodilatation, possibly related to accumulation of adenosine in the basal forebrain.

The temperature continues to fall after sleep onset due to a reduction in physical activity and metabolic rate and to vasodilatation during NREM sleep. The assumption of the supine position also lowers the temperature through a postural reflex. The temperature nadir is usually at 3.00–5.00 AM, which coincides with the phase change in response to light (Fig. 2.9).

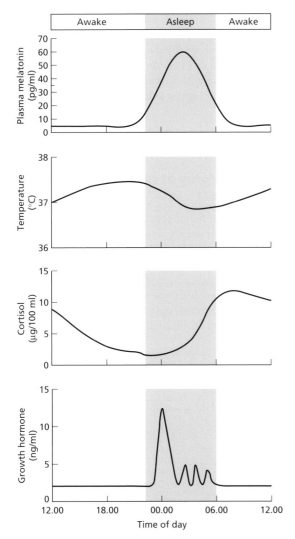

Fig. 2.9 Diurnal changes in melatonin, temperature, cortisol and growth hormone.

The subsequent temperature rise is linked to the increase in duration and density of REM sleep, although thermoregulation is much less precisely controlled in REM sleep than in NREM sleep or wakefulness.

Endocrine cycles

There is an important circadian pattern to the secretion of hormones, many of which are controlled by the hypothalamus [19]. Those needed to adapt the individual to respond to external influences during wakefulness, and which are predominantly catabolic, such as adrenaline and cortisol, are secreted especially during the day, and have a strong circadian influence.

Corticotrophin-releasing hormone (CRH)

This controls release of ACTH. It promotes wakefulness, and inhibits NREM sleep.

Adrenocorticotrophic hormone (ACTH)

The release of ACTH is controlled both by CRH and by arginine vasopressin which also acts on osmoreceptors in the preoptic area of the hypothalamus. Its secretion is inhibited by stages 3 and 4 NREM sleep and changes only slowly with alterations of the timing of circadian rhythms, induced, for instance, by time zone changes (jet lag).

Cortisol

This is secreted in response to ACTH. Its release is closely related to the circadian rhythm but is also slightly influenced by light exposure. Cortisol secretion occurs in several pulses towards the end of the nocturnal sleep episode and peaks around the time of wakening. Its secretion is inhibited by stages 3 and 4 NREM sleep and it also inhibits stages 3 and 4 NREM sleep. In Cushing's syndrome and psychotic depression cortisol secretion occurs continuously throughout sleep and wakefulness, and the dip in secretion at night is absent.

Thyroid stimulating hormone (TSH, thyrotrophin)

TSH secretion starts just before sleep onset, peaks at the onset of sleep and then falls during NREM sleep so that the daytime values are reached by the time of awakening in the morning. Secretion is controlled approximately equally by circadian rhythms and by the state of being asleep, which inhibits its secretion.

Hormones which have a primary anabolic function have a different pattern of secretion, which is predominantly controlled according to the sleep–wake state. These include the following.

Growth hormone

This is normally secreted in pulses during stages 3 and 4 NREM sleep, although its secretion may precede sleep. Between one-half and two-thirds of the total quantity is released during the first NREM sleep episode [20]. Its secretion is inhibited by awakening from sleep. In women the relationship with NREM sleep is less close than in men, probably because of progesterone production in the luteal phase of the menstrual cycle.

Prolactin

There is a slight circadian influence on prolactin secretion, but it is more closely related to the sleep–wake state. Its secretion is promoted by NREM sleep, particularly stages 3 and 4, but its peak plasma concentration is reached later than with growth hormone at around 90 min after sleep onset. It is secreted in pulses throughout the NREM sleep cycles but is suppressed by nocturnal awakenings. Prolactin promotes REM sleep.

Renin and aldosterone

Aldosterone levels rise during REM sleep, whereas renin is secreted mostly in stages 1 and 2 NREM sleep, and it is inhibited by REM sleep.

Luteinizing hormone (LH) and follicle-stimulating hormone (FSH)

These gonadotrophins are secreted in pulses during the night. The serum concentration of LH is low, both during wakefulness and during sleep in prepubertal children, but around puberty there is release of LH in pulses during sleep associated with a corresponding rise in testosterone. By the time that sexual maturation has been reached the secretion of LH during wakefulness is similar to that during sleep. Testosterone blood levels are highest in REM sleep.

Melatonin

See page 35.

Neuroanatomy of sleep and wakefulness

The activity of the cerebral cortex is critical in determining whether sleep or wakefulness occurs, but it does not generate the drive to enter sleep or wakefulness. This is due to the interaction of many influences, some of which are localized to specific areas of the central nervous system and others which are more diffuse (Fig. 2.10). The most important anatomical structures concerned with sleep–wake regulation are as follows.

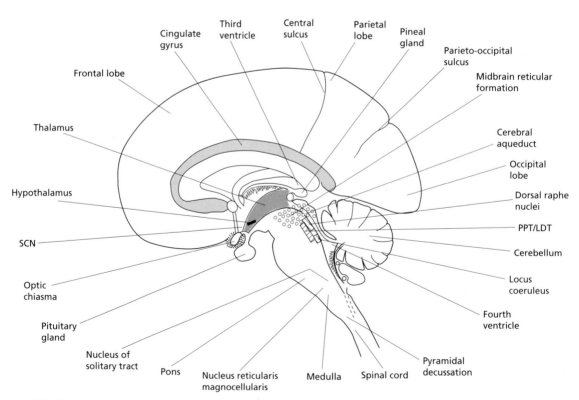

Fig. 2.10 Neuroanatomy of sleep-related structures. SCN, suprachiasmatic nuclei; LDT, laterodorsal tegmental nuclei; PPT, pedunculopontine nuclei.

Ascending reticular activating system (ARAS)

The ascending reticular activating system is a physiological entity which promotes wakefulness when it is active and allows sleep when it is inhibited or inactive (Fig. 2.6). It was originally thought to be a homogeneous system, but the complexity of its structure and function is now realized. It governs the homeostatic drive and many of the reflex components of the adaptive sleep drive, and is closely connected to the circadian sleep rhythms.

The ascending reticular activating system is largely contained in the brainstem reticular formation which is a loosely connected structure with small groups of cells and nuclei, large numbers of short interneurones and complex ascending and descending interconnecting tracts. Most of the reticular formation lies in the central core or tegmentum of the pons and midbrain, but it also extends into the medulla, hypothalamus and thalamus. It has a complex microstructure and GABA is secreted at most of its synapses. It has an extensive influence over the sensory input to the brainstem, motor function of the cranial nerve nuclei and spinal cord, and the state of sleep or wakefulness. It also has close links, through the hypothalamus, with endocrine control.

Nucleus of the solitary tract

This is located in the medulla and is noradrenergic. It has connections throughout the pons, hypothalamus and thalamus. It is more active in NREM sleep than in wakefulness and electrical stimulation in animals promotes sleep.

Locus coeruleus

This is situated in the upper dorsal pons and is noradrenergic. It has widespread connections in the brainstem, thalamus and basal forebrain. It is most active in wakefulness, partially suppressed in NREM sleep and inactive in REM sleep. It inhibits the activity of the LDT/PPT and is itself inhibited by GABA-ergic neurones.

Raphe nuclei

These are situated in the midline in the midbrain and are serotonergic. The most important is the dorsal raphe nucleus. The raphe nuclei are most active in wakefulness, partially suppressed in NREM sleep and inactive in REM sleep. They are inhibited by GABA-ergic neurones. They inhibit the activity of the LDT/PPT and project to the hypothalamus. They may

contribute to the autonomic and motor responses to arousal from sleep and to the emotional state.

Laterodorsal tegmental and pedunculopontine tegmental (LDT/PPT) nuclei

These are situated in the dorsal pontine tegmental reticular formation and their neurones are cholinergic. They are inhibited by the locus coeruleus, raphe nuclei and tubero-mammillary nuclei. They connect to widespread areas in the brainstem and to the thalamus. They are the primary REM sleep generator [21] and when active inhibit both the locus coeruleus and the raphe nuclei. They are also involved in generation of REM sleep atonia and contribute to visual components of dreams and hallucinations.

Mesolimbic system

This arises in the midbrain ventral tegmental area and projects to the prefrontal cerebral cortex, and to the limbic system including the amygdala and hippocampus, and particularly to the thalamic reticular nucleus. It is dopaminergic and appears to cause arousal in response to specific stimuli rather than sustained wakefulness.

Tubero-mammillary nuclei (TMN)

These nuclei are situated in the posterior hypothalamus and are histaminergic. They only receive afferent input from the ventrolateral preoptic nucleus (VLPO) and the orexin system in the lateral hypothalamus. They inhibit particularly the VLPO and the LDT/PPT. The TMN are most active in wakefulness, partially suppressed in NREM sleep and inactive in REM sleep. The TMN promote wakefulness and suppress both NREM and REM sleep.

Perifornical nuclei

These are located in the lateral hypothalamus and their neurones secrete orexins (hypocretins). They project to the brainstem aminergic centres, particularly the locus coeruleus, but also the raphe nuclei. They are excitatory at these sites, but lead to inhibition of the LDT/PPT. They are most active in wakefulness, which they promote, and they limit the duration of REM sleep, but have direct effect on the VLPO.

Suprachiasmatic nuclei (SCN)

The SCN are responsible for circadian rhythms (page 33) and promote wakefulness. Lesions of the SCN are associated with excessive sleepiness.

Preoptic area of hypothalamus (POA)

This important anterior thalamic area is the main site of integration of homeostatic and circadian drives. It includes the VLPO and VMPO, which are close to the SCN, as well as osmoreceptors which secrete arginine vasopressin (AVP).

Ventrolateral preoptic nuclei (VLPO)

These are situated inferiorly to the SCN and lateral to the third ventricle, adjacent to the ventromedial preoptic nuclei (VMPO). Their neurones secrete both GABA and galanine which are inhibitory neurotransmitters. They inhibit all the aminergic brainstem arousal nuclei, including the locus coeruleus, raphe nuclei, mesolimbic system and also the tubero-mammillary nuclei.

The dorsal part of the VLPO promotes NREM sleep, and its medial extension, which projects particularly to the LDT/PPT, induces REM sleep. The VLPO activity is not related to circadian rhythms, but increases with sleep deprivation. The VLPO is active in sleep and inactive during wakefulness. Its widespread inhibitory connections give it the potential to cause a synchronized reactivation of the sleep promoting centres, but it is inhibited by the aminergic arousal systems, particularly the tubero-mammillary nuclei, as well as the cholinergic basal forebrain.

Ventromedial preoptic nuclei (VMPO)

These are particularly involved with temperature control, but also modify sleep–wake function.

Median preoptic nucleus (MPN)

This is located in the hypothalamus, dorsal to the third ventricle, and is GABA-ergic. It receives input from the SCN and projects to the cholinergic neurones in the basal forebrain and to the perifornical nuclei. It is active during sleep, particularly stages 3 and 4 NREM sleep.

Subparaventricular zone

This is close to the SCN and input from this is integrated with other influences which modify circadian rhythms of sleep, temperature (via the VMPO), behaviour and endocrine control.

Dorsomedial nucleus

This receives fibres from the subparaventricular zone and inhibits the VLPO. It is particularly involved with temperature control and feeding behaviour, as well as

arousal. It also projects to the paraventricular nucleus and the perifornical nuclei.

Basal forebrain (substantia innominata)

This lies just anterior to the preoptic area of the hypothalamus. It contains groups of neurones which have important influences on sleep.

Basal nucleus of Meynert

Its neurones are activated by glutamatergic neurones from the pons as well as the locus coeruleus, raphe nuclei and perifornical nuclei. They are cholinergic and are inhibited by accumulation of adenosine.

Neurones related to the amygdala, nucleus accumbens and ventral putamen

These are heterogeneous. Some are GABA-ergic neurones which are active particularly in stages 3 and 4 NREM sleep and project to the LDT/PPT. Others secrete glutamate or galanine as transmitters.

They project widely to the SCN and to the limbic system. This area of the basal forebrain acts as an ascending pathway of the reticular activating system and provides a ventral extra-thalamic relay to the cerebral cortex. It is active in wakefulness and in REM sleep, but inactive in NREM sleep. Adenosine accumulates in the extracellular spaces, attaches to A1 receptors and hyperpolarizes (inhibits) the cholinergic basal forebrain neurones, promoting NREM sleep.

Limbic system

The limbic system regulates both the autonomic nervous system and emotional reactions to external stimuli and memories, thereby making these systems more flexible and adaptive. It regulates mental state, motor activity – for instance related to fight or flight – and sexual activity, and responds to other stimuli such as those associated with thirst and hunger.

The most important areas within the cerebral cortex are the anterior cingulate gyrus, the para-hippocampal gyrus and the hippocampal formation in the temporal lobe, as well as the orbitofrontal region of the pre-frontal cortex. The limbic cortex gives representation for autonomic function such as cardiovascular and gastro-intestinal control and is involved in behaviour related to emotion. It is inactive in NREM sleep, but active in REM sleep.

The non-cortical components of the limbic system include the amygdala, nucleus accumbens, part of the basal forebrain (basal nucleus of Meynert), and parts of the hypothalamus and some thalamic nuclei. In the midbrain the limbic system comprises the peri-aqueductal grey matter whose descending impulses influence motor nuclei, respiratory activity and cardiovascular aspects of autonomic function, particularly sympathetic responses.

Thalamus

The thalamus is the final common path for most of the information reaching the cortex from receptors, apart from olfaction, and from the brainstem. The thalamus modifies these inputs, in effect acting as a gate determining which of the stimuli reach the cortex and in what form, although thalamic activity is itself regulated by the cerebral cortex. As the homeostatic drive to sleep wanes, the ability of the thalamus to block transmission to the cortex weakens and arousals occur.

The thalamic reticular nucleus is especially important in interacting with the cerebral cortex and determining the state of arousal. It has groups of excitatory neurones, which release glutamate, and inhibitory neurones, which release GABA at their synapses. Intrathalamic relay neurones modify the thalamic activity whereas other neurones form the thalamocortical projection fibres. There is reciprocal activity between the thalamus and cerebral cortex through these fibres and thalamic excitation is followed by inhibition by corticothalamic impulses. Their timing determines the frequency of the bursts of thalamic stimulation of the cortex which varies from 0.6 to 1 Hz [22].

The thalamus filters and modifies activity from the ascending reticular activating system and other systems passing through the midbrain. It modifies midbrain spindle activity and through its widespread projections to the cerebral cortex is able to integrate and synchronize cortical activity. Synchronization of cortical activity initiates and maintains the state of NREM sleep. It effectively disconnects the cerebral cortex from brainstem and other influences, although this is reversible through the mechanism of arousal. The thalamus not only protects the cortex from other incoming electrical impulses, so that it is deafferented or sensorily deprived, but also, through its GABA-secreting neurones, it inhibits brainstem centres that are capable of leading to an arousal. It also influences REM sleep through its projections to the LDT/PPT. Although the thalamic arousal inhibiting mechanism responsible for NREM sleep has a global projection to the cerebral cortex there are also specific thalamic effects during NREM sleep, for instance on primary sensory areas [19].

Cerebral cortex

The cerebral cortex is an extensive heterogeneous structure, which has correspondingly complex effects on the initiation, maintenance and cessation of sleep. The activity of different areas of the cortex during NREM and REM sleep is described on pages 23 and 27. The cerebral cortex is responsible for most aspects of the adaptive sleep–wake drive, and it enables the homeostatic and circadian influences on sleep to be more precisely adjusted to optimize responses to environmental changes. Cortical synchronization during NREM sleep is essential for the maintenance of this state, but its activity during REM sleep is more similar to that during wakefulness than to that during NREM sleep.

Neurophysiology of sleep and wakefulness

The neurophysiology of sleep and wakefulness is complex, but is the result of the superimposition of higher neurological control over lower functions [23, 24, 25] (Figs 2.11, 2.12, 2.13). This hierarchy and mutually interacting system can be broken down into the following components.

Brainstem wakefulness promoting centres

1 The aminergic nuclei, particularly the locus coeruleus, raphe nuclei and tubero-mammillary nuclei (TMN), are all most active during wakefulness, partly suppressed in NREM sleep and inactive in REM sleep. They all promote wakefulness, inhibit the REM sleep promoting action of the LDT/PPT, and project rostrally to the thalamus, hypothalamus and basal forebrain as the ascending reticular activating system.

2 Cholinergic LDT/PPT nuclei. These promote REM sleep and are active in this state and in wakefulness, but inactive in NREM sleep [26]. The activity of the LDT/PPT nuclei is probably the source of the high-frequency thalamocortical bursts which result in the desynchronized EEG characteristic of REM sleep. The LDT/PPT also influence sleep-related eye movements, which are controlled by the oculo-motor nuclei, and the loss of muscle tone in REM sleep (Table 2.4).

The difference in the combination of activity of the LDT/PPT and the aminergic nuclei between wakefulness and REM sleep is that although the LDT/PPT are

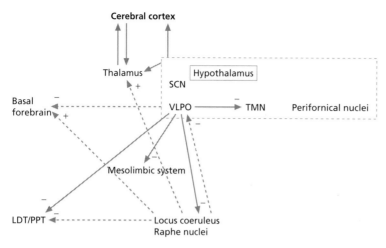

Fig. 2.11 Main pathways involved in NREM sleep.

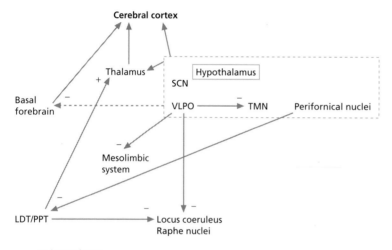

Fig. 2.12 Main pathways involved in REM sleep.

active in both, the aminergic nuclei are only active in wakefulness and inactivated in REM sleep. In contrast both the aminergic and cholinergic nuclei are partially and approximately equally suppressed in NREM sleep.

Wakefulness promoting higher centres

1 The perifornical hypothalamic orexin-releasing neurones have an excitatory effect on the aminergic nuclei, promoting wakefulness, and inhibit LDT/PPT, thereby limiting the duration of REM sleep.
2 The mesolimbic dopaminergic system projects to the prefrontal cortex and limbic system, promoting wakefulness.

3 Cholinergic neurones in the basal forebrain promote wakefulness and REM sleep.
4 The suprachiasmatic nuclei have a wakefulness promoting effect, in addition to providing a circadian influence on sleep and wakefulness.

Sleep promoting higher centres

1 The ventrolateral preoptic nucleus (VLPO) in the anterior hypothalamus inhibits the aminergic nuclei through GABA-ergic neurones. It also has separate projections to the LDT/PPT.

The VLPO and TMN have mutually inhibitory actions so that as the VLPO activity builds up during wakefulness its inhibition of the TMN progressively

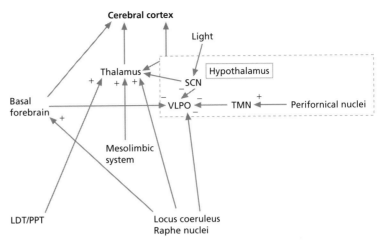

Fig. 2.13 Main pathways involved in wakefulness.

——— Active pathway
- - - - Partially inactivated pathway

Table 2.4 Activity of brainstem centres in sleep and wakefulness.

Nucleus	NREM sleep	REM sleep	Wakefulness
Locus coeruleus	↓	–	+
Raphe nuclei	↓	–	+
Tubero-mammillary nuclei	↓	–	+
LDT/PPT	–	+	+

+ = active; ↓ = reduced activity; – = inactive.

increases and eventually reaches the point at which the TMN becomes inactive. The VLPO at this time also inhibits the other aminergic nuclei and initiates NREM sleep, and subsequently allows REM sleep. As the homeostatic drive to sleep gradually wanes, the VLPO inhibition of the TMN decreases, allowing it to become active again and to inhibit VLPO activity. This releases the other aminergic nuclei from inhibition and enables wakefulness to appear.

This reciprocal inhibition functions as a bistable oscillator or flip-flop mechanism which leads to rapid changes between sleep and wakefulness, minimizing the duration for which a mixed sleep–wake state persists [27].

2 Adenosine accumulation in the extracellular spaces in the basal forebrain inhibits the cholinergic neurones in this region, which would otherwise promote wakefulness and REM sleep. Adenosine may have more widespread actions within the brainstem and influence the VLPO, and may form a component of the homeostatic sleep drive mechanism.

Pathways to cerebral cortex

1 Thalamus. This is the main gate for sensory information, other than olfaction, and for the ascending reticular activating system, comprising mainly the aminergic nuclei reaching the cerebral cortex. Thalamic synchronization protects the cerebral cortex from these influences and effectively deafferentates it during NREM sleep.

2 Basal forebrain and hypothalamus. These closely linked areas integrate sleep/wake drives, circadian influences and neural activity related to external stimuli. The complexity of these centres has been described above and they also interact with the thalamus, particularly the reticular nucleus which is an extension of the ascending reticular activating system. The output of the basal forebrain and hypothalamus is widespread within the cerebral cortex including the limbic cortex.

Cerebral cortex

The cerebral cortex does not initiate sleep, but its impact on the adaptive drive allows sleep to occur or it may delay its onset. Its activity is determined by the combined input from the thalamus, basal forebrain and hypothalamus. Histaminergic and dopaminergic mechanisms are particularly important in maintaining wakefulness and both these and REM sleep are supported by cholinergic activity.

Arousals from sleep

Although the mechanisms of sleep–wake control tend to promote either the state of sleep or the state of wakefulness, neither of these conditions is stable. The level of alertness fluctuates constantly, mainly due to factors affecting the adaptive drive. There may also be an ultradian tendency to enter REM sleep during the day, leading to, for instance, a predisposition to daydream during wakefulness. During sleep, arousal mechanisms are continually active and may lead the subject to awaken in response to any stimulus, especially in stages 1 and 2 NREM sleep and in the elderly [28]. Arousals are heterogeneous, and while many are endogenous, some are triggered, or at least facilitated, by external stimuli.

The tendency towards arousal is a normal feature of sleep and is usually reversible in that a deeper level of sleep is then re-entered. Arousals are more frequent in infants and adults than in young children, and are most common in the elderly, particularly arousals from NREM sleep. They are also more frequent at times when NREM sleep is lightening rather than becoming deeper.

In NREM sleep there is a regular periodicity when arousals are most likely to occur. This is known as the cyclic alternating pattern (CAP) [29]. Arousals occur at intervals of 10–60 s, usually 20–40 s. The neurological basis for this may be an instability in the thalamocortical synchronization, or the failure of this mechanism to filter or suppress impulses reaching the thalamus. The K-complexes and spindles that are seen in arousals are attempts to re-establish NREM sleep. Although the CAP is not detectable in REM sleep some of the aspects of phasic activity characteristic of this state may be analogous to it.

Stimuli that may lead to arousals from sleep do so more frequently if they are combined, such as an increase in noise and simultaneous physical stimulation, and when they coincide with the moment of arousal within the CAP [30]. This probably applies to conditions as diverse as arousal disorders from stages 3 and 4 NREM sleep, such as sleep walking, arousals from obstructive sleep apnoeas, bruxism, and periodic limb movements. Interictal spikes and epileptic seizures both occur particularly at the time of CAP arousals. The

failure to arouse appropriately probably contributes to nocturnal enuresis, and possibly to the sudden infant death syndrome (SIDS).

The arousals may be manifested only by autonomic responses such as an increase in heart rate or blood pressure, but other features of brainstem activity may be seen, such as an increase in respiratory rate or depth, and gross body or limb movements. Subcortical arousals due to activation of aminergic and other brainstem nuclei increase the activity in the ascending reticular activating system but do not cause any electroencephalogram changes. They may or may not lead to a cortical arousal. These can be detected by an abrupt increase in the frequency of the electroencephalogram, alpha waves, high-voltage delta bursts or the appearance of K-complexes and spindles in NREM sleep. In REM sleep cortical arousal may be detected by the reappearance of muscle tone. Arousals, by definition, are transient and are followed by restoration of sleep.

Neurochemistry of sleep and wakefulness

The theory that sleep and wakefulness are determined by the balance of activity in various nuclei and tracts within the brain only partially explains how these states are controlled. There is a continual flux in the relative importance of the various areas concerned in sleep–wake control as well as in the activity within each of these areas. This instability is largely controlled by chemical influences. The long-standing theory of a neurotransmitter as a single compound liberated by the presynaptic membrane passing across the synaptic cleft and inducing depolarization of the postsynaptic membrane has required modification. Some neurones produce two or more chemicals which influence the depolarization of the postsynaptic membrane. One of these (a cotransmitter) may also alter the responsiveness of the membrane to the other transmitter by, for instance, modifying the sensitivity of the receptors. The cotransmitter may also control the synthesis or release of the main transmitter (neuromodulation).

Many of these chemicals are amines, amino acids or peptides, and have other important, but often less clearly defined, effects. They may act as growth factors, altering the pattern of formation of dendrites, remodelling synapses and influencing neurological development. Many of these chemicals secreted in the brain also play a role in the immune system, whose control is closely linked to the control of sleep and wakefulness. Growth, tissue repair and immune func-

Table 2.5 Comparison of neurotransmitter amines.

Effect	Noradrenaline	Acetylcholine	5HT	Dopamine	Histamine	Melatonin
Promotes	Wakefulness	Wakefulness, REM	Wake	—	Wakefulness	NREM
Inhibits	REM	—	REM	—	REM	—
Other actions	Influences mood and behaviour	Motor inhibition in REM	Influences mood, behaviour and motor control	Influences thoughts, emotions, behaviour and motor control	—	Regulates circadian rhythms and immune function

NREM, non-rapid eye movement; REM, rapid eye movement.

tion are closely related and all three are facilitated by the metabolic and endocrine changes during sleep that promote anabolic processes.

The effects of locally released chemicals overlap with the concept of sleep factors (hypnotoxins, somnogens, sleep regulatory substances), which are chemicals found in the brain and cerebrospinal fluid which promote sleep and which increase in concentration during wakefulness. Some of these sleep factors are cotransmitters which are released into synapses, but others may be secreted either by neurones or glia to act as local neurohormones which influence the threshold for depolarization of the postsynaptic membranes. Some systemically released classical hormones probably also cross the blood–brain barrier and have similar effects on the control of sleep and wakefulness.

These chemicals all interact with the recognized nuclei and pathways which influence sleep and wakefulness, and are capable of controlling each of these locally and of altering widespread patterns of neuronal activity and sensitizing to or protecting neurones from other influences. Some are released in response to synaptic activity and then induce new synapses through their growth factor action, modify the ways in which information is processed and change the activity in neuronal networks. These coordinated effects may form a major component of the homeostatic drives to sleep and wake, and the activity of the ascending reticular activating system.

The details of these neurochemical influences on sleep are poorly understood, but the chemicals can be grouped into the following categories.

Amines

Most of the classical neurotransmitters are amines (Table 2.5).

Noradrenaline (norepinephrine)

This promotes wakefulness and inhibits REM sleep through its alpha adrenergic actions.

Neurones in the locus coeruleus release noradrenaline and project widely throughout the brainstem and to the hypothalamus and thalamus. They inhibit the LDT/PPT nuclei and the VLPO and also reach the limbic system where they influence mood and behaviour. There is also a dense noradrenergic innervation in the medulla of nuclei, such as the nucleus of the solitary tract, which control the autonomic nervous system and cranial nerve nuclei.

Acetylcholine

There are two main groups of cholinergic neurones.

LDT/PPT nuclei in the pontine reticular formation
These promote REM sleep and wakefulness through their ability to induce thalamocortical desynchronization. They also project to the hypothalamus and basal forebrain. They contribute to loss of skeletal muscle activity in REM sleep.

Basal forebrain cholinergic neurones
These are located in the basal nucleus of Meynert and radiate to the whole cerebral cortex. They promote REM sleep and wakefulness. They are inhibited by local extracellular accumulation of adenosine.

Acetylcholine is also involved in movement control in the basal ganglia where its action is opposed by dopamine.

Disorders of cholinergic activity within the central nervous system are important factors in depression, dementia, narcolepsy, and REM sleep behaviour disorder.

5-Hydroxytryptamine (5HT, serotonin)

5HT is synthesized through L-tryptophan to 5-hydroxytryptophan and then to 5-hydroxytryptamine (5HT). Around 15 5HT receptors have been identified of which 5HT 1_A and 5HT 2_A have most impact on sleep. Stimulation of 5HT 1_A receptors reduces the duration of REM sleep, elevates the mood and reduces anxiety. 5HT 2_A reduces the duration of stages 3 and 4 NREM sleep, promotes awakenings from sleep, and also leads to vasoconstriction.

The actions of 5HT are complex, not only because of the large number of receptors, but also because of their multiple and often mutually antagonistic interactions. In general, however, they promote wakefulness rather than sleep and are involved with sensory processing and motor activity, particularly related to mood. They may also be involved in the control of respiration and in thermoregulation and hallucinatory states. 5HT-secreting neurones are most active in wakefulness, partially suppressed in NREM sleep and inactive in REM sleep.

Most serotonergic neurones are in the raphe nuclei, particularly the dorsal raphe nuclei. These inhibit the LDT/PPT nuclei in the pons, promote wakefulness through excitation of the thalamic reticular nucleus and also inhibit the VLPO. They project to the SCN, basal forebrain, medulla and spinal cord.

Disorders of 5HT activity within the central nervous system are important factors in depression.

Dopamine

Dopamine is synthesized by phenylalanine being converted to L-tyrosine and then to L-dopa which is converted to dopamine which can then be metabolized to noradrenaline and then to adrenaline. Two major dopamine receptors, D1 and D2, are both coupled to G protein complexes. D1, which is similar to D5, controls mainly motor and cardiovascular activity, whereas D2, which is similar to D3 and D4, is also involved with motor function but particularly influences behavioural responses, and control of prolactin secretion.

Dopamine has complex effects on sleep and wakefulness because of its multiple interactions with other neurotransmitter systems in many areas of the brain. Dopaminergic neurones arise in the midbrain ventral tegmental area and form two systems.

Nigro-striatal pathway

Neurones from the substantia nigra radiate to the striatum, nucleus accumbens, and indirectly to the prefrontal cortex. They increase alertness, modify motor activity and have sympathetic-like effects, including an increase in heart rate and blood pressure, a reduction in appetite and sphincter constriction. Its terminations have both D1 and D2 receptors.

Mesolimbic tract (mesocorticolimbic pathway)

This projects to the prefrontal cortex and limbic cortex, particularly the amygdala and hippocampus, and is associated with arousal, cognitive and emotional function. It has D1 receptors.

In addition, neurones arising in the arcuate nucleus of the hypothalamus project to the pituitary gland and regulate its activity. They are also involved in the response of the carotid body to increase ventilation in the presence of hypoxia. Dopamine in the basal ganglia regulates movements of the skeletal muscles.

Disorders of dopamine activity within the central nervous system are important factors in Parkinsonism and the restless legs syndrome, and in excessive daytime sleepiness.

Histamine

There are H1, H2 and H3 receptors within the central nervous system, but the latter are the most important. Histamine promotes wakefulness and arousal and inhibits both NREM and REM sleep. It is released from neurones in the tubero-mammillary nucleus of the posterior hypothalamus, which project widely, particularly to the VLPO, locus coeruleus, raphe nuclei and LDT/PPT. The mutual inhibition of the VLPO and TMN is responsible for the oscillation between sleep and wakefulness. Histaminergic inhibition of LDT/PPT inhibits REM sleep. The histaminergic neurones that project to the cerebral cortex not only promote arousal but also planning and creative cognitive functions.

Melatonin

See page 35.

Amino acids

The importance of these chemicals as neurotransmitters has probably been underestimated (Table 2.6). They fall into two groups.

Excitatory

Glutamate

Glutamate promotes wakefulness and is the main excitatory neurotransmitter in the central nervous

Table 2.6 Effects of amino acid and other neurotransmitters on sleep.

Wake promotion	NREM sleep promotion	REM sleep inhibition
PGE2	GABA PGD2 Adenosine ?Nitric oxide	GABA

GABA, gamma-aminobutyric acid; NREM, non-rapid eye movement; PGD2, prostaglandin D2; PGE2, prostaglandin E2; REM, rapid eye movement.

system. It is the transmitter of the thalamocortical projection fibres which are responsible for synchronizing cortical activity during NREM sleep, and of the corticospinal pathway which arises from the pyramidal cells in the cerebral cortex. Glutamatergic neurones are also present particularly in the ascending reticular activating system of the brainstem, projecting to the LDT/PPT nuclei and to the basal forebrain.

There are four receptor subtypes including the N-methyl-D-aspartate (NMDA) receptor, which is inhibited by ethanol.

Excess glutamate activity may be responsible for some forms of psychosis.

Aspartate

The role of this excitatory neurotransmitter in sleep–wake control is uncertain.

Inhibitory

Gamma aminobutyric acid (GABA)

This is synthesized from glutamate. $GABA_A$ and $GABA_C$ receptors are linked to chloride channels and the $GABA_B$ receptor is coupled to a G protein complex. $GABA_A$ receptors are primarily involved in promoting sleep.

GABA is present in over 30% of synapses within the central nervous system. GABA-ergic neurones are widespread in the brainstem reticular formation, basal ganglia, hypothalamus and thalamus. GABA is secreted by SCN neurones and in the thalamus it influences sensory transmission and appears to oppose the action of glutamate. GABA release from the VLPO inhibits the aminergic wakefulness promoting nuclei.

Galanine

This is an inhibitory peptide secreted by neurones of the VLPO. It promotes sleep.

Glycine

This is located mainly in the brainstem and spinal cord, where it is released at synapses of the reticulospinal tract with alpha motor neurones. These are inhibited and this leads to the muscle atonia of REM sleep.

Taurine

This is one of the most widely distributed amino acids in the brain. Its postsynaptic inhibitory action is blocked by strychnine, a central nervous system stimulant.

Peptides

This important group of chemicals includes most of the sleep factors and cytokines which, like melatonin, also have an important influence on the immune response (Table 2.7).

Pituitary hormones and related compounds

Growth hormone releasing hormone (GHRH) promotes NREM sleep and the synthesis of growth hormone (GH) through two separate populations of hypothalamic neurones. GHRH secretion is reduced in the elderly, but increases during infections, probably through the influence of IL-1.

GH promotes REM rather than NREM sleep and inhibits GHRH release. Its metabolite, insulin-like growth factor (IGF-1) promotes wakefulness.

Somatostatin is present as a 14 and 28 peptide chain. It is released in the hypothalamus and through the portal system inhibits GHRH release and GH release in the pituitary gland. It reduces the duration of NREM sleep, but promotes REM sleep, probably by an action within the brainstem. Corticostatin is a similar peptide which increases NREM sleep and reduces GH secretion.

Ghrelin is structurally similar to GH, but is produced by the stomach in response to gastric distension. It may promote NREM sleep, but indirectly leads to an increase in REM sleep by stimulating GH secretion.

Table 2.7 Effects of peptide neurotransmitters on sleep.

NREM sleep promotion	NREM sleep inhibition	REM sleep promotion	REM sleep inhibition
GHRH	Nil known	Somatostatin	Opioids
DSIP		VIP	IL-1
CCK		Prolactin	TNF-α
Insulin			
IL-1			
TNF-α			
IFN			

CCK, cholecystokinin; DSIP, delta sleep inducing peptide; GHRH, growth hormone releasing hormone; IFN, interferons; IL-1, interleukin-1; TNF-α, tumour necrosis factor alpha.

Corticotrophin-releasing hormone (CRH) is structurally similar to somatostatin. It promotes wakefulness and inhibits NREM sleep. Adrenocorticotrophic hormone (ACTH) increases the duration of time awake and the lighter stages of NREM sleep, reduces the duration of stages 3 and 4 NREM sleep, and probably has little effect on REM sleep. Glucocorticoids, such as cortisol and alpha melanocyte stimulating hormone (αMSH) inhibit NREM sleep.

Vasoactive intestinal peptide (VIP)-containing neurones are present in the core of the SCN and elsewhere in the hypothalamus. They project to the median eminence where VIP acts as a releasing factor for prolactin. Vasoactive intestinal peptide is structurally similar to GH and increases REM sleep. Prolactin is also chemically similar to growth hormone and, similarly, promotes REM sleep.

Oestrogens
Oestrogens act in the hypothalamic preoptic area to increase arousal, inhibit REM sleep and stimulate motor and sexual activity.

Hypocretins (orexins)
Hypocretins are peptides derived from a pre-hypocretin protein which splits to form two related peptides, hypocretin 1 and hypocretin 2 (orexin A and B). These are located in the synaptic vesicles of neurones in the perifornical area of the lateral hypothalamus. They are excitatory neurotransmitters with specific hypocretin 1 and 2 receptors, although hypocretins appear to interact with noradrenaline, dopamine and acetylcholine.

The neurones in the lateral hypothalamus project widely, particularly to the aminergic brainstem arousal centres, especially the locus coeruleus and the LDT/PPT. They also connect to the limbic system, thalamus and cerebral cortex, but not significantly to the VLPO.

Hypocretin-containing neurones tend to stabilize wakefulness and limit the duration of REM sleep. They also increase motor activity, particularly to increase food intake and for defence, and alter the blood flow to skeletal muscles. In REM sleep hypocretins appear to enhance motor inhibition rather than activity.

Narcolepsy is associated with loss of hypocretin-secreting neurones, but the hypocretin level is raised in the restless legs syndrome, where there is an increase in motor activity.

Delta sleep inducing peptide (DSIP)
Delta sleep inducing peptide increases NREM sleep and may inhibit secretion of ACTH.

Cholecystokinin (CCK)
Cholecystokinin is secreted as a 33-amino acid peptide (CCK33) from the duodenum and jejunum in response to distension. It stimulates pancreatic enzyme secretion and gall bladder contraction. It is also present in the central nervous system as an 8-amino acid peptide (CCK8) fragment of CCK33 and both these types of CCK induce NREM sleep, reduce motor activity and mediate satiety after food intake.

Cholecystokinin-8 is present in the reticular formation, for instance, in the raphe nuclei and in the hypothalamus. It is an excitatory neurotransmitter, usually acting as a cotransmitter either with 5HT, as in the raphe nuclei, or elsewhere with dopamine.

Insulin
Insulin is secreted in response to a rising blood glucose and promotes NREM sleep, but does not affect REM sleep. NREM sleep is often reduced in duration in diabetes mellitus.

Opioid peptides

These interact with endorphins, enkephalins and dynorphins, which are located particularly in the medulla, hypothalamus, thalamus, basal ganglia and limbic system. They tend to inhibit REM sleep partly through their action on the LDT/PPT nuclei.

Substance P

This peptide is released at 40% of the synapses with LDT/PPT neurones. Its role in sleep is unknown but may be related to control of sensory transmission through the brainstem.

Cytokines

These are peptides which are chemically similar to peptide hormones such as growth hormone, but are produced by helper T-lymphocytes and other cells including microglia in the brain in response to a specific stimulus. They modify the immune response and within the brain act on nearby cells. Several of the cytokines are recognized to act as sleep factors.

Interleukin-1

This is produced in the hypothalamus and other areas of the brain in response to endotoxin, tumour necrosis factor alpha (TNF-α) and muramyl peptides derived from peptidoglycans in bacterial cell walls. Its production is inhibited by prostaglandin E2 (PGE2) and glucocorticoids, both of which inhibit sleep.

Interleukin-1 increases the duration of NREM sleep through an action on the anterior hypothalamus, and slightly inhibits REM sleep. These actions may be mediated by IL-1's augmentation of GABA receptor function and its ability to increase GHRH secretion, but it also increases adenosine production and affects prostaglandins. Its actions are inhibited by corticotrophin-releasing hormone (CRH) and alpha melanocyte stimulating hormone (α-MSH).

Interleukin-1 is also a neuronal growth factor. It acts as a pyrogen to raise the body temperature, controls CRH release, has immunological effects, and blocks the metabolism of anandamide, the receptor for tetradihydrocannabinol.

Other interleukins such as IL-2 and IL-6 have little or no effect on sleep.

Tumour necrosis factor alpha

This cytokine, which is produced by macrophages, is released mainly at night. It increases stages 3 and 4 NREM sleep and reduces REM sleep. It acts mainly in the preoptic hypothalamus and on the locus coeruleus.

Interferons (IFN)

Interferons such as IFN alpha 2 are produced by leucocytes in response particularly to viral infections. They enable phagocytes to kill infected cells. The peak gamma interferon level is seen at around 10.00 PM with the minimum at 6.00 AM. Interferons increase NREM sleep.

Neurotrophin-2

This cytokine acts as a sleep and growth factor, enhancing the development and activity of GABA-releasing neurones. Its production and release are increased by acetylcholine and glutamate.

Nerve growth factor (NGF)

This promotes both NREM and REM sleep.

Brain-derived neurotrophic factor (BDNF)

This promotes NREM sleep and possibly REM sleep.

Other neurotransmitters

Prostaglandins

Prostaglandins are polyunsaturated fatty acids with a 5-carbon ring structure and are derived from arachidonic acid.

Prostaglandin D2 (PGD2) acts in or near the VLPO of the hypothalamus to induce both NREM and REM sleep and reduce body temperature. It is secreted by the leptomeninges and the choroid plexus and reaches the cerebrospinal fluid. It appears to increase adenosine release in the basal forebrain.

PGE2 acts in or near the posterior hypothalamus to promote wakefulness and raise body temperature. It inhibits IL-1 production.

Progesterones are chemically similar to prostaglandins and increase NREM sleep.

Oleamide

This is an endogenous sleep-producing polyunsaturated fatty acid which is synthesized from arachidonic acid, and has similar actions to anandamide, an endogenous cannabinoid. It promotes NREM sleep and reduces motor activity. Its concentration in the cerebrospinal fluid increases during sleep deprivation.

Cannabinoids

There are two types of endogenous cannabinoid receptors, CB1 and CB2, both of which are coupled to G proteins. CB1 receptors are widespread within the central nervous system. Anandamide, a fatty acid, is the best recognized endogenous cannabinoid. It appears to promote NREM sleep but its effects are blocked by interleukins.

Adenosine

This is a purine nucleoside which is produced from adenosine triphosphate (ATP) and adenosine diphosphate (ADP) and is converted into inosine and then to hypoxanthine. There are A1, A2A, A2B and A3 adenosine receptors. A1 receptors are antagonized by xanthines.

Adenosine is a vasodilator. It promotes NREM sleep, especially stages 3 and 4, by inhibiting the basal forebrain cholinergic neurones. It may also have an effect on the pontine cholinergic neurones. Adenosine accumulates extracellularly during wakefulness as a result of the metabolic activity of brain cells, particularly astrocytes. Astrocytes provide a readily available supply of glucose for local neurones from their glycogen stores, but their metabolic activity consumes ATP and releases adenosine. This binds particularly to the A1 receptor, leading to inhibition of basal forebrain cholinergic neurones. During sleep the concentration of adenosine falls and this enables the neurones to become active again and promote wakefulness. These cyclical changes in adenosine concentrations probably contribute to the homeostatic sleep drive [31].

Uridine

This nucleoside has been proposed as a sleep promoting neurotransmitter [32].

Nitric oxide

This is a highly lipid soluble gas which acts as a cotransmitter with 5HT in the dorsal raphe nuclei, and is unusual in that it spreads from the point of its release to influence and coordinate neuronal function over a wide region. It is able to alter the intrinsic rhythm of the SCN. It appears to promote REM sleep and may have an effect on NREM sleep as well. It is also a vasodilator and integrates local cerebral blood flow with neuronal metabolic activity.

References

1 Jouvet M. Paradoxical sleep as a programming system. *J Sleep Res* 1998; 7: 1–5.

2 Cipolli C, Fagioli I, Mazzetti M, Tuozzi G. Incorporation of presleep stimuli into dream contents: evidence for a consolidation effect on declarative knowledge during REM sleep? *J Sleep Res* 2004; 13: 317–26.

3 Smith C. Sleep states and memory processes in humans: procedural versus declarative memory systems. *Sleep Med Rev* 2001; 5(6): 491–506.

4 Schabus M, Gruber G, Parapatics S, Sauter C, Klosch G, Anderer P, Klimesch W, Saletu B, Zeitlhofer J. Sleep spindles and their significance for declarative memory consolidation. *Sleep* 2004; 27(8): 1479–85.

5 Stradling JR, Chadwick GA, Frew AJ. Changes in ventilation and its components in normal subjects during sleep. *Thorax* 1985; 40: 364–70.

6 Zoccoli G, Walker AM, Lenzi P, Franzini C. The cerebral circulation during sleep: regulation mechanisms and functional implications. *Sleep Med Rev* 2002; 6(6): 443–55.

7 Orr WC. Gastrointestinal functioning during sleep: a new horizon in sleep medicine. *Sleep Med Rev* 2001; 5(2): 91–101.

8 Bertini M, Gennaro L de, Ferrara M, Curcio G, Romei V, Fratello F, Cristiani R, Pauri F, Rossini PM. Reduction of transcallosal inhibition upon awakening from REM sleep in humans as assessed by transcranial magnetic stimulation. *Sleep* 2004; 27(5): 875–82.

9 Douglas NJ, White DP, Pickett CK, Weil JV, Zwillich CW. Respiration during sleep in normal man. *Thorax* 1982; 37: 840–4.

10 Orem J, Lovering AT, Dunin-Barkowski W, Vidruk EH. Tonic activity in the respiratory system in wakefulness, NREM and REM sleep. *Sleep* 2002; 25(5): 488–96.

11 Johns M. Rethinking the assessment of sleepiness. *Sleep Med Rev* 1998; 2: 3–15.

12 Horne JA. REM sleep – by default? *Neurosci Biobehav Rev* 2000; 24: 777–97.

13 Franken P. Long-term vs. short-term processes regulating REM sleep. *J Sleep Res* 2002; 11: 17–28.

14 Cajochen C, Krauchi K, Danilenko KV, Wirz-Justice A. Evening administration of melatonin and bright light: interactions on the EEG during sleep and wakefulness. *J Sleep Res* 1998; 7: 145–57.

15 Monk TH, Welsh DK. The role of chronobiology in sleep disorders medicine. *Sleep Med Rev* 2003; 7(6): 455–73.

16 Russell N, Gelder V. Recent insights into mammalian circadian rhythms. *Sleep* 2004; 27(1): 166–71.

17 Brzezinski A. Melatonin in humans. *N Engl J Med* 1997; 336: 186–95.

18 Gilbert SS, Heuvel CJ van den, Ferguson SA, Dawson D. Thermoregulation as a sleep signalling system. *Sleep Med Rev* 2004; 8: 81–93.

19 Gronfier C, Brandenberger G. Ultradian rhythms in pituitary and adrenal hormones: their relations to sleep. *Sleep Med Rev* 1998; 2: 17–29.

20 Cauter EV, Plat L, Copinschi G. Interrelations between sleep and the somatotropic axis. *Sleep* 1998; 21(6): 533–66.

21 Reinoso-Suarez F, Andres I de, Rodrigo-Angulo ML, Garzon M. Brain structures and mechanisms involved in the generation of REM sleep. *Sleep Med Rev* 2001; 5(1): 63–77.

22 Huguenard JR. Anatomical and physiological considerations in thalamic rhythm generation. *J Sleep Res* 1998; 7 (Suppl. 1): 24–9.

23 Evans BM. Sleep, consciousness and the spontaneous and evoked electrical activity of the brain. Is there a cortical integrating mechanism? *Neurophysiol clin* 2003; 33: 1–10.

24 Espana RA, Scammell TE. Sleep neurobiology for the clinician. *Sleep* 2004; 27(4): 811–20.

25 Pace-Schott EF, Hobson JA. The neurobiology of sleep: genetics, cellular physiology and subcortical networks. *Nat Rev Neurosci* 2002; 3: 591–605.

26 Rye DB. Contributions of the pedunculopontine region to normal and altered REM sleep. *Sleep* 1997; 20(9): 757–88.

27 Saper CB, Chou TC, Scammell TE. The sleep switch: hypothalamic control of sleep and wakefulness. *Trends Neurosci* 2001; 24: 726–31.

28 Halasz P, Terzano M, Parrino L, Bodizs R. The nature of arousal in sleep. *J Sleep Res* 2004; 13: 1–23.

29 Terzano MG, Parrino L. Origin and significance of the cyclic alternating pattern (CAP). *Sleep Med Rev* 2000; 4(1): 101–23.

30 Parrino L, Smerieri A, Rossi M, Terzano MG. Relationship of slow and rapid EEG components of CAP to ASDA arousals in normal sleep. *Sleep* 2001; 24(8): 881–5.

31 Porkka-Heiskanen T, Alanko L, Kalinchuk A, Stenberg D. Adenosine and sleep. *Sleep Med Rev* 2002; 6(4): 321–32.

32 Kimura T, Ho IK, Yamamoto I. Uridine receptor: discovery and its involvement in sleep mechanism. *Sleep* 2001; 24(3): 251–60.

3 Assessment of Sleep Disorders

Introduction

The assessment of sleep disorders requires an understanding of normal sleep and how it may alter in abnormal circumstances, such as following sleep deprivation; and with disorders that affect the nature of sleep. The details of the history obtained at interview with the patient, and often with a member of the family, partner, friend or carer, should be supplemented by a physical examination where this is applicable. The expanding range of investigative techniques is often invaluable, but they should only be used with clear aims. This chapter assesses the use of the sleep history and examination, and examines the principles underlying the most important investigations. The precise indications for these tests in different sleep disorders are discussed in Chapters 5–12.

History

Aims

It can be more difficult to take a history of a sleep disorder than to enquire about a complaint that occurs during wakefulness. The patient often has little or no awareness of the problem and it is important to obtain the bed partner's view of the events during sleep, and where appropriate, during wakefulness as well. The aim is to establish whether or not there is a sleep disorder and to assess the relative contribution of psychological, medical and social factors to the complaint. The exact nature of the symptoms and the sequence of the appearance of the complaints should be recorded. Details of their onset and the nature of any progression should be obtained. Some sleep disorders resolve, others fluctuate or progress.

Content

Detailed sleep questionnaires, such as the Pittsburgh Sleep Quality Index (PSQI) (Appendix 2), have been developed to cover important questions that need to be asked. They can supplement a conventional history

and may even substitute for this if a history is unavailable. A detailed history is, however, preferable and the first step is to assess the patient's complaint or the reason for seeking attention. It should be established whether this is primarily insomnia, excessive daytime sleepiness or abnormal experiences or movements during sleep. The next step is to establish when the sleep problem began and whether there was any relationship to an external factor, which may be physical, such as a head injury, or more subtle and psychological.

These initial questions should enable the more detailed history to remain focused on the patient's problem (Table 3.1). It is often useful to consider the details of events during sleep and wakefulness as a 24-h cycle, and to follow them around the clock (Fig. 3.1). The most important aspects of the sleep history are detailed below.

Sleep–wake patterns

What time does the patient go to bed? What time does he or she go to sleep, wake up in the morning and get out of bed? The regularity or lack of regularity of these schedules and patterns should be noted, for instance during the working week, at weekends, or holidays. Does shift work or travel influence these sleep schedules?

Is there a reason for any delay in the initiation of sleep and if so what is this? Is the sleep environment satisfactory? Is the bedroom used for other activities, such as work? Is the bed comfortable and is the bedroom quiet, dark and neither too hot nor too cold? Is there any difficulty with the partner which disturbs the sleep pattern?

If the patient finally wakes early in the morning, why is this? Is depression a feature or is there pain or discomfort? Is there any difficulty in awakening in the morning? Is an alarm clock needed?

The sleep pattern before the onset of the sleep disorder should also be noted. Was the patient a long sleeper, more alert in the evenings or early in the mornings? Was there any history of insomnia, sleep walking, or other sleep-related problems?

Table 3.1 Important sleep symptoms and their possible implications.

Symptom	Implications
Short sleep time	Short sleeper; sleep deprivation; depression; DSPS; ASPS
Irregular sleep times	Social- or work-induced; circadian rhythm disorder
Delay in falling asleep	DIS – look for cause
Difficult to wake in the morning	Sleep deprivation; sleep inertia; idiopathic hypersomnia
Restlessness at night	Frequent arousals; OSA; PLMS; other behavioural disorder including epilepsy
Complex movements at night	Behavioural disorder including epilepsy
Snoring	Simple snorer; UARS; OSA
Nocturnal choking	OSA; gastro-oesophageal reflux; vocal cord adduction; panic attacks
Unrefreshing sleep	Sleep restriction; poor quality sleep, e.g. OSA, PLMS; circadian rhythm disorder, hyperarousal disorder, e.g. fibromyalgia
Early morning headaches	CO_2 retention; insomnia
Daytime naps	Sleep restriction; poor quality sleep, e.g. OSA, PLMS; narcolepsy; idiopathic hypersomnia; depression
Loss of strength with emotion	Cataplexy
Pre-sleep apprehension	Anxiety; psycho-physiological insomnia; fear of event during sleep
Pre-sleep leg ache and movements	RLS and PLMS

ASPS, advanced sleep phase syndrome; DIS, difficulty in initiating sleep; DSPS, delayed sleep phase syndrome; OSA, obstructive sleep apnoea; PLMS, periodic limb movements in sleep; RLS, restless legs syndrome; UARS, upper airway resistance syndrome.

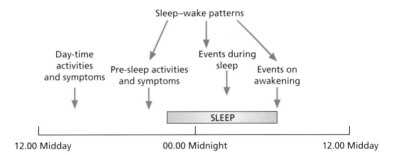

Fig. 3.1 Timing of sleep–wake events and symptoms.

Events during sleep

Does the patient wake during the night? Is he or she aware of this or is it the partner who notices that an awakening has taken place, for instance because of the subject speaking or moving? Why does the awakening happen? Is there any sensation of pain, anxiety, panic, intrusive thoughts or nightmares? What happens when awakening occurs and how long is it before sleep is re-entered?

The frequency, time during the night (or more precisely during the sleep episode), and awareness of any mental or physical activity should be noted. Is there any relationship to other events? For instance, are any limb movements related to snoring and what is the patient's condition after an event such as sleep walking? Is he or she awake or confused, and is there any recall of the episode?

Does the subject dream or are there any nightmares? Is there any significance in the content of the dreams, and are any of these repetitive? Are there either intrusive thoughts or an awareness of thinking for much of the night? Does pain or discomfort lead to arousal from sleep? This may, for instance, be backache whose onset may not be directly related to sleep, or heartburn due to gastro-oesophageal reflux which is exacerbated by sleep.

Are there any abnormal movements, such as sleep walking, periodic limb movements, or nocturnal epileptic fits? Do any of these movements suggest that violence is being directed towards the bed partner?

Does the patient snore, appear to stop breathing, or make snorting noises at the end of an apnoea? These may be associated with jerking movements, suggesting an arousal from sleep. Are there any trigger factors for these problems, such as the position of the patient or alcohol consumption? Is there a sensation of choking during sleep, which may be related to obstructive sleep apnoeas, gastro-oesophageal reflux, vocal cord adduction or panic attacks?

Does the subject have nocturia, nocturnal wheeze, sweating or episodes of being unable to move while awake (sleep paralysis)?

Events on awakening

Is sleep refreshing? Are there any symptoms such as frontal headaches which might be due to carbon dioxide retention caused by hypoventilation during sleep? What is the level of alertness on waking and is there a history of confusional arousals? Has this led to any accidents? How does the subject feel emotionally on waking?

Daytime activities

Are naps taken during the day, and if so when and for how long? Are they refreshing? Is there adequate exposure to light during the day? Is exercise taken and what is the timing and size of meals? Does the type and timing of social activity promote or prevent sleep?

Daytime symptoms

Sensory
Does the subject have any hallucinations which might suggest narcolepsy, schizophrenia, amphetamine-induced psychosis, severe sleep deprivation, or delirium tremens due to alcohol withdrawal? Is there any problem with concentration or memory?

Is there any pain or unpleasant sensations in the legs in the evenings which are relieved by movement, suggesting the restless legs syndrome?

Motor
Are there any abnormal movements to indicate epilepsy or cataplexy or a primary movement disorder, such as Parkinsonism, which may be related to unusual movements during sleep?

Excessive daytime sleepiness
True hypersomnia in which the subject sleeps for an abnormally long duration during each 24-h cycle should be distinguished from hypersomnolence which is the sensation of sleepiness. These two symptoms should also be distinguished from mental fatigue with poor concentration or motivation, physical weariness or fatigue which usually has an organic cause or may be related to insomnia, and the feeling of subalertness which may be due to a reduced wakefulness drive or an increased drive to sleep, as in narcolepsy. The duration, frequency and timing of naps should be noted, and whether or not these are refreshing. Many patients with narcolepsy feel refreshed after a nap of 5–30 min, whereas in idiopathic hypersomnia naps are longer but are unrefreshing.

The severity of daytime sleepiness can be gauged by its frequency and the type of situation in which the subject falls asleep. If it is mild, it only occurs infrequently, at times of day when sleep would be expected, e.g. 2.00–4.00 PM or late in the evening, or at rest or in a monotonous or passive environment, e.g. as a passenger in a car, bus or train, while sitting watching television or reading, or in a meeting. It is likely to be more severe if sleep occurs despite stimulating circumstances, for instance while talking, eating or on exertion, such as walking, and if it occurs frequently and at any time of the day.

Cyclical sleepiness may be due to intermittent sleep deprivation. Patients often sleep too little during the week and catch up their sleep debt at weekends. This leads to a weekly cycle of sleepiness and recovery. Longer cycles of sleepiness are characteristic of other disorders, such as the monthly cycles in premenstrual sleepiness and even longer cycles in the Kleine–Levin syndrome. Elimination of sleepiness when sufficient sleep is allowed, for instance during holidays, suggests that sleep deprivation rather than a primary sleep disorder is the cause.

Pre-sleep activities and symptoms

Is there apprehension about obtaining a poor night's sleep, or of waking, for instance with pain or discomfort? Has the patient been able to wind down mentally prior to the intended time of falling asleep or is mental over-activity and worry about the next day a problem? Are there any physical symptoms preventing sleep or features to suggest the restless legs syndrome, such as an inability to keep the legs still or an unpleasant sensation within the legs?

Other related problems

Symptoms that may be associated with sleep abnormalities should be enquired about. These include, for instance, muscle aches and pains which are a feature of the chronic fatigue syndrome and fibromyalgia, and headaches which may indicate carbon dioxide retention. Poor concentration, reduction in short-term memory and irritability are psychological consequences of sleep deprivation and hypnotic treatment.

Medical disorders which may be relevant to the sleep problem should be noted. These include depression, head injuries, Parkinsonism, nocturnal asthma, angina, prostatic symptoms and arthritis. The symptoms of nocturnal breathlessness, pain or nocturia that these lead to may significantly disrupt sleep.

Social history

Does the patient work regular hours or do shift work? Does he or she cross time zones frequently through international travel? Is there any history of foreign travel which might have predisposed to a sleep disorder, such as trypanosomiasis? What are the patient's housing and sleeping arrangements? Is the bedroom a suitable environment for sleep? Do any pet animals disturb sleep?

General health

Has there been a change in the patient's weight or collar size which might predispose to snoring and obstructive sleep apnoeas? Is the subject depressed?

Medical history

Is there any history of disorders such as acromegaly or hypothyroidism? Is there a history of heart failure, which may cause Cheyne–Stokes respiration and nocturnal pulmonary oedema? Has the patient undergone any relevant surgery, such as a tonsillectomy or palatal surgery for snoring? A developmental history is important in children.

Family history

Is there a family history of any sleep disorders such as narcolepsy, snoring, obstructive sleep apnoeas or the restless legs syndrome? Does the bed partner have a sleep problem which may be disturbing the patient? What is the partner's attitude to the patient's complaint? Do the patient and partner still sleep in the same bed, or same bedroom, and has the sleep disorder caused this to change?

Drug history

Does the patient take any drugs for medical or recreational use which might affect sleep? What are the doses and when are they taken? Could the sleep symptoms be due to withdrawal of one of the drugs or to previous excessive alcohol consumption? What is the caffeine intake in total in each day and what is the timing of this? A stimulant such as caffeine taken shortly before the intended sleep time may cause insomnia, whereas the same amount taken in the morning may not have any effect on night-time sleep. What is the subject's alcohol and nicotine intake, and is he or she taking any 'alternative' or non-prescription medicines which may have effects on sleep which are unknown or at least uncertain?

Physical examination

A general physical examination is often not required to assess the patient with a sleep disorder, but there are specific aspects which should be noted in certain situations (Table 3.2). The degree of sleepiness or alertness, depression or anxiety should be recorded as well as any psychiatric features, for instance, schizophrenia or a personality disorder. The attitudes of the patient and the partner to the sleep complaint are important. The physical appearance may suggest a condition such as hypothyroidism or acromegaly which may be the cause of the sleep disorder.

The weight and neck circumference, examination of the nose and pharynx and the presence of retrognathia are relevant to snoring and obstructive sleep apnoeas. Ground-down teeth are a feature of bruxism, and evidence of physical injuries, which might be either the result of a motor abnormality in sleep or the cause of the sleep disorder, should be sought.

A neurological examination may be required to assess the cause of daytime sleepiness or a motor disorder, and any evidence of a movement disorder such as Parkinsonism should be noted. Examination of other systems such as the respiratory or cardiovascular system is indicated if the clinical picture suggests that these may be implicated in the sleep disorder.

Polysomnography

Electrophysiology

The electrophysiological assessment of sleep enables it to be differentiated from wakefulness, the stage of sleep to be identified, the details of arousals and awakenings to be recorded, and, when it is combined with other physiological measurements, the cause of the sleep disturbance to be investigated. Three signals are required to assess sleep accurately: an electroencephalogram (EEG), an electro-oculogram (EOG) and an electromyogram (EMG). Polysomnography (PSG) (or, more accurately, somnopolygraphy) is the simultaneous acquisition and coordinated analysis of these and other physiological signals during sleep (Fig. 3.2).

Table 3.2 When to examine the patient.

	Situation	Examination
Insomnia	CNS disorder unlikely	Little value
	CNS disorder likely	CNS
EDS	Snoring	Weight, neck, upper airway, jaw
	Features of REM sleep while awake	Little value
	General medical disorder	Relevant system
Behavioural disorder	Epilepsy	CNS
	Disorder of arousal	Little value
	Features of REM sleep	CNS
	Cataplexy	Little value
	Daytime movement disorder	CNS
Respiratory disorder	Breathlessness	Respiratory and cardiovascular systems
	Irregular breathing pattern	CNS, respiratory and cardiovascular systems

CNS, central nervous system; REM, rapid eye movement.

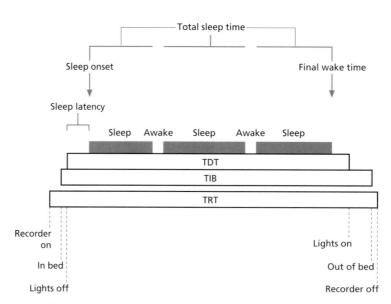

Fig. 3.2 Polysomnography definitions. TRT: total recording time, time from switching on to switching off recording equipment. TIB: time in bed, time from lights out to time of getting out of bed. TSP: total sleep period (SPT: sleep period time), time from sleep onset to end of sleep. TDT: total dark time, time from lights out to lights on in the morning. SO: sleep onset, time of sleep onset. SL: sleep latency, time from lights out until sleep onset. Final wake time: time of final wakening. TST: total sleep time, time from sleep onset to the end of sleep, minus time awake. WT: wake time, time awake between sleep onset and end of sleep. Sleep efficiency: total sleep time divided by time in bed, as a percentage.

Duration of each sleep stage or state in minutes or as a percentage of TST. REM latency: time from sleep onset to onset of REM sleep. REM cycle duration: interval between onset of consecutive REM periods. REM density: percentage of REM epochs containing rapid eye movements. MT: movement time, total time of sleep epochs obscured for greater than 50% by movements or muscle artefact. Awakenings: episodes of longer than 15 s in any 30-s epoch with abrupt changes in EEG frequency and other related features. Arousal: episodes of longer than 3 s with abrupt changes in EEG frequency and other related features.

Table 3.3 Important investigations for sleep disorders.

Symptom	Probable diagnosis	Test
EDS		
– All	Any	Self-assessment scale
+ Snoring	OSA	Respiratory sleep monitoring
+ REM sleep features	Narcolepsy	HLA, polysomnography, MSLT
+ Restlessness	PLMS	Blood tests, actigraphy, polysomnography
+ Complex movements	Neurological disorder	Head CT or MRI, polysomnography
Insomnia		
– All	Any	Sleep diary
– DSPS, ASPS features	Circadian rhythm disorder	Sleep diary, actigraphy, blood and urine tests
– Neurological symptoms	Neurological disorder	Head CT or MRI, polysomnography
– Restlessness	PLMS	Blood tests, actigraphy, polysomnography
Behavioural disorders		
Limb jerks	Hypnic jerks	Nil
Walking	Sleep walking	Nil
Complex movements	Epilepsy etc.	Polysomnography
Vocalization	Frontal lobe epilepsy etc.	Polysomnography
Uncertain nature	Unknown	Polysomnography
Violence	REM sleep behaviour disorder	Polysomnography
Dream related	PTSD, REM sleep behaviour disorder	Polysomnography
Autonomic disorders		Disease-specific investigations
Respiratory disorder	Central sleep apnoeas	EDS self-assessment scale, arterial blood gases
	Cheyne–Stokes respiration	Chest X-ray, ECG lung function tests, respiratory sleep study
	Obstructive sleep apnoeas	EDS self-assessment scale, respiratory sleep study or polysomnography, arterial blood gases if severe
	Snoring	EDS self-assessment scale, respiratory sleep study, localization test, e.g. endoscopy
Combination of 1–5	Any combination	Polysomnography

ASPS, advanced sleep phase syndrome; CT, computed tomography; DSPS, delayed sleep phase syndrome; EDS, excessive daytime sleepiness; HLA, human leucocyte antigen; MRI, magnetic resonance imaging; MSLT, multiple sleep latency test; OSA, obstructive sleep apnoeas; PLMS, periodic limb movements in sleep; PTSD, post-traumatic stress disorder.

Polysomnography has the advantages of being able to determine sleep onset and offset, and the stages of sleep, and correlate these with simultaneous physiological, video and other findings (Table 3.3). It does, however, require the patient to sleep in an unnatural environment, it is dependent on skilled technician time and it is expensive. Portable polysomnography, which can be used in the home, can provide good quality signals and may be useful, not only in avoiding the problems of sleeping in an unfamiliar room, but also in enabling the disabled and those living far from hospital to be investigated [1].

Practical aspects

The EEG, EOG and EMG electrodes are usually silver–silver electrodes and the signals are filtered and amplified before being either recorded on paper by a polygraph or stored and displayed by computer. A recording speed of 10–15 mm/s is most suitable for paper recordings.

Patients are often daunted by the thought or sight of the electrodes and other equipment, and reassurance is important in order to try to help them fall asleep naturally during the study. The quality of sleep may be poor due to anxiety ('first night effect') and the

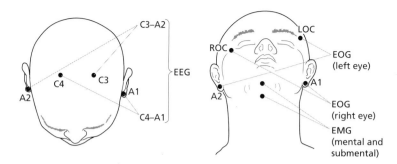

Fig. 3.3 Electrode positions for polysomnography. The left-hand side of the figure indicates the EEG position, and the right-hand side indicates the EOG and EMG. EEG, electro-encephalogram; EMG, electromyogram; EOG, electro-oculogram; LOC, outer canthus of the left eye; ROC, outer canthus of the right eye.

study may occasionally need to be repeated. Checks of the adequacy of the signals should be made once the electrodes are applied and before the subject falls asleep. Artefacts may arise during the study as a result of movement, poor contact of the electrodes due to either displacement or sweating, electrical interference or other problems with the recording system.

Electroencephalogram (EEG) recording

The electrical potentials that are recorded on the scalp reflect the synaptic activity rather than the action potentials of, in particular, the pyramidal cells in the underlying cerebral cortex. These neurones are predominantly radially orientated and generate an electrical field which enables the potential difference between two points on the scalp to be recorded. The orientation of the cortical synapses generates a larger detectable electrical field than that from the spinal cord and brainstem, which is not detectable by scalp electrodes.

The EEG signal in the brain is 10–200 mV which is around one-thousandth of that of the electrocardiogram (ECG). It is also attenuated before reaching the scalp electrodes by 50–95%. The skull filters particularly the higher frequencies.

The EEG provides a continuous and non-invasive monitor of the electrical activity and its oscillation during sleep. The activity of the cerebral cortex is, however, only sampled at the locations where the electrodes are applied, and the resolution for detecting focal abnormalities is low (Fig. 3.3). For this reason, a full 10–20 montage is preferable to diagnose nocturnal epilepsy or to assess focal lesions.

In practice it is usual for only two electrodes to be used, and these monitor the central regions of the brain. Two occipital electrodes can be added to evaluate alpha activity in detail since this is most prominent in this region. Sampling of cortical activity by only two electrodes is probably valid because of the coher-

ence of the whole of its activity due to the widespread projections of the thalamo-cortical fibres which cause synchronized waves of depolarization and hyperpolarization. There is a slight time lag across the cerebral cortex as this wave of activity is propagated, and during NREM sleep the site of maximum activity drifts forwards from the occipital towards the frontal cortex.

Electro-oculogram (EOG) recording

Movements of the eyes are important in diagnosing whether the subject is falling asleep and particularly whether REM sleep or wakefulness is present. The potential difference between the cornea and the retina is measured and it is movement of this electrical dipole, and not the activity of the extra-ocular muscles, that is recorded. One electrode is applied 1 cm above, but close to, the outer canthus of the right eye (ROC) and another electrode 1 cm below the outer canthus of the left eye (LOC). Reference (neutral) electrodes are connected to the contralateral ear (Fig. 3.3).

Electromyogram (EMG) recordings

The presence or absence of muscle activity ('tone') is important in establishing whether the subject is awake, or in NREM or REM sleep. It is usually identified by electrodes on the chin (mentalis) and under the chin (submentalis) (Fig. 3.3).

EEG waveforms

Several patterns of electrical activity are characteristically seen in sleep.

Alpha rhythm

This is normal in relaxed wakefulness, but usually disappears at sleep onset. It may however intrude into sleep, particularly stages 1 and 2 NREM sleep and also stages 3 and 4 (alpha delta rhythm). It is less prominent in the frontocentral rather than occipital areas and has a frequency of 1–2 Hz slower than that during wakefulness. There is a circadian rhythm in alpha activity which is independent of sleep.

Alpha intrusion is thought to be related to arousals or a lower threshold for arousal to stimuli such as pain or noise. It is characteristic of hyperarousal states associated with insomnia, particularly fibromyalgia and the chronic fatigue syndrome.

Alpha intrusion is associated with awareness of thoughts during sleep and with the perception that sleep is unrefreshing. It may be related to the establishment of explicit memory of which the subject is aware, but not implicit memory which takes place subliminally. It may therefore represent an abnormal form of information processing during sleep which is associated with a low threshold for arousal. It may be due to a failure of the thalamocortical projections to modify the activity of the cerebral cortex in the usual way during NREM sleep.

Sleep spindles
Sleep spindles are events lasting > 0.5 s with a frequency of 12–16 Hz which occur only during sleep [2]. They are characteristic of stage 2 NREM sleep, but also occur in stages 3 and 4, in which they are often hidden by delta waves. They are absent in REM sleep.

Sleep spindles are triggered by brainstem activity often in response to stimuli such as noise. They are the result of thalamic hyperpolarization, which is expressed as synchronized cerebral cortical activity. The spindle frequency of 12–16 Hz is determined by the duration of the hyperpolarization of the thalamo-cortical neurones.

Sleep spindles represent a sleep-stabilizing response to a potential arousal. This may arise as a reaction to either internal or external stimuli, but spindles also have an endogenous rhythm and occur around every 10–15 s in stage 2 NREM sleep. They can also be a manifestation of the cyclic alternating pattern (CAP), indicating subcortical arousals which are self limiting and followed by a return to sleep.

Sleep spindles appear in children at the age of around 4 weeks and become less numerous in the elderly. Their frequency is inversely related to the melatonin level during the night. They also have a reciprocal relationship to delta waves and unlike these are less frequent following sleep deprivation.

K-complexes
K-complexes are biphasic events in which the positive wave represents synchronized depolarization and excitation of cortical neurones, and the negative wave is due to synchronized hyperpolarization and inhibition of cortical neurones [3]. They have a frequency of < 1 Hz and while they are a characteristic feature of stage 2 NREM sleep they also appear in stages 3 and 4, where they have a slightly higher frequency. They are bilaterally symmetrical and predominantly fronto-parietal.

K-complexes can be spontaneous events arising in the cerebral cortex and propagated by intracortical circuits. They also arise in response to sensory input to the thalamus, particularly when the monoaminergic brainstem arousal systems are inactivated and the cerebral cortex is deafferented. In addition to responding to internal and external stimuli in this way they are also a feature of the endogenous cyclic alternating pattern (CAP).

K-complexes represent a sleep-maintenance mechanism in response to potential arousals. They often occur with sleep spindles and with these coalesce into delta waves as sleep is re-established and the thalamo-cortical projections become more intense and sensory input to the cortex is gated [4].

K-complexes are also precursors of paroxysmal spike and wave complexes associated with epilepsy. Thalamic depolarization increases in amplitude and becomes briefer, leading to EEG spikes, while the increase in synchronization of the cerebral cortex facilitates propagation of the epileptic discharge from an unstable focus.

Vertex sharp waves and transients
These are represented both by spikes (< 70 ms duration) and sharp waves (> 70 ms duration).

Sleep staging
Sleep stages are conventionally scored according to recommendations set out in 1968 (Fig. 3.4) [5]. These have proved useful, but only characterize the dominant sleep stage at any one time and do not show the dynamic structure of sleep adequately. The criteria have been validated for healthy young adults, but not in other situations. The recording is divided into units (epochs) of 30 s. The sleep stage during each epoch is designated according to which stage is present for over half of the time. This makes it insensitive to rapid changes in sleep state and ignores the microstructure of sleep. The criteria for diagnosing events during sleep are inflexible and no attention is paid to differences in, for instance, the alpha wave frequency or the types of sleep spindle. There is considerable

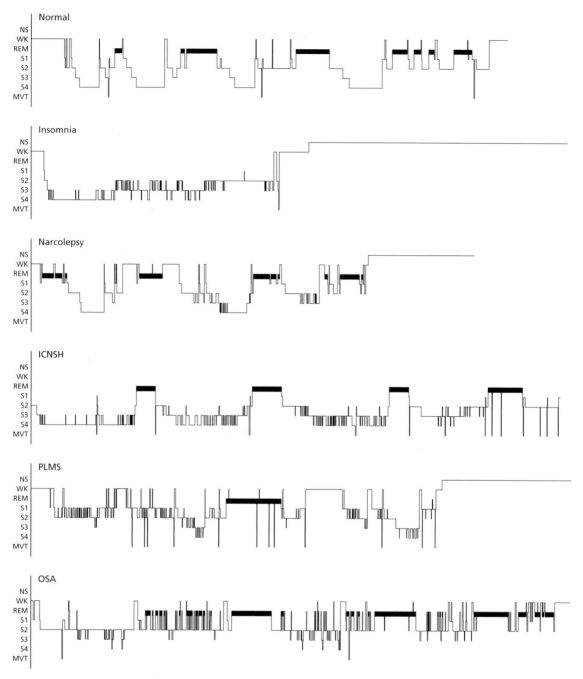

Fig. 3.4 Hypnograms showing differences between (from top to bottom): normal subject; insomnia (prolonged period awake at the end of the night); narcolepsy (sleep-onset REM and frequent sleep-stage shifts); idiopathic hypersomnia (prolonged episodes of stages 3 and 4 NREM sleep); periodic limb movement syndrome (frequent arousals early in the night with difficulty in establishing stages 3 and 4 NREM sleep); and OSAs (frequent arousals and lack of stages 3 and 4 NREM sleep). MVT, movement artefact; NREM, non-rapid eye movement; NS, no signal; OSA, obstructive sleep apnoea; REM, rapid eye movement; S1–4, stages 1–4 NREM sleep; WK, wakefulness.

inter-observer variation in the conventional reporting of sleep staging, although this is more accurate than the computerized reporting systems that have been developed. Newer approaches using computerized analysis of the continuous trends in frequency and amplitude and the analysis of sleep microstructure are being developed, but are not yet in general use [6].

Wakefulness, NREM and REM sleep can be distinguished by a combination of their EEG, EOG and EMG features. The EEG rhythms are identified and classified primarily by their frequency, but also by their amplitude (Tables 3.4 and 3.5, Fig. 3.5). As sleep is entered, the frequency of the EEG slows, with a loss of alpha, increase in theta and then of delta waves. Sleep

Table 3.4 EEG waveforms during sleep and wakefulness.

Waveform	Frequency or duration	Amplitude	Location	Main sleep–wake state and stage
Beta	Unstable frequency, > 13 Hz	10–20 μV	Frontal and prefrontal	Alert wakefulness, stage 1 NREM and REM
Alpha	8–13 Hz	20–50 μV	Occipital	Relaxed wakefulness
Theta	4–8 Hz	10–30 μV	Generalized	Wakefulness, stage 1 NREM
Delta	0.5–4 Hz	> 75 μV	Generalized	Stages 2, 3 and 4 NREM
Vertex sharp waves	0.05–0.2 s duration	30–200 μV	Vertex	Stage 1 NREM
K-complexes	1 Hz, > 0.5 s duration	> 75 μV	Generalized, maximum at vertex	Stage 2 NREM
Sleep spindles	12–16 Hz, > 0.5 s duration	20–40 μV	Generalized	Stage 2 NREM
Sawtooth waves	2–5 Hz, > 0.25 s duration	20–100 μV	Generalized, especially vertex	REM

Table 3.5 Common causes of sleep-stage abnormalities on polysomnography.

Sleep state and stage	Increased	Reduced
NREM stages 3 and 4	Sleep deprivation Drugs Idiopathic hypersomnia Neurological hypersomnias Thyrotoxicosis Fever	First night effect Old age Sleep fragmentation, e.g. OSA, ventilatory failure, PLMS, pain Drugs Degenerative cerebral disorders Depression
REM latency	REM sleep suppressant drugs Idiopathic hypersomnia RLS and PLMS CSA and CSR	REM sleep deprivation Infancy REM sleep fragmentation, e.g. OSA, pain Drugs Narcolepsy Depression Mania Circadian rhythm disorders
REM	Infancy After REM sleep deprivation Drugs	REM sleep deprivation REM sleep fragmentation, e.g. OSA, ventilatory failure, pain Drugs Degenerative cerebral disorders

CSA, central sleep apnoea; CSR, Cheyne–Stokes respiration; OSA, obstructive sleep apnoeas; PLMS, periodic limb movements in sleep; RLS, restless legs syndrome, REM, rapid eye movement.

NREM

Stage 1

Stage 2

Stage 3

Stage 4

Alert

Relaxed

REM

α-intrusion

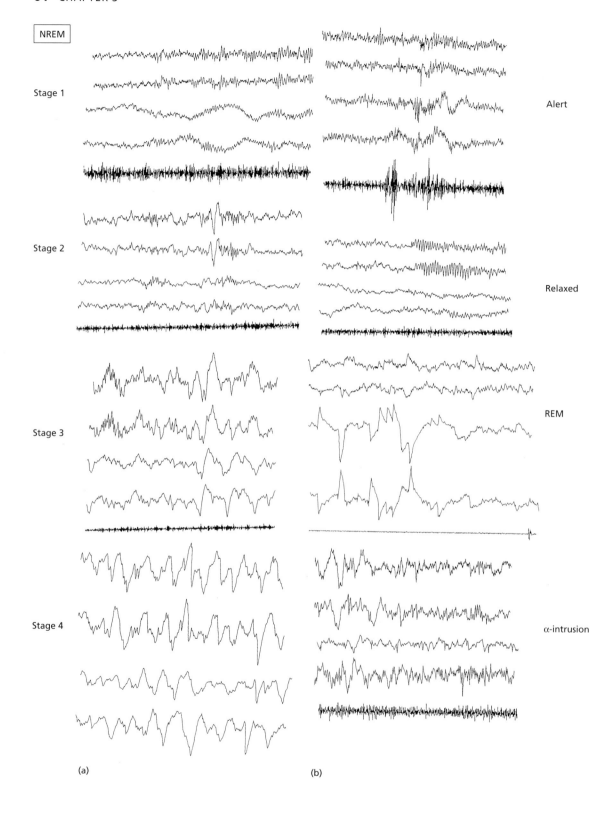

(a)   (b)

onset is taken either as the first of three consecutive epochs of stage 1 NREM sleep, the first epoch of any other sleep stage, or the first epoch of stage 1 NREM sleep which is contiguous with another sleep stage.

Stage 1 NREM sleep is best regarded as a transitional phase between sleep and wakefulness rather than a stage of sleep. It probably has very little recuperative role. Sensory stimulation leads to a return of alpha activity, which is usually seen in relaxed wakefulness rather than in sleep. Stage 2 NREM sleep, however, has characteristic features, such as sleep spindles and K-complexes, which represent cortical synchronization. Sensory stimulation in this stage of sleep intensifies spindle and K-complex activity which are sleep-maintaining mechanisms. Stages 3 and 4 NREM sleep represent more intensive cortical synchronization, appear to be more recuperative than stage 2 and are often regarded as a single phase (slow wave sleep), because of their similarities.

The characteristic EEG features of wakefulness and sleep stages and arousals in adults are as follows.

Alert wakefulness. With the eyes open and when the subject is alert, the EEG tracings show a dominant rhythm of up to 30–50 Hz with a low amplitude. There is a high level of muscle tone and blinking is detectable in the EOG channel.

Relaxed wakefulness. When relaxed with the eyes closed the frequency of the dominant rhythm falls to around 8–13 Hz (alpha rhythm), although this can be

Fig. 3.5 *(opposite)* The EEG, EMG and EOG appearances. (a) Stage 1 NREM sleep: high-frequency EEG activity with slow rolling eye movements. Stage 2 NREM: K-complex with spindles. Stage 3 NREM: delta waves present in EEG for 20–50% of tracing and conducted to the EOG tracings, less chin EMG activity than in stages 1 and 2 NREM. Stage 4 NREM: the EEG shows slow high-amplitude delta waves throughout with no chin EMG activity. (b) Alert wakefulness: high-frequency EEG recording with eye movements and considerable chin EMG activity. Relaxed wakefulness: conspicuous alpha rhythm (8–13 Hz) on EEG tracing and chin EMG activity present. REM sleep: irregular mixed frequency EEG with frequent eye movements and absence of chin EMG activity. Alpha intrusion into stage 3 NREM: alpha waves, superimposed on delta waves in EEG tracing and conducted to EOG recordings. EEG, electro-encephalogram; EMG, electro-myogram; EOG, electro-oculogram; NREM, non-rapid eye movement; REM, rapid eye movement.

abolished by opening the eyes. The alpha rhythm is most easily detected in the occipital region. Muscle tone is less prominent than during alertness.

Stage 1 NREM sleep. In stage 1 NREM sleep, alpha activity diminishes and is replaced by 2–3 s runs of slower waves at a frequency of 4–8 Hz (theta rhythm) and vertex sharp waves. These are seen particularly in children and young adults. Muscle tone is reduced further and horizontal, slow rolling eye movements lasting 2–4 s are detectable [7].

Stage 2 NREM sleep. In stage 2 NREM sleep, spindles appear often at a rate of 3–8 per minute, with K-complexes (often 1–3 per minute). High-amplitude slow-frequency delta waves appear, but occupy less than 20% of each epoch. There is less muscle tone than in stage 1 and no eye movements.

Stages 3 and 4 NREM sleep. The deeper stages of NREM sleep (stages 3 and 4) are characterized by the presence of delta waves. They are known as slow waves because of their low frequency (0.5–4 Hz) and at least some of the delta waves are due to the low firing frequency of the thalamo-cortical projection neurones. These waves occupy 20–50% of each epoch in stage 3 and over 50% of the epochs in stage 4 NREM sleep. Their amplitude is greater than 75 mV in young adults, but this falls in the elderly. Sleep spindles and K-complexes may also be present but can be difficult to distinguish from, and may be masked by, the delta waves. There is some 30–50 Hz activity, but this is much less prominent than in REM sleep. Muscle tone is less than in stages 1 and 2 and eye movements are absent.

REM sleep. The EEG of REM sleep is very similar to that of relaxed wakefulness with a wide range of frequencies of low and irregular amplitude. These largely reflect the 30–50 Hz (gamma band) activity in the cerebral cortex which is characteristic of REM sleep, and which is thought to be a feature of attention in the cerebral cortex, whether this is occurring during sleep or while the subject is awake. This high frequency is also seen in the basal ganglia when they are focusing attention on a movement. This 30–50 Hz activity is driven by the burst frequency in the thalamo-cortical projection neurones.

This high-frequency activity in REM sleep is more localized than the projection of electrical activity during NREM sleep so that the surface EEG appears to be 'desynchronized'. The vertex sharp waves of stage 2 are replaced in REM sleep by sawtooth waves of 2–5 Hz, which often precede rapid eye movements.

In REM sleep the EMG recording appears flat because of lack of muscle activity, except for sporadic bursts of phasic muscle twitches, especially in the facial and limb electrodes. The EOG shows intermittent bursts of rapid eye movements. The frequency of epochs which contain these movements determines the 'density' of REM sleep. Ponto-geniculo-occipital (PGO) waves can be detected in some animals, especially cats, and when deep, rather than surface, electrodes are used. They are said to be characteristic of REM sleep but are not detectable with surface electrodes in humans.

Arousals. Cortical arousals from sleep are detected on the EEG as a sudden increase in frequency lasting more than 3 s which are terminated by a return to sleep. These changes are difficult to identify in REM sleep, in which the transient reappearance of EMG activity indicates an arousal. K-complexes and sleep spindles also represent mechanisms to overcome arousals and to maintain sleep.

Subcortical arousals do not lead to any EEG changes. They may be detectable by observation or video recording through the gross body movements and movements of the limbs and facial muscles which they cause, and changes in respiratory frequency. They also cause autonomic activation which may be detectable as changes in heart rate or blood pressure.

Sleep EEG changes during childhood
The EEG features during sleep change considerably with age as the brain matures. Normal values are less well established in young children than at other ages.

Beta–delta complexes are present from around 26–38 weeks' gestation and are irregular 0.3–1.5 Hz waves of moderate to high amplitude superimposed on bursts of low-amplitude faster activity. They are a mark of prematurity, together with temporal theta bursts which appear at 26–33 weeks and temporal alpha bursts which follow them.

Sleep spindles appear at around 4 weeks post delivery. They may be asynchronous between the two hemispheres until the age of 1 year. Quiet (NREM) sleep in the neonate is shown by very slow (0.5–1.5 Hz) activity with superimposed low-voltage theta and beta activity. The pattern in active (REM) sleep is similar to that seen in wakefulness, which is low voltage up to 8 Hz activity with both slower and faster frequencies. The posterior dominant or alpha rhythm becomes apparent at around 4 months with a frequency of at least 4 Hz, which increases steadily to 8 Hz by the age of 3 years.

Separate stages of NREM sleep can be identified after the age of 6 months. K-complexes appear between 8 and 12 weeks after birth, and occipital delta activity is superimposed on normal occipital alpha activity from around 2 years of age. It is most obvious between 8 and 14 years and disappears by the age of 30 years.

Body position monitoring
Body position monitors are attached to the chest continuously to record whether the subject is upright, supine, prone or on the right or left side. These monitors usually employ piezo-electric crystals which generate an electric current. A tilt switch modifies their activity according to their orientation. Video recordings may also be used to assess body position. Abrupt changes may be due to arousals from sleep or motor abnormalities of sleep.

Limb movement monitoring
This is particularly valuable in assessing whether the patient is awake or asleep and, in conjunction with other monitoring, in assessing abnormal movements during sleep. Arousals from any cause can be detected, but, especially in the elderly, movements during sleep also occur as a result of disorders such as periodic limb movements and obstructive sleep apnoeas, and conversely immobility is frequent during wakefulness.

There are various methods of recording movements, detailed below.

Video recording
This is usually used in conjunction with an audio recording and sleep-stage monitoring. It can detect not only movements of the limbs and respiratory movements, but also the position of the patient. The movements may be difficult to quantify by video recordings, but a combination of video and audio recordings can be useful in assessing the frequency of obstructive sleep apnoeas and hypopnoeas.

Electromyogram electrodes
These are conventionally applied to the anterior tibialis muscle of both legs and ideally these are recorded separately, although often they are combined to give a single EMG input to the recording system. This technique is particularly useful for diagnosing periodic

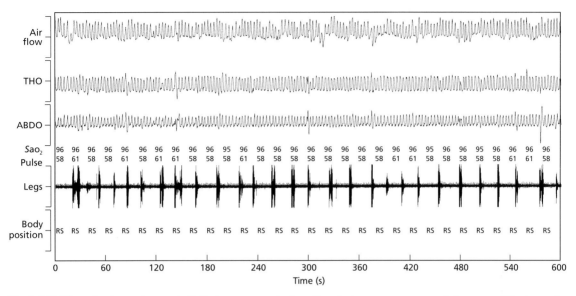

Fig. 3.6 EMG monitoring to show periodic limb movements in sleep. Regular leg movements recorded at around 20-s intervals throughout the tracing. ABDO, abdominal movement; RS, right side; Sao_2, arterial oxygen saturation; THO, thoracic movement.

limb movements (Fig. 3.6), but these may be hard to distinguish from arousal movements associated with obstructive sleep apnoeas, and occasionally from phasic twitches during REM sleep.

Actigraphy

This uses an accelerometer in which small movements are transduced into electrical signals which can be recorded and analysed. It identifies small accelerations, in contrast to the EMG which records the electrical activity of the muscles. Actigraphy can be used on a domiciliary basis and modern actigraphs can record and store data from several nights [8].

Actigraphy can be used as an indirect indicator of whether the subject is awake or asleep. It may be useful in circadian rhythm disorders [9], insomnia and excessive daytime sleepiness, as well as to identify, for instance, the degree of suppression of periodic limb movements with treatment.

Respiratory monitoring

Most of the physiological measurements of respiration during sleep are semiquantitative at best. The most important components of respiratory function that are monitored during sleep are described below.

Respiratory sounds

The normal sounds of respiration and those of snoring, obstructive sleep apnoeas, snorting, grunting, wheezing and stridor can be sensed by a microphone placed either close to the upper airway or over the trachea. Frequency analysis and estimation of the loudness of the noise can be carried out.

Airflow

Airflow can be measured using oral, nasal or oronasal thermistors which detect changes in temperature between the inspired and expired air (Fig. 3.7). These give a semiquantitative estimate of airflow, but can become displaced. An end tidal Pco_2 monitor is an alternative, but nasal pressure transducers can be better quantified than either of these techniques. The pressure profile during each breath indicates whether there is flow limitation due to upper airway narrowing, but a blocked nose, mouth breathing or dislodgement of the cannulae can make interpretation difficult.

Airflow can also be measured using a pneumotachograph connected to an oral, nasal or oronasal mask. In practice these are often poorly tolerated and their use has been largely confined to research situations.

The forced oscillation technique may also detect upper airway flow limitation. High-frequency, low-amplitude pressure waves are applied to the airway and, if this narrows, the amplitude of the pressure oscillation falls. Air leaks through the mouth may produce similar findings but this technique can be useful in detecting upper airway narrowing or temporary

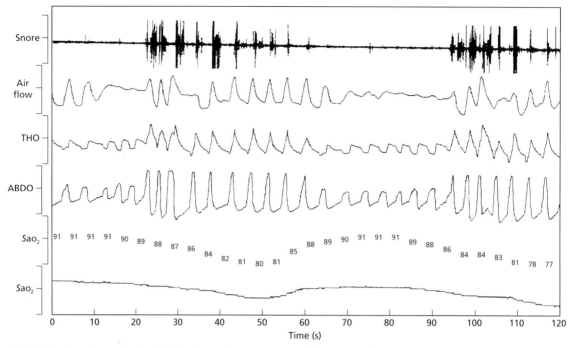

Fig. 3.7 Respiratory monitoring in OSA. Obstructive sleeps apnoeas demonstrated by cessation of airflow associated with paradoxical thoracic and abdominal movement and terminated with snoring sounds, followed by an increase in oxygen saturation. ABDO, abdominal movement; Sao_2, arterial oxygen saturation; THO, thoracic movement.

occlusion in the titration of continuous positive airway pressure (CPAP) treatment for obstructive sleep apnoeas.

Respiratory movements

Respiratory movements can best be measured by inductance, but also by impedance or magnetometry methods, or by using mercury strain gauges. Normally the inspiratory thoracic and abdominal expansion is almost synchronous but when there is an increased upper airway resistance or obstruction, the thorax moves inwards and the abdomen outwards during inspiration, and in expiration this pattern is reversed (paradoxical rib cage and abdominal movements). This represents a complete phase shift of movements from the normal pattern, but if the upper airway is only partially obstructed there may only be a change in the phase angle and timing of the movements of the thorax and abdomen. These are detectable by movement monitors. Although they are all only semi-quantitative they can identify minor degrees of upper airway narrowing as well as distinguishing central from obstructive apnoeas when used in conjunction with recordings of airflow.

Respiratory muscle activity

Respiratory effort can be estimated by measuring oesophageal pressure which reflects the intrapleural pressure. This is an indicator of the activity of the chest wall muscles. The pressure swings increase during, for instance, obstructive sleep apnoeas and the upper airway resistance syndrome in order to overcome the high airflow resistance. This technique is invasive in that it requires swallowing a balloon or catheter into the oesophagus. Arousals from sleep usually occur in normal subjects when the oesophageal pressure exceeds -15 cmH2O, irrespective of the cause of this.

An indirect estimate of pleural pressure swings can be obtained from continuous monitoring of the blood pressure to derive the pulse transit time. This is the time taken for the arterial pulse to travel through the peripheral circulation [10]. It is usually measured as the interval between the R wave of the electrocardiogram, which corresponds to aortic valve opening, and the onset of the pulse wave, on a pulse oximeter applied to the finger.

The pulse transit time is reduced if the blood pressure rises, for instance in response to changes in the intrathoracic pressure during obstructive sleep apnoeas.

It is, in effect, a non-invasive equivalent of measuring the oesophageal pressure, and has the additional advantage of detecting 'autonomic arousals' at the end of each apnoea at which time the pulse transit time increases suddenly. Interpretation is difficult in the presence of cardiac dysrhythmias, left ventricular dysfunction or with beta blockers.

Electromyogram recordings of the diaphragm and other respiratory muscles show whether they are active during respiration, but do not give an indication of the force that they develop.

Oxygen saturation

Pulse oximetry gives a continuous non-invasive record of oxygen saturation. It uses a spectroscopic technique identifying oxyhaemoglobin at the wavelength of 660 nm and reduced haemoglobin at the 940 nm wavelength. Most oximeters are accurate to within 3% when the saturation is above 70%. The extent of desaturation differs according to the initial arterial Po_2 because of the sigmoid shape of the oxyhaemoglobin dissociation curve. Larger desaturations occur more readily, for instance, if the initial Po_2 is around 8 kPa than if it is around 12 kPa. Oximetry is therefore insensitive in detecting changes in oxygenation if the initial Po_2 is nearly normal.

Pco_2

The transcutaneous Pco_2 can be recorded continuously and non-invasively using a heated electrode applied to the skin, usually the arm. It is, however, slowly responding and requires calibration with the Pco_2 measured by arterial blood gas analysis. The alternative is to measure the end tidal Pco_2, but this is technically difficult during sleep, and is only accurate if the function of the lungs is normal and if the respiratory rate is not rapid.

Pco_2 monitoring is not usually required to assess obstructive sleep apnoeas, but it is needed if hypoventilation during sleep is being considered.

Information derived from these types of monitoring enables several concepts and indices to be derived.

Sleep apnoeas

These are defined as a cessation of airflow for 10 or more seconds, although this is in practice usually taken as a reduction in airflow by more than 80% from the previous stable baseline. The duration of 10 s has been widely used, but it has no physiological basis, and in children, in particular, briefer apnoeas appear to be significant.

In central apnoeas there is no detectable chest wall muscle activity on respiratory movement or respiratory muscle activity monitoring. In obstructive sleep apnoeas chest wall movement occurs, as detected by the movement monitors and signs of respiratory muscle effort, but the upper airway obstruction prevents any airflow from occurring. In mixed sleep apnoeas there is an initial central phase followed by upper airway obstruction before arousal occurs.

Hypopnoeas

There has been considerable variation in the use of this term, but it usually implies a reduction in airflow or respiratory movements by over 50% for 10 s or more from the baseline, associated with either oxygen desaturation or evidence of an arousal. It therefore requires more complex monitoring than is needed to identify a sleep apnoea.

A reduction in the airflow signal by more than 50% does not necessarily imply that airflow has fallen to this extent, because of the non-linearity of the monitors. The same applies to respiratory movement. Movement monitoring is also complicated because the reduction is usually taken to be relative to the baseline movements but an unstable baseline may make assessment of both airflow and movement changes difficult. The reduction of 50% applies to the sum of the thoracic and abdominal movement signals.

A reduction in oxygen saturation by 4% or occasionally 3% is taken as sufficient to diagnose a hypopnoea. Arousals may be either subcortical as shown by changes in heart rate or pulse transit time, or cortical as identified by EEG.

Hypoventilation

Hypoventilation is conventionally defined as a reduction in airflow for more than 60 s leading to an EEG arousal. There is often a gradual desaturation, usually from a low baseline. This is seen particularly in chronic lung disease and neuromuscular and skeletal disorders affecting the thorax.

Desaturation index (DI)

Oxygen desaturations are conventionally regarded as a fall in saturation of 4% or more, although often 3% or even 2% is used [11]. None of these values has, however, any specific biological significance. The degree of desaturation depends on the position of the baseline oxygen saturation on the oxyhaemoglobin desaturation curve, as described above. Small desaturations may be difficult to distinguish from variations in oxygen saturation due to, for instance, alterations in body position and ventilation–perfusion matching. Small desaturations often follow hyperventilation during wakefulness at night, leading to a return to a normal oxygen saturation during sleep. This does not represent an abnormal sleep apnoea or sleep desaturation.

The desaturation index is the number of desaturations per hour of sleep. This is ideally determined from EEG monitoring, but in simpler respiratory studies usually calculated by assuming that the duration of sleep is the same as the study.

Visual inspection of the pattern of the oximetry tracing during sleep is often of more value than using unvalidated indices, such as the desaturation index. In obstructive sleep apnoeas each desaturation is slower than the resaturation, but the pattern is more symmetrical in central sleep apnoeas and Cheyne–Stokes respiration, which often also have a more uniform frequency and minimum desaturations during the night. In chronic obstructive pulmonary disease the desaturations are more prolonged and occur particularly in REM sleep.

Apnoea index (AI)

The apnoea index is the number of apnoeas divided by the duration of sleep and expressed as the number per hour of sleep. Either the sleep period time or the total sleep time can be used as the denominator, and both require EEG monitoring.

Apnoea/hypopnoea index (AHI)

This is analogous to the apnoea index but includes hypopnoeas. The respiratory disturbance index (RDI) is usually used synonymously with the apnoea/hypopnoea index and is usually related to the total sleep time.

An AHI of less than 5 per hour is conventionally taken as normal, 5–20 per hour as showing mild obstructive sleep apnoeas, 20–40 per hour as moderately severe and more than 40 per hour as indicating severe sleep apnoeas. These cut-off points are, however, arbitrary. There is also considerable inter-night variability in the AHI. The normal values are higher in the elderly than in younger subjects.

Arousal index (AI)

This is the number of arousals divided by the hours of sleep expressed either as the sleep period time or total sleep time. As with the AHI and apnoea index it requires EEG monitoring.

Cardiovascular monitoring

The heart rate can be monitored continuously using a pulse oximeter. Rapid fluctuations suggest frequent arousals from sleep, which are often due to obstructive sleep apnoeas, but may result from other causes, such as central apnoeas or periodic limb movements during sleep.

An electrocardiogram gives additional detail about the nature of electrical conduction of the cardiac impulse. A three-lead electrocardiogram is usually used in polysomnography but this may be inadequate to define dysrhythmias accurately, in which case conventional 24-h cardiac monitoring may be required. Continuous monitoring of inter-beat heart rate variability can be useful in assessing sympathetic activity due, for instance, to sleep deprivation or sleep fragmentation. Correlation of heart rate with respiratory events can give useful information about central sleep apnoeas and Cheyne–Stokes respiration in cardiac failure.

Blood pressure can be monitored continuously or intermittently, and non-invasively, both during sleep and during wakefulness, and the pulse transit time may be useful in detecting autonomic arousals (see page 68). The pulmonary artery pressure can also be continuously recorded during sleep.

Oesophageal pH monitoring

Oesophageal pH can be recorded continuously from a pH sensor in the oesophagus and is used particularly to identify episodes of gastro-oesophageal reflux. Their significance depends on the frequency, duration and extent of the fall in pH, which relate to the degree of acid reflux and the ease with which it is cleared from the oesophagus.

Penile erection monitoring

The increase in penile circumference can be measured with a mercury-filled strain gauge whose electrical resistance is proportional to the length of the gauge. The circumference is measured by gauges at the base and at the coronal sulcus. The rigidity of the penis is recorded by assessing the force that is needed to cause it to buckle.

Normal values have been obtained for the frequency of erections during sleep, the total duration of the erections and the increase in penile circumference. Knowledge of the sleep structure is required to interpret these measurements, which should therefore only be carried out as part of polysomnography. Severe fragmentation of REM sleep, as in obstructive sleep apnoeas, may prevent erections from taking place.

Penile erection monitoring has been used to distinguish organic from psychogenic causes of impotence. In the latter, erections during sleep are retained, in contrast to organic disorders. Different patterns of abnormalities are seen in vascular and neuropathic disorders.

Assessment of daytime sleepiness

Neuroradiology

A skull radiograph, head computerized tomograph (CT) or magnetic resonance imaging (MRI) scan may be indicated to assess whether there is an organic cause for excessive daytime sleepiness (EDS), insomnia, abnormal movements, or other events occurring during sleep. Functional MRI utilizes alterations in the extent of oxygenation of haemoglobin in the blood to indicate areas of neuronal activity. Positron emission computerized tomography (PET) scans detect the decay of radioisotopically labelled molecules which are functionally important, such as glucose, and can provide 'metabolic imaging' [12]. Single photon emission computerized tomography (SPECT) is a similar technique, and both may give information about the activity of various regions of the brain during sleep.

These functional neuro-imaging techniques give information about either blood flow or metabolic activity, but not at a neuronal level. The degree of resolution varies with each technique, and images can be quantified only by comparison with other sleep–wake states. It may also be difficult for the subject to fall asleep in the scanner.

Sleep diaries

These are usually completed for two weeks, and the subject should record all episodes of sleep, whether these are during the day or at night, together with any other relevant events, such as taking caffeinated drinks, alcohol, meals and exercise (Fig. 3.8). They are of value in patients with irregular sleep–wake patterns and in assessing circadian rhythm disorders and the cause of excessive daytime sleepiness and insomnia.

Self-assessment scales

These are subjective or introspective tests which depend on the accuracy of the subject's perception of sleepiness and the ability to record this precisely. The subject's attitude can influence whether the sleep problem is denied or exaggerated, and the degree of motivation to stay awake may affect the results. Nevertheless these are simple tests which should be used regularly in the assessment of excessive daytime sleepiness. There are two types of scales.

Generic questionnaires

These focus on general health and may thereby give an indication of the impact of any sleep disorder on the quality of life. The Short Form 36 Health Survey (SF36 (Appendix 3)) has been most widely used. Normal values are available for males and females and different age groups and social classes in the USA, UK and other countries. The SF36 is sensitive to some sleep disorders, such as obstructive sleep apnoeas, but is probably less so than the sleep-specific questionnaires. The Functional Outcomes of Sleep Questionnaire (FOSQ) (Appendix 4) and the Medical Outcome Study Sleep Scale (MOS) (Appendix 5) assess the effects of sleep on quality of life more specifically.

Sleep-specific questionnaires

These assess the individual's perception of how sleepy he or she feels [13]. The degree of sleepiness felt at the time that the questionnaire is completed can be assessed by a visual analogue scale in which the degree of sleepiness or alertness is scored from 1–10. Alternatives are the Karolinska Sleepiness Scale (KSS), which has nine items, and the Stanford Sleepiness Scale [14] (Appendix 6), which is a seven-item questionnaire. These tests are repeatable and easy to administer, but are poor at assessing chronic sleepiness.

Other questionnaires are available to assess the overall degree of chronic sleepiness. The best known is the Epworth Sleepiness Scale (ESS) (Appendix 7), which assesses the probability of falling asleep in certain situations rather than how sleepy the subject feels [15, 16]. It has eight items, which the subject grades from 0–3 according to the likelihood of falling asleep. Some of the situations are passive and some active, and it includes situations of which the subject may have no experience. Nevertheless it is a simple test which is repeatable and widely used in the assessment of excessive daytime sleepiness. Like the other self-administered assessment scales it correlates poorly with sleepiness as assessed by the MSLT and MWT (pages 73, 74), and in addition the wording of the questions of the ESS is imprecise.

Behavioural performance tests

Laboratory tests of performance have not been widely used because of the lack of normal values, the improvement with practice and their uncertain sensitivity and specificity for detecting sleepiness. The more complex

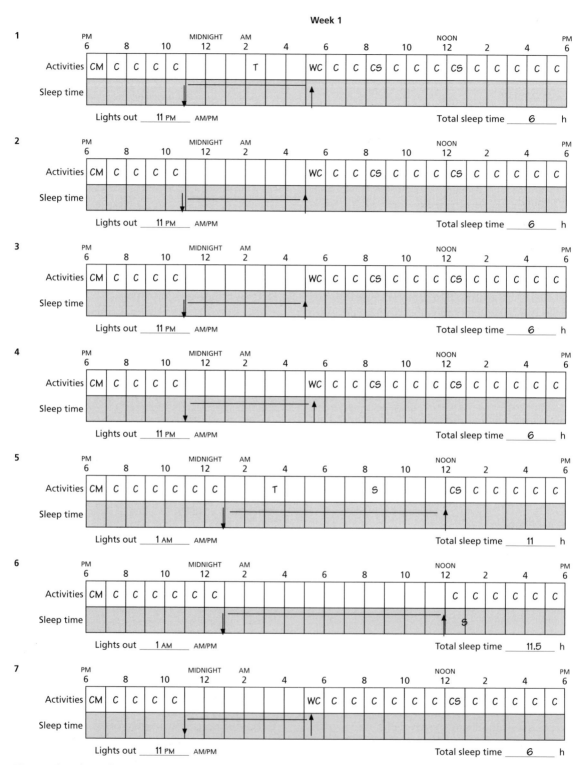

Fig. 3.8 Sleep diary of a patient with EDS showing irregular sleeping times, intermittent sleep restriction and frequent caffeinated drinks, as indicated by 'C' in activities line. M, meals; S, snacks; T, use of toilet in sleep time; W, wake-up time.

tests are also more interesting and may test the degree of motivation rather than the severity of excessive daytime sleepiness. The best recognized tests are described below.

Reaction times

The principle of these tests is that patients who are sleepy have a reduced ability to maintain attention. Their main value is in assessing responses to treatment by serial testing. Repetitive and unpredictable stimuli, such as flashing lights, are presented to the subject who has to respond as rapidly as possible. Delays or failure to respond to these stimuli are recorded. These tests require the subject's cooperation and are influenced by the degree of motivation. Reaction times are longest between 2.00 and 4.00 PM when there is an increased circadian tendency towards sleepiness.

The psychomotor vigilance test (PVT) scores the number of lapses and long response times. The normal value is 250–350 msccs, but if the subject is sleepy the number of longer response times increases as the subject attempts to maintain accuracy [17]. Lapses are more frequent, but the results depend not only on vigilance but also on experience with the test and coping strategies.

Driving simulators

These have been used extensively, particularly in the USA, in order to assess the risk of the subject causing a road traffic accident. The most widely used is the Steer Clear Test. These tests are, however, as much a computer game as an estimate of sleepiness or safety while driving, and the results depend on the aptitude and interest of the subject.

Psychological tests

Simple tracking tests and tests of higher cognitive function, such as planning and decision making, have been used to assess the degree of daytime sleepiness the ability to maintain attention, and other aspects of cortical function.

Pupillometry (pupillography)

This test depends on the principle that the pupil diameter is determined by the balance of sympathetic and parasympathetic tone and that this is influenced by the state of arousal. During sleep the parasympathetic discharge dominates and the pupil constricts, whereas it dilates if the subject is alert, especially in a darkened environment. The test measures the degree of sleepiness or the presence of sleep, but not its cause.

During pupillometry the subject is kept in infrared light for at least 10 min and if he or she is alert the diameter of the pupil should be stable and greater than 7 mm diameter. During sleepiness the pupil fluctuates in size and when the subject falls asleep it becomes smaller.

This test is equivalent to the maintenance of wakefulness test, but uses a peripheral marker of pupil size, instead of EEG criteria. The problems with pupillometry include difficulties in the subject collaborating, closure of the eyelids when he or she becomes sleepy, darkness of the iris which may make it difficult to determine the pupil size (although the use of infrared pupillography has reduced this difficulty), and ocular and neurological disorders, particularly those affecting the autonomic nervous system, which may hinder interpretation of the test.

Pupillometry is being increasingly used but requires carefully controlled conditions, technical skill and better defined normal values. These vary with the time of day. The pupils are, for instance, normally less reactive between 2.00 and 4.00 PM, when there is an increased circadian tendency to be sleepy.

Multiple sleep latency test (MSLT)

This is an objective test which assesses the ease with which the subject can fall asleep during the day in the artificial environment of a sleep laboratory. Subjects should ideally have been following a normal sleep–wake routine for two weeks, without night or shift work and without taking any medication that might affect sleep. The sleep pattern can be documented by a sleep diary or actigraphy, but ideally polysomnography is carried out on the night before the MSLT to establish that the duration of sleep is adequate and to look for any signs of sleep deprivation or a sleep disorder.

The first MSLT begins either 2 h after waking or at around 9.00 AM and the test is repeated at 2-h intervals. Four tests are carried out during the day, plus a fifth if one of the first four has shown sleep-onset rapid eye movement sleep (SOREM) and the possibility of narcolepsy is being considered.

During each MSLT the subject is asked to lie down in a quiet, darkened room and to try to fall asleep. The test is terminated after 20 min if sleep has not been documented electrophysiologically, or at 15 min after the first appearance of sleep. The onset of sleep is the interval from the time that the lights are switched off until the appearance of stage 1 NREM sleep for a single epoch of 30 s. This differs from the criteria for sleep onset during polysomnography. Rapid eye movement sleep arising within 15 min of sleep onset is scored as sleep-onset REM sleep.

Exact normal values have not been determined for the MSLT [18]. They are longer in prepubertal children and vary during the day according to fluctuations in the circadian rhythm and sleep and wake drives, being shortest between 2.00 and 4.00 PM.

The mean of the four or five MSLTs is taken as the value of the test. In general this is greater than 10 min in normal subjects. A mean MSLT of 8–10 min is indeterminate, but 5–8 min is probably mildly abnormal, and less than 5 min is definitely abnormal. An MSLT of less than 5 min is seen in 80% of subjects with narcolepsy, and less than 8 min in 95%, but the feature which distinguishes this most clearly from other causes of excessive daytime sleepiness is the presence of sleep-onset REM in two out of four or five of the MSLTs. If one SOREM period is documented in the first four tests, a fifth MSLT should be performed. Sleep-onset REM may also occasionally be seen in severe obstructive apnoeas, depression, severe sleep deprivation, and following withdrawal of REM sleep suppressant drugs, and in infants.

Multiple sleep latency tests are based on the assumption that the degree of sleepiness is related to the time that it takes to enter sleep as judged by EEG criteria. This has not been demonstrated and MSLTs do not correlate closely with other measures of sleepiness. They are insensitive at documenting serial changes with, for instance, drug treatment, and may not give an accurate representation of the degree of sleepiness in daily life, let alone in a sleep laboratory [19].

Multiple sleep latency tests have the advantage that they are quantitative, objective and repeatable tests, but they are difficult to standardize, time consuming and require technical experience and expensive equipment. They need careful interpretation if the subject has not been able to follow the ideal sleep–wake routines before the test or has remained on drugs that may influence the results. Microsleeps are not scored in MSLTs and normal values are hard to establish, particularly because of the changing phases of the circadian rhythm during the test. It is common for REM sleep to appear during the first MSLT when the physiological drive to enter REM sleep is greatest, and for anxiety about the need for the patient to leave hospital at the time of the last test to prevent sleep from being entered.

Maintenance of wakefulness test (MWT)

The MWT is similar to the MSLT except that the subject is asked to sit in a comfortable chair in a quiet darkened room for 20–40 min and to resist falling asleep. It is a measure of the ability to remain awake in a non-stimulating environment and more closely simulates real life situations than the MSLT which measures the ease with which the subject can fall asleep. The onset of sleep is assessed as in the MSLT.

The mean of four MWTs at 2-h intervals is taken as the value of the test. A normal MWT is greater than around 18 min, although precise normal values have not been established [20]. The mean MWT for untreated patients with narcolepsy is around 10 min.

The MWT can detect acute and severe sleep deprivation, but it is as much a test of will power as of sleepiness. Its role in the assessment of excessive daytime sleepiness is unclear, but it may be useful in monitoring changes with, for example, drug treatment [21].

The Osler test is equivalent to the maintenance of wakefulness test, but the end point is a failure to respond to seven successive flashing lights at 3 s intervals, rather than EEG criteria [22].

Evoked potentials

The degree of sleepiness influences the EEG evoked potential that can be detected after various stimuli, particularly auditory [23]. The responses are of lower amplitude and longer latency when the subject is sleepy. This technique has been used mainly in research rather than clinical practice.

References

1 Mykytyn IJ, Sajkov D, Neill AM, McEvoy RD. Portable computerized polysomnography in attended and unattended settings. *Chest* 1999; 115: 114–22.

2 Gennaro L de, Ferrara M. Sleep spindles: an overview. *Sleep Med Rev* 2003; 7(5): 423–40.

3 Amzica F, Steriade M. The functional significance of K-complexes. *Sleep Med Rev* 2002; 6(2): 139–49.

4 Davies RJO, Bennett LS, Stradling JR. What is an arousal and how should it be quantified? *Sleep Med Rev* 1997; 2: 87–95.

5 Rechtschaffen A, Kales A, eds. *A Manual of Standardized Terminology, Techniques and Scoring System for Sleep Stages of Human Subjects.* Los Angeles: Brain Information Service/Brain Research Institute, 1968.

6 McKeown MJ, Humphries C, Achermann P, Borbely AA, Sejnowski TJ. A new method for detecting state changes in the EEG. Exploratory application to sleep data. *J Sleep Res* 1998; 7 (Suppl. 1): 48–56.

7 Porte HS. Slow horizontal eye movement at human sleep onset. *J Sleep Res* 2004; 13: 239–49.

8 Sadeh A, Acebo C. The role of actigraphy in sleep medicine. *Sleep Med Rev* 2002; 6(2): 113–24.

9 Pollak CP, Tryon WW, Nagaraja H, Dzwonczyk R. How accurately does wrist actigraphy identify the states of sleep and wakefulness? *Sleep* 2001; 24(8): 957–65.

10 Greenwald SE. Pulse pressure and arterial elasticity. *QJ Med* 2002; 95: 107–12.

11 Oeverland B, Skatvedt O, Kvaerner KJ, Akre H. Pulse oximetry: sufficient to diagnose severe sleep apnea. *Sleep Med* 2002; 3: 133–8.

12 Maquet P, Phillips C. Functional brain imaging of human sleep. *J Sleep Res* 1998; 7 (Suppl. 1): 42–7.

13 Olson LG, Cole MF, Ambrogetti A. Correlations among Epworth Sleepiness Scale scores, multiple sleep latency tests and psychological symptoms. *J Sleep Res* 1998; 7: 248–53.

14 Hoddes E, Zarcone V, Smythe H, Phillips R, Dement WC. Quantification of sleepiness: a new approach. *Psychophysiology* 1973; 10: 431–6.

15 Johns MW. A new method for measuring daytime sleepiness: the Epworth Sleepiness Scale. *Sleep* 1991; 14(6): 540–5.

16 Chervin RD, Aldrich MS. The Epworth Sleepiness Scale may not reflect objective measures of sleepiness or sleep apnea. *Neurology* 1999; 52: 125–31.

17 Balkin TJ, Bliese PD, Belenky G, Sing H, Thorne DR, Thomas M, Redmond DP, Russo M, Wesensten NJ. Comparative utility of instruments for monitoring sleepiness-related performance decrements in the operational environment. *J Sleep Res* 2004; 13: 219–27.

18 Arand D, Bonnet M, Hurwitz T, Mitler M, Rosa R, Sangal RB. The clinical use of the MSLT and MWT. *Sleep* 2005; 28(1): 123–44.

19 Sangal RB, Thomas L, Mitler MM. Maintenance of Wakefulness Test and Multiple Sleep Latency Test. Measurement of different abilities in patients with sleep disorders. *Chest* 1992; 101: 898–902.

20 Doghramji K, Mitler MM, Sangal RB, Shapiro C, Taylor S, Walsleben J, Belisle C, Erman MK, Hayduk R, Hosn R, O'Malley EB, Sangal JM, Schutte SL, Youakim JM. A normative study of the maintenance of wakefulness test (MWT). *Electroencephalogr Clin Neurophysiol* 1997; 103: 554–62.

21 Poceta JS, Timms RM, Jeong D-U, Ho S-L, Erman MK, Mitler MM. Maintenance of wakefulness test in obstructive sleep apnea syndrome. *Chest* 1992; 101: 893–7.

22 Krieger AC, Ayappa I, Norman RG, Rapoport DM, Walsleben J. Comparison of the maintenance of wakefulness test (MWT) to a modified behavioral test (OSLER) in the evaluation of daytime sleepiness. *J Sleep Res* 2004; 13: 407–11.

23 Bastuji H, Garcia-Larrea L. Evoked potentials as a tool for the investigation of human sleep. *Sleep Med Rev* 1999; 3: 23–45.

4 Drugs and Sleep

Introduction

The main indications for pharmacotherapy in sleep disorders are as follows.

1 To modify circadian rhythms.

2 To promote alertness and wakefulness (e.g. central nervous system (CNS) stimulants). The most frequent use is in excessive daytime sleepiness.

3 To promote and improve the quality of sleep (hypnotics). The most frequent use is in insomnia.

4 To treat the large group of sleep disorders which lead to abnormal experiences, autonomic and immunological activity, and motor activity during sleep, usually by modifying the nature or duration of individual sleep stages.

Two other groups of drugs also have important effects on sleep although these are usually not the primary indication for their prescription.

1 Drugs used to treat psychiatric or neurological disorders. These are used to influence, for instance, mood or thought processes and behaviour (psychotropic drugs), but can have a profound effect on the state of wakefulness and sleep.

2 Drugs used for non-psychiatric or non-neurological disorders. Most of these agents affect sleep and wakefulness by altering neurotransmitter function within the brain.

In this chapter these major groups of drugs will be considered. No distinction is made between drugs that have a licence for medical disorders, 'over the counter' preparations, drugs in commonly used foods and drinks, socially used drugs such as alcohol and nicotine, and illicit (recreational) drugs such as lysergic acid diethylamide. The aims are to:

1 describe the principles of action of each class of drug;

2 give examples of important individual drugs;

3 highlight the advantages and disadvantages of each drug;

4 provide a brief indication of the use of the drugs in sleep disorders.

Details of the use and effectiveness of the drugs in individual sleep disorders are given in later chapters. It is important to emphasize that drug treatment should only be used after the sleep disorder has been assessed and a working diagnosis made, and as part of the total management plan. Insomnia, for instance, may respond to analgesics or antidepressants to relieve pain or depression rather than to a hypnotic to promote sleep.

Circadian rhythm modifiers

Introduction

The range of drugs which can modify circadian rhythms is very limited. Melatonin is the only one that has a significant effect that is sustained. The lack of available drugs is unfortunate since disorders of circadian rhythms are frequent, especially those due to shift work, and effective treatment could have widespread application.

Antidepressants and hypnotics

Lithium and some monoamineoxidase inhibitors delay the sleep phase. Short-acting benzodiazepines can entrain the circadian rhythm, but usually only for a few days. These drugs are rarely prescribed for the primary purpose of altering circadian rhythms.

Melatonin

Melatonin is produced in the pineal gland and its effects are described in Chapter 2. This section is restricted to the administration of exogenous melatonin.

Pharmacology

Melatonin is rapidly absorbed from the gastrointestinal tract and the peak plasma concentration is reached within around 60 min. It has a half-life of 30–45 min. It is lipid soluble and therefore enters most tissues, including the brain. It is inactivated in the liver.

Effects on sleep

Melatonin has two effects on sleep.

Sleep-phase alteration

Endogenous melatonin is secreted in the absence of light exposure and influences the timing of the suprachiasmatic nuclei. Exogenous melatonin has an identical action and acts on the circadian sleep rhythm like an episode of darkness. If it is taken late in the evening it advances the next phase of sleep and of endogenous melatonin secretion. It causes a delay of the next sleep phase if it is taken in the morning since it is superimposed on the endogenous secretion. Exogenous melatonin taken in the middle of the day retains its soporific effect, but has little influence over circadian rhythms or the total sleep time.

Hypnotic effect

Melatonin is a mild hypnotic when given in the day at the time when endogenous melatonin levels are low. This effect is detectable within 1 h of administration, lasts for 1–2 h and is dose related. Melatonin also causes a fall in body temperature. This is usually associated with sleep onset, but its soporific effect is present before any change in body temperature, suggesting that this has a different mechanism.

Other actions and side-effects

Melatonin is a vasoconstrictor, has a slight hypotensive effect, and inhibits reproduction. Daytime sedation is not a problem with melatonin administered in the evening.

Problems with use

Preparations of melatonin

The availability of melatonin varies between countries. It is taken regularly by several million people in the USA where it is classed as a nutritive or dietary supplement. This does not require review of the quality of the preparations by the Food and Drug Administration (FDA) and one study showed that one-third of the brands contained no melatonin and in 75% there was significantly less than advertised. Most melatonin is synthesized, but some is prepared from bovine pineal glands.

Uncertainty about dose

The recommended dose of melatonin ranges from 0.1 mg to 5–10 mg daily [1]. Doses up to 0.5 mg give plasma levels similar to those generated by endogenous secretion and doses of 1–5 mg give blood levels around 10–100 times the physiological values. Only 0.03 mg is normally secreted every 24 h, but these high doses may be needed to elevate cerebrospinal fluid and brain tissue concentrations to physiological levels.

A dose of around 0.5 mg appears to be sufficient to entrain the circadian rhythm when taken on a regular basis, but 5 mg is probably more effective in making acute changes to the sleep phase. This dose may also increase the total sleep time slightly.

Lack of data

There is little data regarding the safety or efficacy either in the short term or with long-term use of melatonin, probably because of its variable status as a drug in different countries.

Drug interactions

There are no known drug interactions with exogenous melatonin, but its effect also depends on the endogenous secretion which can be increased by selective serotonin re-uptake inhibitor antidepressants and antipsychotic drugs and reduced by beta blockers, benzodiazepines, sodium valproate, gabapentin and nonsteroidal anti-inflammatory drugs.

Effects on reproduction

Melatonin is recognized to affect reproduction, inhibiting ovarian function and reducing prolactin and luteinizing hormone levels. The importance of these effects is uncertain, but because of them it should be avoided in children, in women wishing to conceive and whilst breastfeeding.

Effects on inflammation

Melatonin enhances the immune response and although there is little data regarding this it should be avoided in autoimmune diseases which may deteriorate during melatonin treatment.

Indications in sleep disorders

Some of the claims for the efficacy of melatonin have been exaggerated and there have been few controlled studies, particularly of its long-term use. Different doses and timing of administration of melatonin have been used in these reports, and some of the results are conflicting.

It has two main indications as described below.

Chronobiological (chronobiotic) agent

This relies on its ability to reset the sleep phase. Its efficacy depends more on the timing than the size of the dose, although 5 mg is usually recommended initially. A fast release preparation is required to advance the sleep phase and is given 1–2 h before the time of the previous night's onset of sleep. It can be used in the short and long term.

Short term. It accelerates the adaptations of the circadian rhythms to time zone changes causing jet lag. It should be taken in the evening before and after the flight on eastward travel in order to cause a phase advance, and in the morning with westward flights to delay sleep onset. Similar principles underlie its use in shift workers and it may also be useful in re-establishing sleep patterns after withdrawal from drugs, such as alcohol and cocaine.

Long term. Melatonin can promote more regular sleep–wake cycles in those who are blind and experience insomnia or excessive daytime sleepiness due to the failure to entrain their circadian rhythms to environmental light exposure. It can also be used to advance the sleep phase when it is taken in the evening in the delayed sleep-phase syndrome, and to retard sleep when it is taken in the morning in the advanced sleep-phase syndrome. Disorders of the pineal gland, such as pineal tumours, are usually associated with low endogenous melatonin secretion, and melatonin administration may be of benefit, acting as a hormone replacement or supplement treatment.

Hypnotic
Melatonin is a weak hypnotic, but can cause sleepiness during the day. It may have a use in treating the early morning wakening pattern of insomnia when there is a deficient secretion of endogenous melatonin. Sustained release preparations may be effective in the elderly, in whom melatonin levels are often low, and have been proposed for treating early morning wakening in depression.

Melatonin agonists

Several melatonin agonists, such as ramelteon, are being developed, but are not yet available for clinical use. They have the potential advantages over melatonin of higher standards of preparation and of confidence in their purity, that they will have undergone superior safety and efficacy studies, and that their dose ranges would have been better established. Their potential physiological advantages over melatonin may be a longer half-life, and increased bio-availability.

Central nervous system stimulants and wakefulness-promoting drugs

Introduction

The most commonly taken CNS stimulants to combat excessive daytime sleepiness are caffeine and nicotine which are usually self-administered. Of the prescribed drugs, amphetamines, which have been available since around 1930, have been the most widely used. The ideal drug would have a completely selective action on the CNS so that it only increased alertness and reduced sleep. None of the stimulants are this specific [2]. They all influence other aspects of neurological function, particularly the older drugs such as strychnine and ephedrine which are now hardly ever prescribed for excessive daytime sleepiness. Caffeine, the amphetamines and related drugs also have several unwanted effects due to generalized CNS stimulation. Modafinil is more specific in promoting wakefulness.

The use of stimulants is also limited by the risk of drug dependency, withdrawal symptoms, tolerance, side-effects, drug interactions and the dangers of overdose. The risks of each of these unwanted effects vary between the different drugs. The issues that determine the choice of stimulant are discussed in detail in Chapter 6.

Caffeine and other xanthines

Pharmacology
Xanthines are alkaloids and while caffeine (1, 3, 7-trimethylxanthine) is a trimethylxanthine, theophylline and theobromine are dimethylxanthines. They are all well absorbed from the gastro-intestinal tract. The peak blood level of caffeine is reached 30–60 min after ingestion. It has a plasma half-life of 3–4 h although there is considerable inter-individual variability. It is prolonged in pregnancy and with the oral contraceptive pill.

Caffeine crosses the placenta, enters breast milk and readily crosses the blood–brain barrier to reach the CNS. It is metabolized in the liver by the cytochrome P-450 microsomal enzymes and its metabolites are excreted in the urine. One of these, paraxanthine, can be detected in the serum and can be used as marker of caffeine intake.

Dose
The usual dose of caffeine in tablet form is 50–200 mg. Caffeine is a constituent of a wide range of food and drinks, such as tea, coffee, cola and other soft drinks,

Table 4.1 Doses of caffeine in food and drinks.

Food and drink	Quantity	Caffeine (mg)
Tea	1 cup (150 ml)	25–50
Instant coffee	1 cup (150 ml)	60–80
Brewed or percolated coffee	1 cup (150 ml)	100–150
Decaffeinated coffee	1 cup (150 ml)	3
Cocoa	1 cup (150 ml)	15
Cola drink	330 ml	40–60
Plain chocolate	100 g	40
Milk chocolate	100 g	15
White chocolate	100 g	0

drinking chocolate and cocoa, and is also present in many analgesic preparations, appetite suppressants and tonics. The quantity of caffeine in some of these preparations is shown in Table 4.1.

Mechanisms of action

Xanthines competitively inhibit phosphodiesterase which degrades cyclic 3–5 AMP (adenosine monophosphate) and thereby increases its intracellular concentration. They act as antagonists at adenosine receptors widely within the CNS, and thereby stimulate it at all levels. Their effect on wakefulness is mainly via A1 receptors in the basal forebrain. The results of activating A2a receptors in the striatum are opposed by dopamine. In high doses xanthines also stimulate the medullary vagal, vasomotor, and respiratory centres.

Caffeine has a greater effect on the CNS and skeletal muscle than other xanthines, but other drugs in this group such as aminophylline, theophylline and theobromine (which is present in cocoa) have greater effects on other systems.

Effects on sleep

Caffeine and other xanthines reduce the total sleep time, increase the sleep latency, and reduce the duration of stages 3 and 4 NREM sleep and of REM sleep [3]. They cause insomnia, particularly if they are taken in the evening, by the elderly, or if the total daily dose is greater than 500 mg. This may worsen daytime sleepiness so that more caffeine is taken which further worsens the insomnia.

Effects on wakefulness

Caffeine and other xanthines can prolong wakefulness, increase mental activity, improve attention and vigilance and performance of complex logical mental tasks, especially if the subject is fatigued. They do not improve mental function requiring originality, but increase psychomotor coordination, except in high doses, or if they have caused sleep deprivation or anxiety.

Other actions and side-effects

1 Respiratory effects. Theophylline is a respiratory stimulant and bronchodilator.
2 Diuresis. This is due to an increase in the renal blood flow and glomerular filtration rate.
3 Tachycardia, cardiac dysrhythmias and hypertension.
4 Nausea, vomiting, abdominal pain and gastro-oesophageal reflux.
5 Tremor and muscle twitching.

Problems with use

1 Tolerance to CNS effects.
2 Withdrawal symptoms. Withdrawal may cause headaches, irritability, anxiety and dizziness.
3 Drug interactions. Smoking and drugs that induce microsomal enzymes in the liver, such as phenytoin, increase the clearance of caffeine and reduce its half-life.
4 Insomnia.

Indications in sleep disorders

Excessive daytime sleepiness

Caffeine is a moderately effective CNS stimulant which is widely available and is frequently used to relieve excessive daytime sleepiness due to sleep deprivation, irregular sleep–wake patterns, shift work and jet lag, and to prevent and relieve sleepiness during driving. The alerting effect of 500 mg caffeine is approximately equivalent to 5 mg dexamphetamine. It is usually ineffective in excessive daytime sleepiness due to primary neurological disorders, such as narcolepsy and idiopathic hypersomnia.

Central sleep apnoeas and Cheyne–Stokes respiration
Aminophylline 225–450 mg bd is the most effective of the xanthines for these conditions.

Nocturnal asthma
Theophylline or aminophylline, which is metabolized to theophylline, are effective bronchodilators. Sleep fragmentation due to nocturnal asthma is reduced, but the stimulant effect of these drugs may cause insomnia.

Nicotine

Pharmacology
Nicotine is a pyridine alkaloid which is rapidly absorbed when inhaled or chewed. Approximately 1 mg is absorbed from smoking each cigarette. It has a half-life of 1–2 h.

Mechanisms of action
Nicotine acts on nicotinic cholinergic receptors in autonomic ganglia and at the neuromuscular junction as well as within the CNS. In low doses it is excitatory but in higher doses it inhibits these receptors. It also increases central nervous system 5HT and dopamine release, particularly in the striatum and nucleus accumbens.

Its alerting effects are probably due to stimulation of cholinergic neurones in the basal forebrain, but in high doses it can also activate the hypothalamic-pituitary-adrenal axis.

Effects on sleep
There has been surprisingly little research into the effects of nicotine on sleep, but it reduces the total sleep time, increases sleep latency, and reduces sleep efficiency and the duration of REM sleep.

Effects on wakefulness
Nicotine in a low dose leads to mental relaxation, is a mild sedative, and anxiolytic, and promotes sleep, but in higher doses it acts as a stimulant, increasing arousal, and it may cause agitation. It can improve motor performance, but commonly causes muscle tremors and in overdose leads to dizziness, fits and delirium.

Other actions and side-effects
1 Loss of appetite and nausea.
2 Tachycardia.

Problems with use
1 Tolerance.
2 Withdrawal symptoms. Nicotine is addictive and its withdrawal may cause irritability, arousals and insomnia.

Indications in sleep disorders
Smokers commonly have fragmented sleep, possibly due to the stimulant effect of nicotine, or to regular nicotine withdrawal effects each night. Nicotine reduces the total sleep time and is a mild stimulant in higher doses. Nicotine is rarely prescribed for excessive daytime sleepiness, but is usually taken in tobacco or occasionally as a gum or skin patches.

Glucocorticoids
These increase alertness and motor activity in the day and reduce the total sleep time, increase the number of awakenings from sleep, especially NREM sleep, and may slightly reduce the duration of REM sleep and increase the duration of stage 2 NREM sleep. These effects are probably mediated through interactions with cytokines.

Glucocorticoids are rarely specifically prescribed as CNS stimulants. They occasionally cause depression or a steroid psychosis which, when it occurs, is dose related. The insomnia that they cause is usually well tolerated because of the increased alertness and hyperactivity that compensates for it.

Strychnine
Strychnine is an alkaloid extracted from the seeds of *Strychnos nux-vomica*. It was the most commonly prescribed drug in the UK until the early 1920s and was used as a 'tonic' to improve alertness, sensory acuity and wakefulness. It has fallen out of use and is almost never prescribed.

Strychnine abolishes CNS inhibitory postsynaptic potentials due to the release of taurine as a neurotransmitter and thereby reduces inhibition of reflexes. In overdose it causes muscle spasms, fits and death, although these actions can be antagonized by barbiturates. It has a poor toxic to therapeutic ratio and is usually fatal in a dose of 60–90 mg.

Sympathomimetics
These include adrenaline and ephedrine. They reduce the duration of sleep and improve alertness, but also cause tachycardia, hypertension, anxiety and tremor. Ephedrine in a dose of 30–60 mg orally, 2–4 hourly, was used to treat narcolepsy before amphetamines

became available, but it is now rarely prescribed because of its side-effects.

Pemoline

This stimulant is structurally unrelated to amphetamines. It has a long half-life of 9–14 h and its clinical effects last for 8–10 h. Sixty per cent of pemoline is metabolized in the liver and 40% excreted unchanged in the urine. The usual dose is 40–120 mg. It increases mental alertness, has a mild euphoric action and increases motor activity, possibly through its action as a dopamine agonist. It causes relatively little peripheral nervous system stimulation, but can lead to insomnia and is an effective appetite suppressant.

A rise in the liver enzymes is common and acute liver necrosis, which may be fatal, occasionally occurs. This has led to its withdrawal from the UK market, although it is effective in treating mild and moderate daytime sleepiness.

Mazindol

This is an imidazole derivative which differs chemically from the amphetamines. It is readily absorbed, has an onset of action within 30–60 min and its peak effect is at around 2 h. It is excreted in the urine. The usual dose is 2–12 mg daily given either as one or two doses. Two milligrams are equivalent in effectiveness to around 10 mg dexamphetamine.

Its mechanism of action is uncertain, but it may inhibit noradrenaline and dopamine re-uptake, particularly in the limbic system. It has little effect on total sleep time, but reduces REM sleep. It increases alertness and may cause insomnia, but not euphoria. Loss of appetite, nausea, abdominal pain, constipation, hypertension, tremor and urinary retention may occur. Tolerance and abuse are also recognized.

Mazindol is an effective stimulant with an anticataplectic action but its side-effects have limited its use, and it is now hardly available.

Selegiline

This is a selective, irreversible inhibitor of monoamine oxidase type B which is responsible for dopamine catabolism. It therefore increases dopamine levels, particularly in the thalamus and brainstem, but its stimulant action is probably mainly due to its metabolism to levo-amphetamine and levo-metamphetamine. It does not have an antidepressant effect because of its lack of type A action. It has been used as a stimulant and as an anticataplectic in narcolepsy in a dose of 10 mg daily, but may provoke vivid dreams and hallu-

cinations. It should not be used in conjunction with a selective serotonin re-uptake inhibitor antidepressant.

Amantadine

Amantadine acts at dopamine and possibly NMDA synapses. It leads to release of preformed dopamine and inhibition of its re-uptake and therefore resembles amphetamines in its mode of action. The usual dose is 100–400 mg daily. It has been used to improve alertness in neurological disorders, but is only slightly effective. It has also been used to relieve fatigue, for instance in multiple sclerosis and after brain injuries.

Amphetamines and related drugs

Pharmacology

Amphetamines are well absorbed through the gastrointestinal tract. Approximately 50% is hydroxylated in the liver and oxidized to benzoic acid, and 50% excreted in the urine as glucuroxide or glycine conjugates.

Mechanisms of action

All the amphetamines enhance activity at dopamine, noradrenaline and 5HT synapses. They cause presynaptic release of preformed transmitters, and also inhibit the re-uptake of dopamine and noradrenaline. These actions are most prominent in the brainstem ascending reticular activating system and the cerebral cortex. Amphetamines also cause release of noradrenaline from peripheral nerve terminals which leads directly to enhanced sympathetic activity.

The alerting effects of amphetamines are probably due either to noradrenaline or 5HT release or to both of these. Their effects on motor function are probably mainly due to potentiation of dopamine activity in the basal ganglia and limbic cortex, but their action in relieving cataplexy may also be due to their noradrenergic effects (Table 4.2).

Individual drugs

Amphetamines are listed under Schedule 2 of the Misuse of Drugs Act 1971, and prescriptions have to comply with controlled drug requirements. The most important individual drugs are as follows.

Amphetamine
This was the first amphetamine to be used clinically. It is a racemic mixture of dextro- and levo-amphetamines. It has relatively more central than peripheral actions compared to ephedrine, but fewer central and more

Table 4.2 Effects of CNS stimulants on neurotransmitters.

Drug	Noradrenaline	Acetylcholine	5HT	Dopamine	GABA	Adenosine	Cytokines	Taurine
Caffeine	–	–	–	–	–	†	–	–
Nicotine	– –	*low dose †high dose	–	–	–	–	–	–
Glucocorticoids	–	–	–	–	–	–	†	–
Strychnine	–	–	–	–	–	–	–	†
Sympathomimetics	*	–	–	–	–	–	–	–
Pemoline	–	–	–	*	–	–	–	–
Mazindol	*	–	–	*	–	–	–	–
Selegiline	*	–	*	*	–	–	–	–
Amphetamines and related drugs	*	–	*	*	–	–	–	–
Modafinil	–	–	–	–	†	–	–	–

*promotes action of neurotransmitter; † inhibits action of neurotransmitter; 5HT, 5-hydroxytryptamine; GABA, gamma-aminobutyric acid.

peripheral actions than dexamphetamine. It has a half-life of 8–16 h. Dose 5–60 mg daily.

Dexamphetamine

This is the dextro- or d-isomer of amphetamine and is three to four times more potent than levo-amphetamine. The peak blood level is reached around 2 h after ingestion. It has a half-life of 8–12 h and a duration of action of 6–10 h. Dose 5–60 mg daily usually taken in two to three divided doses.

Levo-amphetamine

This has no clinical advantage over dexamphetamine. Dose 20–60 mg daily.

Metamphetamine

This is the most rapidly absorbed and potent amphetamine. Its peak blood level is reached 1 h after ingestion and it has a half-life of 12 h. It is lipophilic and has more peripheral actions than dexamphetamine and is rarely used clinically. It is subject to drug abuse and known as methedrine and speed. Dose 5–15 mg daily.

Phenmetrazine

This drug is now rarely used, but can cause euphoria and psychosis. Dose 25–75 mg in one to three divided doses.

Methylphenidate

This is a piperidine derivative which is structurally similar to amphetamine. It binds to the dopamine transporter, and thereby blocks dopamine re-uptake. It has similar but less marked effects on noradrenaline and 5HT re-uptake [4]. It is rapidly absorbed and is de-esterified to an inactive metabolite, ritalinic acid, in the liver and is then excreted in the urine. Its peak blood level is reached within 1–2 h. It has a plasma half-life of 2–4 h and a clinical effect for 3–6 h. Dose 10–60 mg daily in three to four divided doses.

It acts particularly on the thalamus and cerebral cortex, but causes more sympathetic side-effects than amphetamines. It is used to treat attention deficit hyperactivity disorder as well as excessive daytime sleepiness, particularly when this is due to narcolepsy.

Cocaine

This is very similar structurally and in its mechanisms of action to methylphenidate. It potentiates the effects of noradrenaline and adrenaline. It increases alertness, relieves fatigue, has a euphoric action and increases motor activity. It reduces the total sleep time, increases sleep latency and reduces both stages 3 and 4 NREM and REM sleep.

In overdose it may lead to fits and delirium, and chronic use causes sleep deprivation. Abrupt withdrawal leads to depression and prolonged sleep with REM sleep rebound, especially if it has been used in high dose for a prolonged time. Tolerance frequently develops and chronic use is associated with death from cardiac dysrhythmias, myocardial infarction and strokes.

Ecstasy

This is chemically related to metamphetamine, NMDA and mescaline, a hallucinogen. It is a stimulant, mood

Table 4.3 Effects of CNS stimulants on sleep.

Drug	TST	SL	Awakenings	1 and 2 NREM sleep	3 and 4 NREM sleep	REM sleep latency	REM sleep	Dreams
Caffeine	↓	↑	–	–	↓	–	↓	–
Nicotine	↓	↑	–	–	–	–	↓	↑
Glucocorticoids	↓	–	↑	↑	↓	–	Slightly ↓	–
Mazindol	0	–	–	–	–	–	↓	–
Amphetamines and related drugs	↓	↑	↑	–	Slightly ↓	↑	↓	–
Modafinil	↓	–	–	–	–	–	–	–

NREM, non-rapid eye movement; REM, rapid eye movement; SL, sleep latency; TST, total sleep time.

altering and hallucinogenic drug, which occasionally causes hyperpyrexia. It leads to a reduction in REM sleep and its use may be followed by depression.

Effects on sleep

Amphetamines reduce total sleep time, increase sleep latency, slightly reduce the duration of stages 3 and 4 NREM sleep, increase REM sleep latency and reduce the duration of REM sleep, often to as little as 10%. They cause sleep fragmentation and if taken late in the day cause difficulty in initiating sleep (Table 4.3).

Effects on wakefulness

Amphetamines prolong wakefulness, increase the level of alertness, reduce the sense of fatigue, increase confidence, concentration and loquacity, increase the capacity for physical and mental activity, and lead to euphoria and a sense of excitability. They improve psychomotor and mental performance for simple, but not complex, tasks, particularly when fatigue is present. They can lead to agitation and aggression and to a paranoid psychosis, with auditory hallucinations, which is indistinguishable from schizophrenia. Depression and fatigue often follow the phase of psychic stimulation. The need to sleep usually returns suddenly as the amphetamine blood level is falling, and this 'crash' or rebound sleep is more profound with high doses.

Other actions and side-effects

1 Appetite suppression.
2 Respiratory stimulant.
3 Peripheral sympathetic and motor effects, including a rise in body temperature, tachycardia, palpitations, mild hypertension, nausea, vomiting, abdominal cramps, dry mouth, headaches and tremor. Hypertension may be severe, particularly during exertion, and lead to intracranial haemorrhage. Amphetamines should be avoided in those with hypertension, ischaemic heart disease and cardiac dysrhythmias, but have been used in these situations with beta blockers to minimize the risks of sympathetic side-effects.
4 Growth retardation with prolonged treatment in children.

Problems with use

Short duration of action
Amphetamines give quick relief from sleepiness, but the offset of their action is equally quick and patients frequently find this 'crash' and return of their symptoms unpleasant.

Tolerance
Around 30% of those with narcolepsy become tolerant to amphetamines, especially when doses above 60 mg daily of dexamphetamine are used. 'Drug holidays', which are spells of a few days off amphetamine treatment, have been used to try to minimize tolerance. There is little evidence that they help, and they may cause recurrent episodes of withdrawal symptoms.

Dependency
The euphoria of amphetamines has led to their widespread use and abuse. Withdrawal causes fatigue, depression, hypersomnia, an increase in appetite and occasionally paranoia and agitation. The total sleep time increases, and REM sleep rebound may be present for up to 2 months after cessation of amphetamines.

Drug interactions
Amphetamines are metabolized by hepatic microsomal enzymes and any drug that influences these will alter the rate of their metabolism. Tricyclic and MAOI antidepressants inhibit their metabolism, potentiate

Table 4.4 Precautions with amphetamines.

Patient problems	Drug effects
Addictive personality	Tolerance
Psychiatric disorders	Dependency
Ischaemic heart disease	Overdose
Hypertension	Drug interactions
Children	Psychosis

their effects and require the amphetamine dose to be reduced by around one-third. Beta blocking agents, such as propranolol, and lithium may antagonize the effects of amphetamines.

Overdose
This causes intense sympathetic nervous system stimulation with hypertension, tachycardia, hyperthermia and a toxic psychosis, often with paranoid delusions and violence accompanied by epileptic fits, and occasionally a stroke due to hypertension, particularly during exercise. Amphetamines cross the placenta, reach the fetus and also enter breast milk. They should be discontinued during pregnancy and while breastfeeding.

Indications in sleep disorders
Amphetamines are effective stimulants, but their use is limited by their side-effects, abuse potential, tolerance and withdrawal symptoms (Table 4.4).

Excessive daytime sleepiness
Amphetamines have been used to relieve excessive daytime sleepiness due to unavoidable sleep restriction for social reasons, to increase performance at work and in competitive sport, both in humans and in animals (such as horses and greyhounds), but their medical indications are in treating the following.

Excessive daytime sleepiness due to central nervous system disorders. These include narcolepsy and idiopathic hypersomnia. Amphetamines are effective, but their short action leads to a rapid return of sleepiness. Little benefit is obtained by increasing the dose above 60 mg dexamphetamine daily, and tolerance to amphetamines occurs in around one-third of subjects with narcolepsy. Their use is limited by side-effects, including psychosis and insomnia. There has been less experience of using amphetamines in neurological disorders other than narcolepsy, but they are probably as effective in idiopathic hypersomnia.

Excessive daytime sleepiness due to opiate treatment. Amphetamines may be of value through increasing wakefulness during treatment with opiates without antagonizing their analgesic action.

Cataplexy. Amphetamines have a mild anticataplectic action, possibly due to their noradrenergic effects, which is often useful in treating narcolepsy.

Modafinil

Pharmacology
Modafinil (2-[(diphenylmethyl)sulphinyl]acetamide) is well absorbed from the gastro-intestinal tract. The peak blood level is reached at 2–3 h, although this can be delayed by food. Its half-life is 10–15 h. It is metabolized in the liver to modafinil acid and sulphone, both of which have little activity. Ninety per cent of the drug is excreted through the kidneys in these forms and 10% as unchanged modafinil.

Dose
The initial dose is 100–200 mg daily, often increasing to 400–600 mg daily. It is usually given twice daily with around two-thirds of the total dose on waking and one-third in the middle of the day. The dose should be reduced in the elderly and in the presence of severe renal and hepatic impairment. A lower dose of 100–200 mg daily is usually optimal in treating fatigue rather than sleepiness.

Mechanisms of action
Modafinil is not known to have a direct action on any neurotransmitter system. It does not influence the suprachiasmatic nuclei or melatonin secretion. It does not have any direct effect on hypocretin-containing neurones in the lateral hypothalamus, although their activity increases indirectly as a consequence of the wakefulness induced by modafinil. In vitro in high doses it inhibits the dopamine re-uptake transporter, but this is probably of little clinical significance. Modafinil has a very low affinity for dopamine receptors and does not lead to dopamine release. Its action requires an intact alpha 1 adrenergic system, and there is some evidence that it selectively activates the locus coeruleus, leading to pupillary dilatation but not to other sympathetic effects such as tachycardia or hypertension.

Modafinil increases the activity of histaminergic neurones in the tubero-mammillary nuclei of the posterior hypothalamus, which promote wakefulness.

This is partly through a direct effect but mainly through inhibition of the ventrolateral preoptic (VLPO) area of the anterior hypothalamus which inhibits the tubero-mammillary nuclei. There is some evidence that modafinil inhibits the VLPO by increasing its noradrenergic input, possibly as a result of an increase in locus coeruleus activity [5].

Effects on sleep

Modafinil has little effect on sleep if it is taken in the morning [6], but taken later in the day it can cause insomnia. It has no effect on circadian rhythms, or cortisol or growth hormone secretion [7], but it does abolish the normal fall in core body temperature during sleep.

Effects on wakefulness

Modafinil promotes alertness and wakefulness, but, unlike amphetamines, it does not increase motor activity or have any effects on the sympathetic nervous system. It does not lead to a sleep debt with sleep rebound as occurs with amphetamines. Recovery sleep is, if anything, slightly shortened by modafinil. It does not cause euphoria or any other mood change and is not hallucinogenic.

Other actions and side-effects

1 Headaches, nausea and a dry mouth may occur early in treatment, but are usually transient.
2 Mental hyperactivity, anxiety and nervousness occur with high doses.

Problems with use

Tolerance

This has not been well documented, but may develop in some narcoleptics.

Dependency

Modafinil has little potential for drug dependency since it does not cause any euphoria. Cessation of treatment does not lead to any withdrawal symptoms or sleep rebound.

Drug interactions

Modafinil causes reversible inhibition and induction of some of the cytochrome P-450 enzymes and on theoretical grounds care should be taken if it is administered with anticoagulants and anticonvulsants, such as phenytoin. It may increase the blood level of tricyclic antidepressants such as clomipramine. Modafinil does not interact with amphetamines, but it may cause oral and other steroidal contraceptives to be less effective. Alternative methods of contraception should be employed.

Indications in sleep disorders

Excessive daytime sleepiness

Modafinil is a selective wakefulness promoting drug which appears to be effective in relieving excessive daytime sleepiness whatever its cause (Table 4.5). It is indicated when this persists after sleep hygiene advice and treatment of the cause, and if there has not been any response to first-line stimulant treatments such as caffeine. It is preferable to amphetamines and related drugs, because although they are equally effective, it has a more specific effect on sleep–wake control, fewer side-effects, low potential for dependence, no withdrawal symptoms, few drug interactions and is safer in overdose. Its main indications are as follows.

Neurological disorders. Modafinil has been most widely used in narcolepsy, but it is probably equally effective in idiopathic hypersomnia and excessive

Table 4.5 Comparison of amphetamines and modafinil.

	Amphetamines	Modafinil
Efficacy	+	+
Duration of action	Short	Long
Specificity of action	Low	High
Dependency	Moderate risk	Low risk
Withdrawal symptoms	Common	Absent
Tolerance	30% narcoleptics	Unknown
Side-effects	Multiple, often serious	Few, mild
Contraindications	Multiple	Few
Drug interactions	Occasional	Rare
Effects of overdose	May be fatal	Insomnia

daytime sleepiness due to other conditions such as myotonic dystrophy and Parkinson's disease. It may also be useful in relieving excessive daytime sleepiness due to multiple sclerosis and occasionally in periodic limb movements in sleep. It does not improve cataplexy, which therefore may worsen if patients with narcolepsy are transferred from dexamphetamine to modafinil.

Excessive daytime sleepiness that persists despite optimal treatment of the cause. Modafinil is indicated if excessive daytime sleepiness persists despite optimization of treatment of obstructive sleep apnoeas with nasal continuous positive airway pressure (CPAP).

Drug-induced sleepiness. Modafinil is effective in relieving sleepiness due, for instance, to opiates or atypical antipsychotics.

Depression. Excessive daytime sleepiness may persist in depression despite effective treatment of the mood changes with antidepressants. Modafinil may be of benefit in this situation but the evidence regarding its efficacy is limited.

Chronic shift-work sleep disorder. Modafinil is effective in relieving sleepiness if taken 30–60 min before the start of the night shift, but should only be prescribed if other counter-measures are ineffective.

Severe and unavoidable sleep deprivation. Modafinil has been used by military organizations and others in civilian life to overcome prolonged episodes of sleep deprivation, but it is not a substitute for obtaining sufficient sleep. It improves both subjective and objective alertness, improves simple objective cognitive and performance tests, and it may improve executive function such as planning and critical reasoning.

Fatigue
There is some evidence that modafinil may reduce fatigue rather than excessive daytime sleepiness in certain conditions, such as multiple sclerosis and after brain injuries.

Cognitive enhancer
Modafinil has been proposed as a cognitive enhancer, but it only reverses the transient cognitive defects associated with sleepiness. It has been used by athletes as a performance enhancer, but it probably has little benefit other than to slightly increase their alertness and speed of awareness of their situation.

R-Modafinil
Modafinil is a racemic mixture of l- and r-enantiomers. R-Modafinil contains only the r-enantiomer and has a longer duration of action than modafinil. Its mechanism of action and indications are likely to be similar to those of modafinil although these have not been clearly established.

Hypnotics
Introduction
Synthetic hypnotic drugs were developed in the nineteenth century. Bromides became available in 1857, chloral has been used since 1869 and barbiturates were introduced in 1903. These were largely superseded by the benzodiazepines in around 1960 and, despite doubts about their effectiveness and advisability for long-term use, they have continued to be used in increasing quantities. World-wide sales of hypnotics are increasing by around 8% per year, particularly in the USA and many European countries. Within Europe the sales are least in the UK, Holland and Belgium, and greatest in France, Germany and Italy.

The main use of hypnotics is in the treatment of insomnia [8]. The aim of treatment should not be simply to increase the quality and duration of sleep, but also to improve alertness during wakefulness. The balance between these two effects is difficult to achieve with the currently available hypnotics. The ideal drug would promote sleep but not result in any residual sleepiness during the next day, or cause any other features of CNS depression. None of the available drugs have this combination of actions. Most have other effects such as respiratory depression or a muscle relaxant effect and they usually interact with other hypnotics. The issues that determine the choice of a hypnotic are described in detail in Chapter 7.

Mechanisms of action

GABA receptor modifiers
Most of the well-established hypnotics fall into this group. Gamma aminobutyric acid (GABA) is a widely distributed inhibitory amino acid transmitter which is secreted particularly by interneurones. These hypnotics interact with $GABA_A$ rather than $GABA_B$ receptors (Fig. 4.1). The $GABA_A$ receptor consists of a GABA

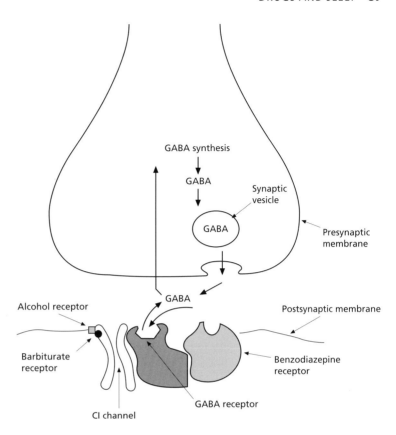

Fig. 4.1 GABA$_A$ receptor and hypnotics. Cl, chloride; GABA, gamma-aminobutyric acid.

binding site on the cell membrane close to the chloride channels which are opened by GABA so that the post-synaptic membrane becomes hyperpolarized. This inhibits the activity of the neurone and reduces its firing frequency.

Benzodiazepines bind to this macromolecular GABA receptor chloride ionophore complex close to the GABA binding site and at a location close to but distinct from the binding site for barbiturates, alcohol, chloral and clomethiazole. Zopiclone, eszoplicone, zolpidem, zaleplon and indiplon all bind to a further receptor site. Binding to each of these three sites promotes the affinity of GABA to the GABA receptor and leads to opening of chloride channels.

The group of hypnotics including barbiturates and alcohol bind directly to the GABA receptor as well as to their own receptor in high concentrations. This reduces their safety when they are taken in overdose or combination.

The only hypnotic which binds solely to the GABA receptor is gaboxadol. It increases the duration of stages 3 and 4 NREM sleep, but has no effect on REM sleep. It does not alter the duration of stage 2 or sleep spindles, but improves sleep maintenance.

GABA re-uptake inhibitors

Tiagabine is an anticonvulsant as well as a hypnotic. It impairs the function of the GABA transporter protein and the re-uptake of GABA. It increases the duration of stages 3 and 4 NREM sleep, but has no effect on stage 2 or sleep spindles.

Other GABA-related mechanisms

Gabapentin increases the GABA content of neurones. Pregabalin has an effect on GABA transmission through its action on voltage-gated calcium channels. Both these drugs increase stages 3 and 4 NREM sleep, they are anticonvulsants and analgesics, and they improve the subjective quality of sleep.

5HT antagonists

5HT2 antagonists such as ritanserin and atypical antipsychotics increase stages 3 and 4 NREM sleep. This is also a feature of noradrenergic and specific serotonergic antidepressants (NaSSAs), such as mirtazapine.

Antihistamines

These antagonize the wakefulness promoting effects of the tubero-mammillary nuclei and increase the total sleep time.

Melatonin

This is a mild hypnotic as well as a circadian rhythm modifier.

Herbal and homeopathic treatments

The mechanisms of action, if any, of most of these preparations are unknown. Valerian acts on GABA receptors, lettuce contains lactucarium, an opiate, and St John's Wort, which is a mild antidepressant and sedative, probably acts through 5HT mechanisms.

Benzodiazepines

Pharmacology

The benzodiazepines contain a benzene ring linked to a seven-member diazepine ring. They are rapidly absorbed from the gastro-intestinal tract, although this is slowed by food and particularly by antacids. Most of the benzodiazepines are lipophilic, cross the blood–brain barrier readily and have a wide distribution within the body. A clinical effect is apparent with most of these drugs within 1 h and the peak plasma level is usually reached between 1 and 3 h after ingestion.

All the benzodiazepines are metabolized by hepatic microsomal enzymes and are conjugated with glucuronic acid to form water-soluble metabolites which are excreted in the urine. Some benzodiazepines such as triazolam and midazolam have few active metabolites, but diazepam, for instance, is metabolized to desmethyldiazepam which is active and has a half-life of 50–100 h. This metabolite is not produced by lorazepam, oxazepam or temazepam. The metabolism of benzodiazepines is slower in the elderly, in whom there is also a greater neurological sensitivity because of the ageing processes within the brain.

Despite these similarities, there are quantitative differences between the individual benzodiazepines which have important implications for the timing and extent of their effects. They only have a hypnotic action if their level in the brain and cerebrospinal fluid is above a threshold which differs for each drug. This threshold may vary according to the balance of the

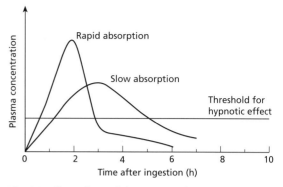

Fig. 4.2 Effects of rate of absorption on hypnotic action.

sleep–wake drives, circadian rhythm and if tolerance to the drugs develops, but it is mainly affected by pharmacokinetic issues. The most important factors are as follows.

Rate of absorption

Rapidly absorbed drugs exceed the hypnotic threshold level quickly and have an early onset of action. Triazolam and diazepam are the most rapidly absorbed and have a quick effect, but oxazepam, which is the most slowly absorbed, has a slower onset of hypnotic effect (Fig. 4.2).

Distribution

The volume of distribution of the benzodiazepines varies considerably. Lipophilic drugs, such as diazepam, cross the blood–brain barrier readily and the brain and plasma concentrations quickly equilibrate. Lipophobic drugs, such as oxazepam, lorazepam and clonazepam, have a smaller volume of distribution. The rate of equilibriation and volume of distribution are important in determining the effects of a single dose. Drugs that cross the blood–brain barrier have a quick onset of action, but if they also have a large volume of distribution they are removed from the receptors in the brain rapidly and the brain and blood levels soon fall below the threshold for the hypnotic effect so that the duration of action is short (Fig. 4.3).

Elimination

This comprises both metabolism and excretion of the drug. Drugs that are rapidly eliminated reach a low blood level before the next dose is administered, and this prevents them accumulating. A steady state blood level is reached after four to five times the half-life of the drug and if this is sufficiently long for it to fail to be eliminated before the next dose is given there will be a

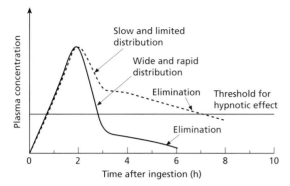

Fig. 4.3 Effects of distribution on hypnotic action.

gradual increase in the blood level with a risk of sedation during the daytime (Fig. 4.4).

Mechanisms of action

The benzodiazepines do not have any direct action on neurological function, but enhance the effects of GABA. Benzodiazepines interact especially with $GABA_A$ rather than $GABA_B$ receptors. They bind to the macromolecular GABA receptor complex close to the GABA binding site and increase its affinity for GABA (Fig. 4.1). This leads to opening of the chloride channels and hyperpolarization of the post-synaptic membrane with inhibition of neuronal activity. Subtypes of the benzodiazepine receptors (e.g. BZ1, omega-1; BZ2, omega-2) have been identified but their significance is uncertain. BZ1 receptors may mediate sedation and BZ2 cognition, memory and psychomotor function. They also increase the affinity of the barbiturate and alcohol receptors for these compounds, and potentiate the effects of these drugs.

The action of benzodiazepines on the GABA receptor complex is most marked in the hypothalamus, thalamus and limbic system, and the inhibition of these regions underlies the sedative and hypnotic effects of the benzodiazepines as well as their anxiolytic, muscle relaxant, and antiepileptic actions.

Individual drugs

Details of the individual benzodiazepines are given in Table 4.6. The drugs are distinguished particularly by their speed of onset, potency, extent of distribution in the body, elimination half-life and ability to accumulate in the body, particularly in the brain. The availability of benzodiazepines varies considerably between different countries. Triazolam, for instance, was withdrawn from use in 1991 in the UK because of its pronounced rebound insomnia and anterograde amnesia, but is still available in the USA. Flunitrazepam has been removed from the list of prescribable drugs under the National Health Service in the UK, but is available in other countries.

Effects on sleep

Benzodiazepines in low dose have a sedative effect and in higher dose induce sleep, and may even lead to coma. They reduce the spontaneous activity and response to afferent stimuli of the ascending reticular activating system and block the electroencephalogram responses that are evoked by its stimulation. The EEG during wakefulness shows a reduction and slowing of the alpha-rhythm with an increase in the beta-rhythm, particularly in the frontal cortex.

Benzodiazepines increase total sleep time, shorten sleep latency, reduce the number of awakenings and provide a sense of deep and refreshing sleep. REM sleep latency is prolonged, and the duration of REM sleep is reduced. There are fewer eye movements and less dreaming during REM sleep, except with

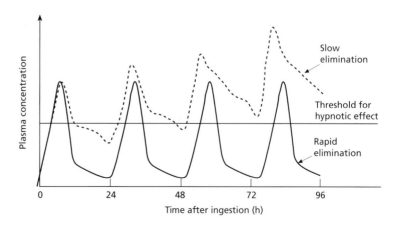

Fig. 4.4 Effects of rate of elimination on hypnotic action.

Table 4.6 Individual benzodiazepines.

Drug	Dose	Effect of single dose on sleep	Effect of regular dose in daytime	Uses
Triazolam	0.125–25 mg	Short acting	Nil	Brief daytime and nocturnal sleep, DIS
Midazolam	7.5–15 mg	Short acting	Nil	DIS
Flunitrazepam	0.5–1 mg	Short acting	Mild sedation	DIS
Diazepam	2.5–10 mg	Short acting	Sedation	Transient DIS, DMS and EMW with anxiety
Temazepam	10–20 mg	Intermediate	Mild sedation	DIS, DMS
Lormetazepam	0.5–1 mg	Intermediate	Nil	DIS, DMS
Oxazepam	15–30 mg	Intermediate	Nil	DMS, EMW with anxiety
Flurazepam	15 mg	Moderately long	Mild sedation	DMS, EMW
Nitrazepam	5–10 mg	Moderately long	Sedation	DMS, EMW with anxiety
Clorazepate	7.5–15 mg	Long acting	Sedation	DMS, EMW with anxiety
Clonazepam	0.5–1 mg	Long acting	Sedation	DMS, EMW with anxiety

DIS, difficulty in initiating sleep; DMS, difficulty in maintaining sleep; EMW, early morning awakening.

Table 4.7 Effects of hypnotics on sleep.

	TST	Sleep latency	1 and 2 NREM sleep	3 and 4 NREM sleep	REM sleep latency	REM sleep
Most GABA receptor-acting drugs	↑	↓	↑	↓	↑	↓
5HT agonists	↑	↓	?↑	↑	Little effect	Little effect
Melatonin	No effect	↓	↑ during day	No effect	No effect	No effect

NREM, non-rapid eye movement; REM, rapid eye movement; TST, total sleep time.

short-acting drugs, such as triazolam, which cause a rebound in REM sleep late in the night. Sleep is consolidated in that there are fewer sleep-stage transitions, but the duration of stages 3 and 4 NREM sleep is reduced in parallel with that of REM sleep. The duration of stage 2 NREM sleep increases. The clinical significance of these changes in sleep architecture is uncertain (Table 4.7).

Withdrawal of benzodiazepines leads to REM sleep rebound, which may be associated with vivid dreams and nightmares for several weeks.

Effects on wakefulness

Daytime sedation is most pronounced with benzodiazepines with a long duration of action, such as flurazepam, particularly if the drugs are given for prolonged periods and in high dose. A steady state blood level is reached at four to five times the half-life, which implies that if the drug has a 72 h half-life it may take up to 15 days before a steady state is reached.

Elimination of the drugs is slowed in the elderly, who are also more predisposed to sedation. The degree of sedation during the day also depends on the balance between the improvement in sleep quality and the 'hangover' effect of persisting sedation. Tolerance to the sedative effect often develops.

The sedative effect of benzodiazepines impairs motor skills, attention, memory and judgement, and if severe may lead to confusion and incoordination. The risk of accidents, including road traffic accidents, is increased, particularly in those who take alcohol as well. Accidents, such as falls, may also occur during the night if the subject becomes confused and leaves the bed.

Other actions and side-effects

The benzodiazepines have little effect on the autonomic nervous system, but can cause the following.
1 Anxiolysis. This is seen with lower doses than are required to induce sedation or sleep and is common

with long-acting hypnotics taken at night. Their anxiolytic effect probably has a similar underlying mechanism to the hypnotic effect. Oxazepam has relatively more anxiolytic and less hypnotic effect than other benzodiazepines.

2 Muscle relaxation.

3 Amnesia. Transient global anterograde amnesia is independent of the level of sedation and is probably mediated by a different mechanism from the hypnotic action of these drugs. It is particularly marked with short-acting drugs such as triazolam and flunitrazepam.

4 Anticonvulsant effect.

5 Depression is common but occasionally disinhibition occurs.

6 Respiratory failure and obstructive sleep apnoeas may be precipitated in susceptible patients, particularly with high doses of benzodiazepines. This complication can be reversed by the specific benzodiazepine antagonist, flumazenil.

Problems with use

Tolerance
This is common and often develops within a few weeks, but occurs to a lesser extent than with barbiturates. The loss of efficacy may require an increase in the dose.

Withdrawal symptoms
Cessation of benzodiazepines may lead to a recurrence of the original symptoms, or even to a transient worsening, or rebound of these. A specific withdrawal syndrome may also appear and is characterized by disturbed sleep, vivid dreams and nightmares, associated with an increase in REM sleep and in stages 3 and 4 NREM sleep. Autonomic effects such as excessive sweating, tachycardia and hypertension, and psychosis, delirium and fits may occasionally be induced.

These problems are most common if the benzodiazepine has been used in high dose, is of high potency and has been used for a long duration. They are often sufficiently intense to lead the subject to return to regular benzodiazepine usage despite the intention to discontinue treatment. They can be minimized by using the lowest effective dose of benzodiazepine, avoiding long-term treatment if possible and gradually withdrawing treatment rather than suddenly stopping it.

This type of physical 'dependency' is distinct from drug addiction in which the subject loses control over the use of the drug, has a compulsive need for it and develops maladaptive drug-seeking behaviour. This type of drug addiction is uncommon, but high dose benzodiazepines, especially temazepam, are taken for their euphoriant effect, with the risk of a fatal overdose.

Interaction with other drugs
The sedative and hypnotic effects of benzodiazepines are accentuated if other drugs acting on the $GABA_A$ receptor, especially barbiturates and alcohol, are taken as well. Each drug increases the affinity of the receptor for the others so that the risk of overdose is greatly increased by combined treatment.

Phenobarbital (phenobarbitone) and spironolactone increase the metabolism of benzodiazepines and reduce their effect, but there is no interaction with oral anticoagulants.

Rebound insomnia
This may occur either during each night of treatment with benzodiazepines or during withdrawal of regular treatment as described above. Rebound insomnia during treatment is associated with short-acting drugs which do not accumulate in the body. The initial hypnotic effect wears off so that towards the end of the night rebound of REM sleep occurs with vivid dreams and frequent awakenings.

Pregnancy
Benzodiazepines cross the placenta and also enter breast milk. It is advisable to avoid benzodiazepines in pregnancy and to discontinue breastfeeding if a benzodiazepine has to be administered.

Indications in sleep disorders

Insomnia
Benzodiazepines are often considered as first-line hypnotic treatment for insomnia, but are similar in many ways to newer drugs such as zopiclone, zolpidem and zaleplon which are preferable in certain circumstances. The advantages of benzodiazepines over older hypnotic drugs are:

1 greater sedation : anxiolysis ratio;

2 less tendency to tolerance and dependency, particularly compared to barbiturates;

3 less abuse potential;

4 safer in overdose, especially compared to barbiturates;

5 fewer drug interactions since they do not induce hepatic microsomal enzyme production.

Despite these advantages, tolerance and dependency do occur and benzodiazepines should be used in courses of less than four weeks whenever possible. Their indications for insomnia are as follows.

Transient insomnia. Drugs such as diazepam or temazepam may be needed for 2–7 days to consolidate the sleep pattern. They may also be used to relieve jet lag and short-acting drugs may be helpful in rotating shift work.

Chronic insomnia. Their use should be limited to one month or less if possible, and towards the end of the course they should be taken on alternate nights so that their withdrawal is gradual. Occasionally patients require long-term treatment, although tolerance to their effects may reduce their efficacy and psychomotor performance and mood changes may develop.

The hypnotic effect is only required intermittently and it is important that the blood and cerebrospinal fluid level falls below the threshold for the hypnotic effect during the daytime, both with single and repeated doses. The exception is if anxiety as well as insomnia requires treatment, in which case symptoms may be helped by a long-acting preparation which retains significant blood levels during the day. In general, short-acting drugs tend to cause more amnesia, rebound insomnia and tolerance than longer-acting preparations, but avoid the difficulties of drug accumulation and daytime sedation.

Details of the choice of benzodiazepine are given in Chapter 7, but in general these drugs should be avoided wherever possible in the elderly. Short-acting drugs should be advised if the patient works with dangerous machinery, has to drive a motor vehicle or needs to be particularly alert at work. Benzodiazepines should be avoided wherever possible in children, in the presence of respiratory impairment, a predisposition to obstructive sleep apnoeas, or liver disease, or if there is a history of drug abuse.

Motor abnormalities in sleep
Benzodiazepines are effective in treating many of the behavioural abnormalities associated with an increase in motor activity during sleep. These include PLMS, REM sleep behaviour disorder, sleep walking and sleep terrors, although benzodiazepines should be avoided in children whenever possible. Their efficacy is partly due to their muscle relaxant activity and also because they suppress stages 3 and 4 NREM sleep which is when many of these disorders arise. Clonazepam appears to be particularly effective.

Epilepsy in sleep
Benzodiazepines, such as clonazepam, have a place in treating nocturnal epilepsy.

Zopiclone

Pharmacology
Zopiclone is a cyclopyrrolone and has a different structure from the benzodiazepines. The peak plasma level is reached within 2 h. It has a short half-life of 4–6 h and a duration of action of 6–8 h. It is metabolized in the liver and excreted in the urine. The usual dose is 7.5–15 mg nocte, but this should be reduced to 3.75 mg in the elderly and in those with significant liver disease.

Mechanisms of action
Zopiclone binds to the $GABA_A$ receptor complex, but at a different site to benzodiazepines.

Effects on sleep
Zopiclone is as effective a hypnotic as the benzodiazepines, but has different effects on sleep architecture. It does not influence REM sleep, but reduces the duration of stage 1 NREM sleep and the number of arousals, and does not significantly alter the duration of stages 3 and 4 NREM sleep.

Other actions and side-effects
Zopiclone is short-acting, but can cause daytime sedation, particularly at high dose. It has similar anxiolytic, muscle relaxant and anticonvulsant actions to the benzodiazepines. It often causes a metallic or bitter taste in the mouth but does not increase the frequency of obstructive sleep apnoeas.

Problems with use

Tolerance
This is probably less than with the benzodiazepines.

Withdrawal symptoms
These may be less than with the benzodiazepines.

Interaction with other drugs
There is said to be less interaction with alcohol and other sedatives than with the benzodiazepines.

Indications in sleep disorders

Insomnia
Zopiclone is similar in its effects to a short-acting benzodiazepine although it does have different consequences for sleep architecture. It should be used for up to one month for insomnia, particularly if this is transient and if there is difficulty in initiating sleep.

To assist with withdrawal from benzodiazepines
Rebound insomnia and other withdrawal symptoms can be reduced by substituting zopiclone.

Eszopiclone
This is a cyclopyrrolone which rapidly induces sleep. It is the l-enantiomer of zopiclone and, unlike the r-enantiomer, it is the active form. The usual dose is 1–3 mg nocte. It has a short duration of action and rarely causes early morning drowsiness. It does not cause any REM sleep rebound, and withdrawal symptoms and tolerance have not been reported.

It is suitable for treating difficulty in initiating sleep, especially when it is important to avoid daytime sedation, for instance in the elderly.

Zolpidem

Pharmacology
Zolpidem is an imidazopyridine derivative which is chemically unrelated to the benzodiazepines. It is rapidly absorbed, and has a half-life of only 1.5–2.5 h in healthy adults, although this is longer in the elderly and in the presence of liver disease. Its onset of action is detectable within 15–30 min, the peak plasma level is reached within 1–2 h of ingestion and its clinical effect lasts 5–7 h. It is metabolized in the liver. The usual dose is 5–10 mg nocte in adults or 5 mg in the elderly.

Mechanisms of action
Zolpidem acts at the $GABA_A$ receptor complex close to but at a different site from the benzodiazepines. Its specificity for the BZ1 receptor may explain its slightly different actions compared to the benzodiazepines which act at both BZ1 and BZ2 receptors.

Effects on sleep
Zolpidem probably has little effect on sleep architecture, in contrast to the benzodiazepines. Its short duration of action occasionally leads to rebound insomnia later in the night.

Other actions and side-effects
Zolpidem is not an anxiolytic, muscle relaxant or anticonvulsant, probably because of its different site of action to the benzodiazepines.

It rarely causes daytime sedation because of its short duration of action, but can lead to nausea, vomiting, diarrhoea, headaches and dizziness.

Problems with use
1 Tolerance. This is said to be less than with the benzodiazepines.
2 Withdrawal symptoms. These are unusual.
3 Mild respiratory depression which may induce obstructive sleep apnoeas.

Indications in sleep disorders
Zolpidem is as effective as a hypnotic as the benzodiazepines and its indications are similar to this group of drugs. It has less effect on sleep architecture, but the clinical value of this is uncertain. Its short duration of action makes it suitable for treating difficulty in initiating sleep in the elderly and in other situations where it is important to avoid daytime sedation.

Zaleplon

Pharmacology
Zaleplon is a pyrazolopyrimidine compound which is rapidly absorbed. Its peak plasma level is reached 1 h after ingestion and its half-life is half an hour. It has a short duration of action, less than 5 h. It is metabolized in the liver, mainly to inactive compounds, but a small amount of desmethylzaleplon, which has a hypnotic effect, is produced. There is some renal excretion. The usual dose is 5–10 mg.

Mechanism of action
Zaleplon binds to BZ1 (omega-1) receptors, in a similar manner to zolpidem.

Effects on sleep
Zaleplon has a dose-related effect in reducing sleep latency, but because of its short duration of action it does not increase the total sleep time. In high doses (40–60 mg) it may reduce the duration of REM sleep. Rebound insomnia later in the night is uncommon.

Other actions and side-effects
Zaleplon is an anxiolytic with muscle relaxant and anticonvulsant actions. It occasionally causes

headaches and dizziness, and may lead to respiratory depression.

It rarely causes daytime sedation because of its short duration of action, and psychomotor impairment is unusual.

Problems with use

1 Tolerance. The risk of this appears to be low.
2 Withdrawal symptoms. These are probably rare.
3 Dependency. This is unlikely.

Indications in sleep disorders

Zaleplon is a very short-acting hypnotic whose main indications are in treating difficulty in initiating sleep and in promoting naps at times of heightened circadian alertness, for instance in night shift workers who wish to sleep during the day. It may also be of use in difficulty in maintaining sleep when there is a limited time left before the desired awakening time in the morning.

Indiplon

This is chemically similar to zaleplon and acts at the same receptor site. It is rapidly absorbed, with a peak plasma concentration at 0.75–1.5 h after ingestion and a half-life of 1.5–2 h. It is metabolized to inactive compounds and only 2% is excreted unchanged in the urine and faeces.

Indiplon reduces the sleep latency and is suitable for the difficulty in initiating sleep type of insomnia. It can also be taken during the night to relieve difficulty in maintaining sleep, as long as this is more than 5 h before driving a motor vehicle. There is no evidence for tolerance or withdrawal symptoms. The usual dose is 10–20 mg.

Barbiturates

Pharmacology

The barbiturates are substituted pyrimidine derivatives with a basic barbituric acid structure. They are well absorbed as sodium salts and have an onset of action of 10–60 min. Their lipid solubility varies and determines how readily they cross the blood–brain barrier. They have a long duration of action, usually 6–8 h, particularly in the elderly and in the presence of liver disease. They are metabolized by hepatic microsomal enzymes and lead to induction of these enzymes which is the basis of the tolerance that develops to them. They are conjugated with glucuronic acid and are excreted in the urine mainly in this form, although some are excreted unchanged.

Mechanisms of action

Barbiturates act on the $GABA_A$ receptor complex at a site close to but different from the benzodiazepines. They have a widespread action within the CNS, but particularly in the midbrain reticular formation, and cause generalized CNS depression.

Individual drugs

Amobarbital (amylobarbitone): dose 60–200 mg nocte.

Butobarbital (butobarbitone): dose 100–200 mg nocte.

Secobarbital (quinalbarbitone): dose 50–100 mg nocte.

Effects on sleep

Barbiturates may cause sedation, sleep, anaesthesia, and even death according to the dose, age, individual susceptibility and interaction with other drugs. They have a similar effect on sleep to the benzodiazepines in that they reduce the sleep latency and the duration of REM sleep, and REM sleep latency increases. The duration of stage 2 NREM sleep is increased, but stages 3 and 4 NREM sleep become shorter and the number of arousals is reduced. Withdrawal of barbiturates after prolonged use leads to REM sleep rebound with nightmares and rebound insomnia.

Other actions and side-effects

1 Daytime sedation. This is common because of the long duration of action. Barbiturates reduce psychomotor skills and may cause mood changes.
2 Anxiolytic.
3 Muscle relaxant.
4 Anticonvulsant.
5 Nausea, vomiting and diarrhoea.
6 Respiratory depression. This is dose dependent and is usually fatal at around 10 times the hypnotic dose [9].

Problems with use

Tolerance
This develops within 2 weeks of treatment because of induction of hepatic microsomal enzymes.

Withdrawal symptoms
These, and addiction to barbiturates, are more frequently a problem than with benzodiazepines. Withdrawal of barbiturates leads to REM sleep rebound and rebound insomnia.

Drug interactions

The metabolism of barbiturates by microsomal enzymes in the liver underlies most of the drug interactions. The rate of metabolism of warfarin, phenytoin, tricyclic antidepressants and the oral contraceptive pill is increased, and conversely MAOIs inhibit these enzymes and reduce the rate of barbiturate metabolism.

Pregnancy

Barbiturates cross the placenta to reach the fetus and a small quantity enters breast milk. They should be avoided in pregnancy.

Overdose

The barbiturates have a lower toxic : therapeutic ratio than benzodiazepines and much more frequently cause death when an overdose is taken.

Indications in sleep disorders

Insomnia

Barbiturates are rarely used nowadays because of their disadvantages relative to the benzodiazepines and related drugs. Their only place is for short-term treatment if benzodiazepines and other modern hypnotics cannot be tolerated or are ineffective, as well as in those patients who have been taking barbiturates regularly for many years without any side-effects. When barbiturate treatment is initiated it should be restricted to 2 weeks because of the risk of tolerance and dependence developing.

Chloral and related drugs

Pharmacology

Chloral is rapidly absorbed and its hypnotic effect is detectable within 30 min. It is widely distributed within the body and has a half-life of 6–8 h. It is metabolized to trichloroethanol by alcohol dehydrogenase, especially in the liver, and this is then conjugated with glucuronic acid and largely excreted in the urine. Trichloroethanol is the active agent of chloral and related drugs and is responsible for their hypnotic effect.

Mechanisms of action

These drugs bind to the $GABA_A$ receptor complex.

Individual drugs

Chloral hydrate: dose 0.5–2 g in adults; 0.03–0.05 g/kg to a maximum of 1 g in children.

Triclofos sodium: dose 1–2 g nocte.
Dichloralphenazone: dose 0.65–1.3 g nocte.

Effects on sleep

These are similar to those of benzodiazepines and barbiturates.

Other actions and side-effects

Daytime sedation is uncommon because of their short duration of action. These drugs have few cardiovascular or respiratory effects except in overdose. They may cause nausea and vomiting.

Problems with use

1 Tolerance.
2 Withdrawal symptoms.
3 Chloral should be avoided in hepatic and renal failure.
4 Drug interactions. Chloral potentiates the effects of alcohol, barbiturates and other sedatives. Alcohol dehydrogenase is responsible for the metabolism of both chloral and alcohol, and chloral acts as a competitive inhibitor increasing the effects of alcohol.

Indications in sleep disorders

Chloral is a mild hypnotic and is an alternative to benzodiazepines, particularly in the elderly.

Clomethiazole (chlormethiazole)

Pharmacology

Clomethiazole is rapidly absorbed from the gastrointestinal tract and its peak plasma level is reached within 15–90 min. It has a brief duration of action and is rapidly metabolized in the liver. Dose: 192–384 mg nocte.

Mechanisms of action

It acts at the GABA receptor complex close to the benzodiazepine receptor site.

Effects on sleep

Its hypnotic effect is dose related.

Other actions and side-effects

1 Daytime sedation is rarely a problem because of its short duration of action.
2 Anticonvulsant.
3 Sneezing and conjunctival irritation.
4 Nausea and vomiting.

Problems with use
Withdrawal symptoms.

Indications in sleep disorders
Clomethiazole is a useful hypnotic in the elderly because of its short duration of action. It should be reserved for transient insomnia because of the risk of dependence, but it is also of value in alcohol and narcotic withdrawal.

Paraldehyde

Pharmacology
This drug is slowly absorbed orally, but is widely distributed and readily crosses the blood–brain barrier. Its half-life is 4–10 h. Eighty per cent is metabolized in the liver to acetaldehyde and then acetic acid, but the remainder is excreted as paraldehyde through the lungs and has a characteristic odour. Dose: 5–10 ml orally, rectally or intramuscularly.

Mechanisms of action
Its hypnotic effect is thought to be due to inhibition of the ascending reticular activating system in the brainstem. It probably acts on the GABA receptor complex.

Effects on sleep
Its effects on sleep are similar to those of the benzodiazepines.

Other actions and side-effects
1 Anticonvulsant.
2 Gastric irritation.
3 Hepatitis.
4 Nephrotic syndrome.

Problems with use

Drug interactions
Its sedative and hypnotic actions are additive to those of other sedative drugs such as alcohol and barbiturates.

Indications in sleep disorders
Paraldehyde is very rarely used in sleep disorders, but is occasionally indicated in status epilepticus and has been used in acute agitation and alcohol withdrawal.

Alcohol

Pharmacology
Ethyl alcohol (ethanol) is rapidly absorbed through the mouth, stomach and small intestine, although this is delayed by food, especially fatty food. It is oxidized in the liver to acetaldehyde and then to acetic acid and to carbon dioxide and water. It is also excreted in the urine and to a lesser extent through the lungs.

Mechanisms of action
Alcohol acts on the GABA receptor complex in a similar way to the benzodiazepines, but at a slightly different site. It also acts as a glutamate inhibitor. It influences particularly the ascending reticular activating system and causes generalized CNS depression.

Effects on sleep

Acute effects
Alcohol is an anxiolytic and a weak hypnotic. It increases the total sleep time, reduces sleep latency, reduces the latency before stages 3 and 4 NREM sleep and increases their duration as well as suppressing REM sleep. It is short-acting so that as the blood alcohol level falls during the night REM sleep rebound occurs, often with vivid dreams, loss of NREM sleep and frequent awakenings. After a large intake of alcohol these withdrawal features are seen on the next night. High doses may also reduce the duration of stages 3 and 4 NREM sleep and its diuretic effect causes awakenings from sleep. It also induces obstructive sleep apnoeas which lead to sleep fragmentation.

Chronic effects
Chronic alcohol ingestion disrupts the sleep–wake cycle, possibly through disturbing the pattern of melatonin secretion. Alcohol is often taken initially in order to promote sleep, but tolerance to its hypnotic effect leads to the quantity being increased and often other hypnotics are taken as well. The pharmacological effects of alcohol are combined with episodes of partial withdrawal and dehydration which lead to difficulty in maintaining sleep. Waking with dreams and headaches is common, especially in older subjects in whom the homeostatic drive to sleep is weaker. The sleep architecture disintegrates with the duration of both stages 3 and 4 NREM and REM sleep being reduced and low-amplitude K-complexes. Frequent sleep stage shifts and arousals lead to both insomnia

and excessive daytime sleepiness. Periodic limb movements in sleep are common.

Effects on wakefulness

Sedation is common if alcohol is taken during the daytime or in large quantity at night. This is partly due to its sedative action and partly to the sleep disruption described above. It impairs judgement, attention and concentration.

Other actions and side-effects

1 Anxiolytic.
2 Diuretic. Its diuretic action is through inhibition of antidiuretic hormone (ADH).
3 Respiratory depression. Alcohol precipitates obstructive sleep apnoeas by reducing respiratory drive and upper airway muscle tone, increasing nasal congestion, and it also reduces the threshold for arousal during apnoeas.
4 Drug interactions. Alcohol potentiates the sedative effect of other hypnotics such as benzodiazepines and barbiturates.
5 Restless legs syndrome and periodic limb movements in sleep. The effect of alcohol has not been studied in detail, but while the sedative effect of acute alcohol intake may prevent arousals from periodic limb movements, chronic alcohol ingestion appears to worsen this condition. This may be due to nutritional deficiencies, particularly iron, or to the development of an alcoholic peripheral neuropathy, or to more direct effects of alcohol on the neurological systems responsible for leg movements during sleep.
6 NREM sleep motor abnormalities. These disorders, including sleep walking, are commonly triggered by acute alcohol consumption, probably because of enhancement of stages 3 and 4 NREM sleep or because of an abnormality in the mode of arousal from them.

Problems with use

Tolerance

This is due to both enzyme induction in the liver and CNS adaptation to its hypnotic effects.

Withdrawal symptoms

Acute withdrawal of alcohol after long-term consumption causes REM sleep rebound with a short REM sleep latency, a reduction in stages 3 and 4 NREM sleep, and sleep fragmentation with an increase in the number of sleep stage shifts and awakenings. Sympathetic hyperactivity underlies the tachycardia, sweating and headaches, and an increase in muscle tone is common. Dreams may be vivid and frightening, and in severe cases merge into delirium tremens. This probably represents intrusion of vivid REM sleep imagery into an alert, but agitated state. Visual hallucinations and paranoid delusions are common. They usually appear around 48 h after withdrawal of alcohol which is at the time that REM sleep rebound would be expected to be most prominent. They may lead to alcohol being restarted, but if abstinence can be maintained for around 2 weeks these symptoms gradually improve.

The sleep pattern may remain abnormal with frequent awakenings for up to 2 years. The total sleep time and duration of stages 3 and 4 NREM sleep are reduced and there are frequent awakenings. The severity of the insomnia is related to the risk of relapsing from abstinence, possibly because taking alcohol again initially improves sleep quality, although this effect is only brief, and possibly also because insomnia exaggerates the mood swings and defects in performance during the period of abstinence.

Indications in sleep disorders

Insomnia

Alcohol is commonly taken to treat difficulty in initiating sleep either on a regular basis or to cope with transient insomnia due to special circumstances such as changes in shift work schedules. It has the disadvantage of causing rebound insomnia later in the night, in doses that are sufficient to induce sleep, and can lead to considerable sleep disruption with long-term use.

Tryptophan

L-tryptophan is an essential amino acid which is present in many proteins and particularly in dairy products such as milk and cheese, and in meat, eggs, bananas and nuts. It is metabolized to 5-hydroxytryptophan and then to 5HT which is thought to mediate its mild hypnotic effect.

It has been taken as a food supplement in a dose of 1–2 g three times daily, but in 1989 was recognized to be associated with the eosinophilia–myalgia syndrome which included fatigue and inflammatory changes in the heart, lungs and liver. It was withdrawn from production in 1991 because of this, but subsequent investigation indicated that this syndrome was probably due to a contaminant rather than to tryptophan itself. A limited licence was reinstated in the UK in 1994. 5-hydroxytryptophan is also available.

Tryptophan is readily absorbed through the gastro-intestinal tract. It crosses the blood–brain barrier and is metabolized in the liver. It can cause nausea, vomiting, headaches and Parkinsonism. It reduces sleep latency, increases the total sleep time, prolongs stages 3 and 4 NREM sleep, but has little effect on REM sleep.

It is a weak antidepressant as well as a mild hypnotic, but should not be taken with an SSRI, since this combination may lead to the 'serotonin syndrome' of confusion, agitation, sweating, tachycardia and a fluctuating blood pressure. This syndrome may also develop with other drugs that increase 5HT availability within the CNS, such as lithium, L-dopa and dopamine agonists, lysergic acid diethylamide (LSD) and ecstasy.

Indole-3-pyruvic acid is similar to tryptophan but may increase the duration of REM sleep as well as acting as a mild hypnotic.

Valerian

Valerian is present in many herbal remedies, and is derived from a dried extract of the rhizome, root, and stolon of *Valeriana officinalis*. The active agents have not been precisely identified, but may include valepotriates, volatile oils such as valerenic acid and other compounds. They probably act on $GABA_A$ receptors in the CNS.

The content and purity of the preparations of valerian vary, but a dose of around 150–500 mg of valerian extract or 1–2 g dried root 30–60 min before the desired onset of sleep is usually taken. Valerian has a mild hypnotic action. It particularly reduces the sleep latency, but may also prolong the total sleep time and reduce the frequency of awakenings. It may be useful in treating difficulty in initiating sleep, and it also has a muscle relaxant effect.

Its long-term safety is uncertain and it has been recognized to be cardiotoxic and can lead to liver damage, probably due to a drug-induced hepatitis. It may also have cytotoxic effects since valepotriates act as alkylating agents in vitro and possibly in vivo.

Herbal preparations

A large number of other herbal remedies have been proposed, particularly extracts of hops (*Humulus lupulus*), passion flower (*Passiflora*), lavender oil (*Lavandula*), lobelia, dogwood, lemon balm (*Melissa officinalis*) and lettuce. There is little evidence regarding the effectiveness or safety of any of these preparations, except that lavender oil may increase the duration of NREM sleep.

Sodium oxybate (gamma hydroxybutyrate, GHB)

This is a Schedule 3 controlled drug under the Misuse of Drugs Act 1971, and prescriptions have to comply with controlled drug requirements.

Pharmacology

Sodium oxybate is a 4 carbon fatty acid. It is the sodium salt of gamma hydroxybutyrate, a naturally occurring compound, which is a metabolite of GABA. Its absorption is rapid, although slightly delayed by food. The peak plasma concentration is attained around 1 h after ingestion, and its half-life is around 45 min. It has extensive first pass metabolism and is eventually metabolized to carbon dioxide and water. Around 5% is excreted unchanged in the urine.

Dose

The dose of sodium oxybate is 3–9 gm, usually prescribed in two equal doses of 1.5–4.5 gm, with the first taken shortly before sleep onset, and the second $2^{1}/_{2}$–4 h later.

Mechanisms of action

The mechanism of action is uncertain. Although it has a short half-life, its effects are prolonged and unrelated to the plasma concentration. Sodium oxybate influences lipid breakdown and the pentosephosphate shunt. These metabolic actions may underlie its combination of effects on sleep and wakefulness.

Sodium oxybate has some affinity for $GABA_B$ receptors, but probably acts mainly through GHB receptors or changes in GHB metabolism to reduce dopamine release.

Effects on sleep

Sodium oxybate is a potent hypnotic which may lead to difficulty in arousing the subject from sleep. It has little effect on sleep latency, but increases the total sleep time. It shortens the REM sleep latency and may reduce the duration of REM sleep. It causes a dose-related increase in NREM sleep, particularly stages 3 and 4. The increase in delta-wave activity is probably due to changes in thalamic or thalamocortical functioning.

Effects on wakefulness

Sodium oxybate may cause short-lived drowsiness on waking in the morning. Work with moving machinery should be avoided for 6 hours after the last dose.

Other actions and side-effects

1 Nausea, abdominal pain, headaches and dizziness are occasional side-effects.
2 Nocturnal confusion and sleep walking.
3 Nocturnal enuresis. This is probably due to the increased arousal threshold, which leads to micturition before wakefulness is restored.
4 Increase in growth hormone, cortisol and prolactin secretion. The increase in growth hormone and prolactin may be related to the increase in stages 3 and 4 NREM sleep.
5 Gradual weight loss.

Problems with use

1 Tolerance. This has not been reported.
2 Dependency. There is little evidence for dependency, although it can lead to euphoria. Cessation of sodium oxybate does not lead to any rebound or withdrawal symptoms.
3 Illicit use. Sodium oxybate has been used illicitly in low doses to induce a sense of euphoria and relaxation, and in high doses as a body building drug, in view of its effect on growth hormone, and as a date rape drug, because of its quick-acting and profound hypnotic effect.
4 Overdose. This causes epileptic seizures, respiratory depression and coma, but sodium oxybate does not exacerbate obstructive sleep apnoeas at therapeutic doses.
5 Pregnancy. There are no data regarding the safety of sodium oxybate in pregnancy. It should be avoided at this time and during breastfeeding.

Drug interactions

Sodium oxybate does not interact with narcotics, tricyclic antidepressants or modafinil, but its hypnotic effect is potentiated by alcohol and benzodiazepines, which should be avoided.

Indications in sleep disorders

Narcolepsy

Sodium oxybate has the unusual combination of properties in narcolepsy of consolidating nocturnal sleep, improving daytime alertness and relieving cataplexy. These effects are dose related and increase gradually over several weeks. There is no rebound worsening of cataplexy after discontinuing sodium oxybate, although it gradually deteriorates over a few days to its original level of severity. The increased alertness during the day may be related to the pro-longation of stages 3 and 4 NREM sleep at night. Its effectiveness in cataplexy may be the result of its ability to cause sustained muscle atonia during sleep. It may also relieve sleep paralysis and hypnagogic hallucinations.

Other uses

Sodium oxybate may have a role in idiopathic hypersomnia, REM sleep behaviour disorder and in reducing pain in fibromyalgia, but there is little evidence regarding these possible indications.

Antidepressants

Mechanisms of action

The biochemical basis of depression is thought to be related to over-activity of CNS cholinergic systems relative to that of the monoaminergic systems. Most antidepressants tend to restore the balance of these two in various ways. They probably act mainly in the pontine reticular formation, hypothalamus, thalamus, limbic system and neocortex and thereby regulate the level of arousal and sensory processing as well as mood.

Monamineoxidase inhibitors (MAOIs), e.g. phenelzine, tranylcypromine

These increase noradrenaline and 5HT activity within the CNS by blocking the activity of monoamine oxidase which normally metabolizes these amines to inactive compounds. These are non-selective drugs with both type A (noradrenaline and 5HT metabolizing) and type B (dopamine metabolizing) actions.

Tricyclic antidepressants (TCAs), e.g. amitriptyline, clomipramine, imipramine, protriptyline

These block the presynaptic re-uptake of noradrenaline and 5HT and also have antihistaminic and anticholinergic effects.

Selective serotonin re-uptake inhibitors (SSRIs), e.g. fluoxetine, paroxetine, sertraline, citalopram, escitalopram

These are more selective in that they reduce 5HT re-uptake, but do not affect noradrenaline.

Serotonin and noradrenaline re-uptake inhibitors (SNRIs), e.g. venlafaxine, milnacipran, viloxazine, sibutramine

These have the theoretical advantage over the SSRIs of increasing activity of both 5HT and noradrenaline.

Sibutramine is also a mild dopamine re-uptake inhibitor. It is usually prescribed as a weight reduction agent because of its effect in promoting satiety and reducing food intake. It was originally developed as an antidepressant and also has an anticataplectic action in narcolepsy.

Noradrenergic and specific serotonergic antidepressants (NaSSAs), e.g. mirtazapine, trazodone

These antagonize alpha 2 autoreceptors and thereby increase the activity of both noradrenaline and 5HT, particularly at the 5HT1 receptor.

Mirtazapine is a 5HT2 and 5HT3 antagonist as well as enhancing 5HT1 actions. It also reacts with H1 receptors. It increases the duration of stages 3 and 4 NREM sleep [10] and may lead to weight gain and daytime sedation.

Trazodone is a 5HT2 antagonist which increases sleep efficiency, reduces time awake, shortens sleep latency, and increases the duration of stages 3 and 4 NREM sleep, but has little effect on REM sleep latency or duration.

Noradrenaline re-uptake inhibitors (NARIs), e.g. reboxetine

These selectively inhibit noradrenaline re-uptake without affecting 5HT or dopamine re-uptake.

Reboxetine's effects on sleep are probably mediated by its action on the locus coeruleus. It may cause insomnia and increase interest, motivation and social function, especially if there is initial psychomotor retardation. It also relieves sleepiness and cataplexy in narcolepsy.

Reversible inhibitors of monoamines (RMAIs), e.g. moclobemide

These newer types of monoamineoxidase inhibitors are more selective and reversible, and enable tyramine to be metabolized.

Moclobemide is a selective reversible type A inhibitor which does not precipitate epileptic seizures. It increases the duration of REM sleep but has no effect on stages 3 and 4 NREM sleep.

Noradrenergic and dopaminergic enhancers, e.g. bupropion

These increase the activity of both these monoamines, but have little effect on 5HT or cholinergic activity.

Bupropion is chemically similar to diethylpropion. Its peak plasma concentration is reached in 3 h and its half-life is 21 h. It is metabolized in the liver. The usual dose is 150–300 mg daily, but there is a dose-related risk of epilepsy and it interacts with antipsychotics, beta blockers and flecainide.

It leads to insomnia and increased alertness during the day as well as acting as an antidepressant. It is indicated in depression and addictive behaviours, such as nicotine addiction, but it may also control cataplexy in narcolepsy. It is the only antidepressant that does not worsen the restless legs syndrome, periodic limb movements in sleep or the REM sleep behaviour disorder, probably because of its dopaminergic action.

Effects on sleep

Almost all the antidepressants increase the REM sleep latency and reduce the duration of REM sleep as well as increasing the duration of stages 3 and 4 NREM sleep [11]. The effects on REM sleep are seen after the first dose of tricyclic and SSRI drugs, but are often delayed with MAOIs. The action is most marked with clomipramine, a 5HT re-uptake inhibitor, and is less so with trimipramine, and tolerance develops with desipramine.

Moclobemide increases the duration of REM sleep without any effect on stages 3 and 4 NREM sleep, bupropion has no effect on REM sleep duration, and while mirtazapine has no effect on REM sleep, it increases the duration of stages 3 and 4 NREM sleep. All the sedating antidepressants also reduce the frequency of arousals and awakenings from sleep in depression, and thereby improve sleep efficiency.

Withdrawal of antidepressant treatment usually causes REM sleep rebound which may be prolonged and leads to frightening dreams and insomnia.

Other relevant actions

Daytime sedation

Many of the antidepressants are sedative and this effect often parallels the anticholinergic properties of the drugs which are most marked with trimipramine and amitriptyline, absent with protriptyline and nortriptyline, and rarely a problem with SSRIs which may increase alertness and even cause agitation. Sedating tricyclic antidepressants should be taken in the evening while SSRIs can be taken in the morning.

Upper airway muscle activity

SSRI antidepressants may reduce the degree of loss of tone in upper airway dilator muscles in NREM sleep and thereby reduce the frequency of obstructive sleep apnoeas. This effect may be due to their action on 5HT release in the dorsal raphe nuclei.

Indications in sleep disorders

1 Insomnia associated with depression.
2 Nightmares. The effectiveness of antidepressants is dependent on their REM suppressing action. Clomipramine is probably the most effective.
3 Cataplexy. The anticataplectic effect of some antidepressants may be mediated by their 5HT promoting action more than their noradrenergic and anticholinergic effects. Tricyclic antidepressants, particularly clomipramine, imipramine and protriptyline, are effective. Although SSRIs may be slightly less effective, they have fewer side-effects. SNRIs, such as venlafaxine and viloxazine, and NARIs, such as reboxetine, are probably as effective as the SSRIs. Bupropion may also be useful in controlling cataplexy.
4 Obstructive sleep apnoeas, snoring and other motor disorders occurring in REM sleep.

Lithium

Lithium increases the synthesis and concentration of 5HT and reduces noradrenaline and dopamine activity. It competes with mono- and di-valent cations to affect the postsynaptic receptor protein sites and to alter sodium and potassium channel function.

It does not alter the total sleep time but reduces the number of arousals, increases the duration of stages 3 and 4 NREM sleep, increases REM sleep latency and reduces the duration of REM sleep. It also has a small, but consistent, effect in delaying circadian rhythms. It interacts with hypnotics, such as alcohol, to cause sedation and confusion.

The main indication for lithium is to stabilize the mood in bipolar (manic-depressive) disorders and in mania.

Antipsychotics (neuroleptics)

Mechanisms of action

The older antipsychotics are dopamine receptor antagonists. Their antipsychotic action is related to D2 and D3 receptors, but most are also D1 antagonists. They inhibit the arousal systems in the brain, including the ascending reticular activating system, limbic system and cerebral cortex. Many also have anticholinergic, antihistaminic, anti-alpha 1 adrenergic and anti-5HT actions. The atypical antipsychotics have an antagonist action particularly on 5HT2 receptors.

Individual drugs

These are of three main types.
1 Phenothiazines including piperazines (e.g. trifluoperazine and perphenazine), alkylamines (e.g. chlorpromazine) and piperidines (e.g. thioridazine).
2 Butyrophenones (e.g. haloperidol).
3 Atypical antipsychotics (e.g. clozapine, risperidone, olanzapine, quetiapine).

Effects on sleep

The phenothiazines and butyrophenones vary considerably in their effects on sleep. In general the total sleep time increases, there is a reduction in sleep latency, a slight increase in the duration of stages 2, 3 and 4 NREM sleep and usually, but not invariably, an increase in the duration of REM sleep. Withdrawal shortens the total sleep time and the duration of REM sleep.

The atypical antipsychotics, especially olanzapine, increase the duration of stages 3 and 4 NREM sleep.

Other relevant actions

1 Daytime sedation. This is a problem with many of these drugs but is less prominent with the butyrophenones. Daytime sleepiness is more common with clozapine and olanzapine than with risperidone.
2 Anxiolytic.
3 Mild antidepressant action.
4 Drug interactions. These drugs potentiate the effects of alcohol, hypnotics, narcotics and antihistamines.
5 Movement disorders. These are mainly extrapyramidal and include akinesia, tardive dyskinesia and akathisia which is an unpleasant need to move the limbs associated with anxiety and agitation and which may be confused with the restless legs syndrome.

Anticonvulsants

Mechanisms of action

The anticonvulsant drugs have several mechanisms of action. These include:
1 Blockage of voltage-dependent excitatory sodium channels, e.g. phenytoin, carbamazepine, sodium valproate, lamotrigine.
2 Modulation of calcium channels, e.g. gabapentin, lamotrigine, pregabalin.
3 Glutamate receptor blockers, e.g. topiramate.
4 Potentiation of GABA inhibition, e.g. benzodiazepines, barbiturates, gabapentin, tiagabine, vigabatrin.
5 Closure of potassium channels, e.g. levetiracetam.

Table 4.8 Effects of psychotropic drugs on sleep.

Drug	TST	SL	Arousals	1 and 2 NREM sleep	3 and 4 NREM sleep	REM sleep latency	REM sleep
Antipsychotics	↑	↓	–	–	Slight ↑	–	Variable
Antidepressants	–	–	↓	–	↑	↑	↓
Lithium	–	–	↓	–	↑	↑	↓
Anticonvulsants							
Sodium valproate	↑	↓	–	–	Slight ↑	–	–
Phenytoin	–	↓	–	–	Transient ↑	–	↓
Carbamazepine	–	–	↓	↑	↑	↑	↓

NREM, non-rapid eye movement; REM, rapid eye movement; SL, sleep latency; TST, total sleep time.

6 Modulation of monoaminergic transmission, e.g. sodium valproate, gabapentin.

Individual drugs

These are a heterogeneous group which includes benzodiazepines (e.g. clonazepam), barbiturates (e.g. primidone), phenytoin, sodium valproate, carbamazepine, vigabatrin, lamotrigine, gabapentin, tiagabine and levetiracetam.

Effects on sleep

Anticonvulsants have two major effects on sleep. First they tend to normalize sleep by suppressing epileptic seizures and interictal epileptic discharges which are often associated with microarousals. Carbamazepine is the only commonly used drug that does not reduce interictal discharges. These actions reduce the time awake after sleep onset and increase the duration of REM sleep, particularly in temporal lobe epilepsy in which REM sleep is most fragmented.

The second effect on sleep is through their direct pharmacological actions (Table 4.8).
1 Benzodiazepines and barbiturates (pages 88, 94).
2 Sodium valproate. This increases total sleep time, reduces sleep latency and reduces the number of sleep stage shifts, and may increase the duration of stages 3 and 4 NREM sleep slightly.
3 Phenytoin. This reduces sleep latency, reduces the duration of REM sleep and causes a transient increase in the duration of stages 3 and 4 NREM sleep.
4 Carbamazepine. This reduces the frequency of arousals, reduces the duration of REM sleep, increases REM sleep latency, and increases the duration of stages 3 and 4 NREM sleep.

5 Gabapentin. This increases sleep efficiency and increases the duration of stages 3 and 4 NREM sleep and REM sleep.
6 Tiagabine. This increases sleep efficiency, reduces time awake after sleep onset, increases the duration of stages 3 and 4 NREM sleep and reduces the duration of REM sleep.
7 Lamotrigine. This reduces the frequency of sleep stage shifts, reduces the duration of stages 3 and 4 NREM sleep, and increases the duration of REM sleep.

Other relevant actions

Most of these drugs cause sedation, especially when used in combination, except for lamotrigine and vigabatrin. The sedative effect of carbamazepine is usually transient and can be minimized by slowly increasing the dose.

Indications in sleep disorders

1 Nocturnal epilepsy.
2 Restless legs syndrome and periodic limb movements in sleep. These respond particularly to gabapentin and occasionally to other anticonvulsants such as carbamazepine, sodium valproate and lamotrigine.
3 REM sleep behaviour disorder. Carbamazepine and possibly gabapentin are occasionally of value.

Other drugs influencing neurotransmitters

Introduction

An increasingly wide range of compounds are now recognized to act as neurotransmitters, cotransmitters or sleep factors, and to influence sleep and wakefulness.

Table 4.9 Drugs that influence NREM sleep.

	Promoter	Suppressant
Stages 1 & 2 NREM sleep	Glucocorticoids (slight) Hypnotics Carbamazepine (stage 1) Baclofen	Zopiclone (stage 1)
Stages 3 & 4 NREM sleep	Tryptophan Antipsychotics (slight) Sodium oxybate Gaboxadol Antidepressants Lithium Phenytoin (transient) Carbamazepine Gabapentin Tiagabine Atypical antipsychotics Clonidine Cyproheptadine Cimetidine Cannabis	Caffeine and other xanthines Amphetamines and related drugs Hypnotics Methyldopa Opiates Aspirin

In this section the effects of agonist and antagonist drugs on the main groups of these chemicals are considered (Tables 4.9, 4.10).

Amines

Noradrenergic and adrenergic drugs and blockers

Alpha agonists

Clonidine is a central alpha 2 agonist as well as an H1 antagonist and an anticholinergic drug. It inhibits the locus coeruleus and causes sedation, increases the total sleep time, increases REM sleep latency, reduces the duration of REM sleep, causes vivid dreams and prolongs stages 3 and 4 NREM sleep.

Methyldopa is also a sedative leading to lethargy, drowsiness and fatigue. It increases REM sleep and reduces the duration of stages 3 and 4 NREM sleep and predisposes to nightmares.

Alpha blockers

These include prazosin which is short-acting and lipid soluble and indoramin, both of which can cause daytime sedation, and thymoxamine which increases REM sleep.

Beta agonists

Isoprenaline stimulates both beta-1 and beta-2 receptors, dobutamine is a selective beta-1 stimulant and salbutamol a selective beta-2 stimulant. There has been little study of their effects on sleep, but, in general, their actions are potentiated by xanthines and amphetamines.

Beta blockers

These drugs increase REM sleep latency, reduce the duration of REM sleep, increase the number of arousals from REM sleep and of nightmares, and cause visual hallucinations. They also suppress melatonin secretion and cause fatigue, at least partly through peripheral effects on skeletal muscle. The lipophilic drugs such as propranolol, metoprolol, labetalol and pindolol have more effects on sleep than lipophobic drugs such as sotalol and atenolol. Withdrawal of beta blockers leads to an increase in REM sleep and nightmares.

Cholinergic drugs and antagonists

Acetylcholine is a neurotransmitter which has muscarinic effects at postganglionic parasympathetic synapses and nicotinic effects in the CNS and at preganglionic synapses. It promotes REM sleep and wakefulness.

Table 4.10 Drugs that influence REM sleep.

	Promoter	Suppressant
REM sleep	Antipsychotics	Caffeine and other xanthines
	Methyldopa	Glucocorticoids (slight)
	Thymoxamine	Mazindol
	Muscarinic agonists, e.g. pilocarpine	Amphetamines and related drugs
	Anticholinesterases, e.g. neostigmine	Hypnotics
	LSD	Antidepressants
	Reserpine	Lithium
	Baclofen	Phenytoin (slight)
	Withdrawal of:	Carbamazepine
	Amphetamines and related drugs	Clonidine
	Hypnotics	Beta blockers
	Alcohol	Beta blockers
	Antidepressants	Opiates
	Beta blockers	Cannabis
	Opiates	Withdrawal of antipsychotics
	Cannabis	

LSD, lysergic acid diethylamide.

1 Muscarinic agonists (e.g. carbachol and pilocarpine). These increase the duration of REM sleep.

2 Nicotinic agonists (e.g. nicotine page 80).

3 Anti-muscarinic agents (e.g. atropine and hyoscine). Both these drugs are CNS stimulants. They delay the onset of REM sleep, and may lead to agitation and excitement and reduce the motor inhibition during REM sleep.

4 Nicotinic antagonists (e.g. succinylcholine, atracurium and tubocurarine).

5 Anticholinesterases (e.g. pyridostigmine and neostigmine). These inhibit the enzymes responsible for the metabolism of acetylcholine and thereby prolong its neurotransmitter action. They reduce REM sleep latency, increase REM sleep duration, are associated with dreams and nightmares and increase the number of arousals from sleep.

6 Cholinesterase inhibitors (e.g. donepezil, galantamine, rivastigmine). These increase the duration of REM sleep both in normal subjects and those with dementia. They are used to improve cognitive function in dementia, but frequently cause insomnia and intense dreams. Galantamine leads to less insomnia than donepezil, which is also associated with hallucinations and agitation. Memantine is an NMDA receptor antagonist and has similar effects.

5HT and anti-5HT drugs

The release of 5HT in the CNS has a complex effect on sleep. Its action can be increased slightly by oral administration of L-tryptophan which is its precursor. 5HT release is increased by amphetamines and its action is also enhanced by most antidepressants which reduce its re-uptake and alter the characteristics of its receptors.

Buspirone is a 5HT receptor agonist which is anxiolytic, but has little sedative or respiratory depressant action.

Cyproheptadine is a 5HT antagonist which increases stages 3 and 4 NREM sleep.

Lysergic acid diethylamide (LSD) is a 5HT2 antagonist and a dopamine (D1 and D2) agonist. It increases the duration of the early REM sleep episodes and interrupts stages 3 and 4 NREM sleep with short bursts of REM sleep. These are associated with frequent body movements and arousals from sleep. Use of LSD may lead to an agitated psychosis with severe sleep disruption which can last for several days.

Atypical antipsychotic drugs are 5HT2 antagonists. They increase the duration of stages 3 and 4 NREM sleep. Ritanserin has a similar mechanism of action and similar effects on sleep.

Dopamine agonists and antagonists

Dopamine release in the CNS promotes alertness.

Dopamine agonists

L-dopa is a precursor of dopamine and synthetic

dopamine receptor agonists include bromocriptine, ropinirole, pergolide, cabergoline and pramipexole. These are primarily D2 receptor agonists, whereas apomorphine is a D1 receptor agonist. Amphetamines, bupropion and amantadine also cause release of preformed dopamine and impair its re-uptake and are therefore indirectly acting dopamine agonists.

Dopamine receptor agonists are rapidly absorbed, and metabolized by the cytochrome P450 enzymes. They cause nausea, which can be relieved by domperidone which does not cross the blood–brain barrier, dizziness and postural hypotension. These side-effects are dose related and are less common if the dose is increased gradually. Dopamine receptor agonists also lead to vivid dreams, nightmares, hallucinations, hyperexcitability, confusion and delusions. Sudden sleep attacks have been reported [12] in patients treated for Parkinson's disease. The tetracyclic ergot derivatives, such as bromocriptine, pergolide, cabergoline and lisuride, can cause serosal inflammation with pleuropulmonary fibrosis, retroperitoneal fibrosis, cardiac valve fibrosis and pericarditis. Ankle oedema, Raynaud's phenomenon and nasal congestion may also occur.

Dopamine antagonists
These include antipsychotics and reserpine which reduces dopamine storage, increases REM sleep, and causes nightmares. Domperidone is a D2 blocker which does not cross the blood–brain barrier and causes little daytime sedation.

Histaminergic drugs and antagonists
H1, H2 and H3 receptors are present within the CNS and their stimulation has a role in arousal from sleep, in increasing vigilance while awake and in inhibiting both NREM and REM sleep.

The earlier H1 antihistaminic drugs (e.g. trimeprazine, promethazine, chlorpheniramine and diphenhydramine) also had antinoradrenaline, anti-5HT and anticholinergic activity. The latter caused their sedative and hypnotic effects, with an increase in stages 3 and 4 NREM sleep. They have been widely used as hypnotics, particularly in children, but have a prolonged action and cause daytime sedation, psychomotor impairment and anticholinergic side-effects. Tolerance develops rapidly and they should not be used continuously for more than 2 weeks.

More selective and less hypnotic antihistamines have now been developed. These include the H1 antagonists cetirizine and terfenadine which do not cross the blood–brain barrier and are non-sedating.

The H2 antagonist cimetidine increases the duration of stages 3 and 4 NREM sleep, but ranitidine has no effect on sleep.

Amino acids

Gamma aminobutyric acid agonists and antagonists
Gamma aminobutyric acid (GABA) is a widespread inhibitory neurotransmitter. Its action is potentiated by many hypnotic drugs and some anticonvulsants which act at the $GABA_A$ receptor. Baclofen is a $GABA_B$ agonist. It increases the total sleep time and the duration of stages 1 and 2 NREM sleep and REM sleep, but does not alter stages 3 and 4 NREM sleep.

The effects of GABA are antagonized by tetanus toxin.

Peptides
Administration of peptide hormones and their analogues can influence sleep and it is likely that more drugs of this type which interact with sleep-controlling peptides will be developed.

Opiates
Most of the older opiates act on all three types of CNS opioid receptor (mu, delta and kappa). Their sedative effect is mainly due to kappa and to a lesser extent mu activity. Opioids reduce total sleep time, increase sleep latency, increase the number of arousals and lead to sleep fragmentation, reduce the duration of REM sleep, and increase stage 2, but decrease stages 3 and 4, NREM sleep. The sleep disturbance is about twice as great with diamorphine as with morphine.

Withdrawal of opioid drugs causes rebound insomnia, rebound increase in REM sleep and, to a lesser extent, a rebound increase in stages 3 and 4 NREM sleep for up to several days.

Opioids lead to a relaxed wakefulness, reducing anxiety and distress. They impair cognitive and psychomotor performance, and in overdose they lead to sedation, respiratory depression, coma and death. Their main use in sleep disorders is in the treatment of the restless legs syndrome and periodic limb movements in sleep.

Cannabinoids
The active component of cannabis preparations is delta-9-tetrahydrocannabinol (THC) [13]. Marijuana is made from the flowering top and leaves of *Cannabis sativa*, and hashish, which is more concentrated, is derived from a dried exudate from the flowers. Around

50% of THC is absorbed into the blood when cannabis is smoked and a subjective effect is detectable within 10 min but disappears after around 2–4 h. Delta-9-tetrahydrocannabinol is metabolized in the liver.

It acts at two types of specific G protein receptor. CB1 is widely distributed within the CNS, and is found especially in immune cells derived from the brain. CB1 is antagonized by an endogenous compound, anandamide, whose metabolism is blocked by interleukin-1. There is also interaction with opiate, GABA, dopamine, glutamate and 5HT systems.

The duration of REM sleep is reduced by THC, which is a sedative, and it disproportionately reduces the number of rapid eye movements. It slightly increases the duration of stages 3 and 4 NREM sleep, but these effects become less marked with long-term THC use. Withdrawal leads to REM sleep rebound and a reduction in REM latency, as well as anxiety and anorexia.

Delta-9-tetrahydrocannabinol causes euphoria and is a mild anxiolytic which may help to induce sleep. In low doses it improves memory, but in higher doses psychomotor and cognitive skills and reaction times are impaired. It is frequently abused and dependency is common. Its effects are potentiated by alcohol and chronic use leads to increased duration of sleep and lassitude.

Anti-inflammatory drugs

Aspirin

Aspirin (acetyl salicylic acid) inhibits prostaglandin synthesis and release and, probably through this mechanism, reduces the duration of stages 3 and 4 NREM sleep.

Montelukast

This leukotriene receptor antagonist leads to insomnia, presumably by opposing the NREM sleep promoting effect of cytokines.

References

1 Zhdanova IV, Lynch HJ, Wurtman RJ. Melatonin. A sleep-promoting hormone. *Sleep* 1997; 20: 899–907.

2 Boutrel B, Koob GF. What keeps us awake: the neuropharmacology of stimulants and wakefulness-promoting medications. *Sleep* 2004; 27(6): 1181–94.

3 Roehrs T, Merlotti L, Halpin D, Rosenthal L, Roth T. Effects of theophylline on nocturnal sleep and daytime sleepiness/alertness. *Chest* 1995; 108: 382–7.

4 Challman TD, Lipsky JJ. Methylphenidate: its pharmacology and uses. *May Clin Proc* 2000; 75: 711–21.

5 Gallopin T, Luppi P-H, Rambert FA, Frydman A, Fort P. Effect of the wake-promoting agent modafinil on sleep-promoting neurons from the ventrolateral preoptic nucleus: an in vitro pharmacologic study. *Sleep* 2004; 27(1): 19–25.

6 Buguet A, Montmayeur A, Pigeau R, Naithoh P. Modafinil, d-amphetamine and placebo during 64 hours of sustained mental work. II. Effects on two nights of recovery sleep. *J Sleep Res*, 1995; 4: 229–41.

7 Brun J, Chamba G, Khalfallah Y *et al*. Effect of modafinil on plasma melatonin, cortisol and growth hormone rhythms, rectal temperature and performance in healthy subjects during a 36 h sleep deprivation. *J Sleep Res* 1998; 7: 105–14.

8 Gillin JC. The long and the short of sleeping pills. *N Engl J Med* 1991; 324: 1735–6.

9 Launois S, Similowski T, Fleury B *et al*. The transition between apnoea and spontaneous ventilation in patients with coma due to voluntary intoxication with barbiturates and carbamates. *Eur Respir J* 1990; 1: 573–8.

10 Aslan S, Isik E, Cosar B. The effects of mirtazapine on sleep: a placebo controlled, double-blind study in young healthy volunteers. *Sleep* 2002; 25(6): 677–9.

11 Sharpley AL, Cowen PJ. Effect of pharmacologic treatments on the sleep of depressed patients. *Biol Psychiatry* 1995; 37: 85–98.

12 Homann CN, Wenzel K, Suppan K, Ivanic G, Kriechbaum N, Crevenna R, Ott E. Sleep attacks in patients taking dopamine agonists: review. *BMJ* 2002; 324: 1483–7.

13 Hall W, Solowij N. Adverse effects of cannabis. *Lancet* 1998; 352: 1611–16.

5 Circadian Rhythm Disorders

Introduction

The endogenous circadian rhythm has a cycle of around 24.2 h, but its fine tuning to the environment is achieved through the influence of external time givers of which the most important is light (Fig. 5.1). The fluctuations in the circadian sleep rhythm alter the threshold of the homeostatic and adaptive drives to initiate sleep. Disturbances in circadian sleep rhythms can therefore cause either insomnia or excessive daytime sleepiness, or both.

The sleep, temperature and hormonal circadian rhythms are usually synchronized and are synergistic in promoting sleep and wakefulness at different points in each circadian cycle. This synchrony can break down in certain situations because each rhythm adapts to changes in external factors at different rates and to different degrees. The circadian sleep rhythm could, for instance, be promoting sleep at a time when the temperature is rising instead of falling as is usual late in the evening, and when catabolic rather than anabolic hormones are being secreted. The conflicting effects of this 'internal desynchronization' disturb sleep and reduce the level of alertness during wakefulness.

Assessment

History

The clinical diagnosis of a circadian rhythm disorder is often difficult because there are no specific features. The main symptoms are insomnia and excessive sleepiness, and the clue to an underlying circadian rhythm disorder is that these symptoms have a distinct pattern, as described below.

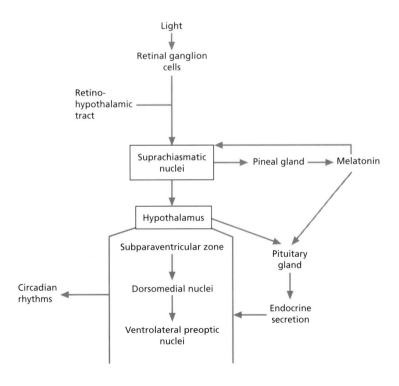

Fig. 5.1 Components of circadian sleep rhythms.

Regular relationship to day and night

There may be a pattern of early onset of sleep and early wake-up time (advanced sleep phase syndrome) or late sleep onset and late wake-up time (delayed sleep phase syndrome).

Cyclical relationship to day and night

The symptoms of excessive sleepiness and insomnia wax and wane as the relationship between the circadian sleep rhythms and light–dark exposure comes in and out of phase. This pattern is typical of non-24 h sleep–wake rhythms.

Irregular relationship to day and night

The symptoms fluctuate with no regular pattern. These irregular sleep–wake rhythms usually do not have an organic cause, but are more commonly due to social or occupational factors, such as rotating shift work.

Circadian rhythm disorders are occasionally due to organic neurological conditions affecting, for instance, the visual pathways or hypothalamus, in which case symptoms related to these lesions should be sought. Depression and the restless legs syndrome also cause sleep phase disorders and should be considered.

Physical examination

Physical examination is only required if an organic neurological lesion or visual impairment is suspected.

Investigations

Investigation of circadian rhythm disorders is difficult because of the multiple confounding factors which interact with circadian rhythms and influence their outcomes. It is usually difficult to control for most of these except in carefully organized 'constant routine' studies. In clinical practice it is difficult, for instance, to separate the effects of sleep/wake rhythms from exposure to light and dark, physical activity, food, stress and posture. Isolation studies where the environment is carefully controlled and exposure to light is carefully regulated give more information. Forced desynchrony studies, in which the circadian rhythms are dissociated from environmental factors, can also give useful information.

In clinical practice the most useful indicators of circadian rhythms are the following.

Sleep–wake or rest–activity patterns as determined by either polysomnography or actigraphy

See Fig. 5.2.

Melatonin estimations

Melatonin is affected by fewer confounding factors than most of the other indicators of circadian rhythms. Its secretion is not affected by sleep, physical activity, food or stress, but is modified by certain drugs and posture which need to be controlled for. Melatonin secretion is suppressed even by low light levels of around 10 lux.

Salivary melatonin levels can be estimated at hourly intervals in the evening and overnight. The subject is exposed to a low light level of less than around 8 lux. The 'dim light melatonin onset' is taken as the point at which 25% of the peak value is reached. Salivary melatonin levels rise around 30 min later than those in the blood. It may be difficult to sleep when the samples are being acquired and diurnal changes may be difficult to detect since the concentration is only around one-third of that in the plasma.

An alternative is estimation of 6-sulphatoxymelatonin concentration in the urine. This runs in parallel with the plasma levels, but around 1 h later. Urine is collected in 4–6-h samples while awake and as a single sample overnight so that the total melatonin production and its diurnal fluctuation can be estimated.

Cortisol levels

Repeated plasma cortisol estimations can be used to assess the amplitude and timing of circadian rhythms, and similar recordings of other hormones which are under circadian control may be of use.

Temperature recording

Continuous temperature recording, usually using a rectal probe, is of value in assessing the circadian temperature cycle, which is usually closely related to the circadian control of sleep and wakefulness.

Causes

The circadian sleep rhythms are largely under genetic control and this contributes to the wide variation among normal subjects. The patterns are also influenced by age. In adolescence the circadian rhythms lead to a delayed sleep phase, but throughout adult life this gradually moves forward until in the elderly an advanced sleep phase is common.

Disorders of circadian rhythms fall into three groups, according to whether the disturbance is due to an endogenous (intrinsic) abnormality, unusual environmental (exogenous) conditions, or a disorder of the linkage between the circadian rhythms and

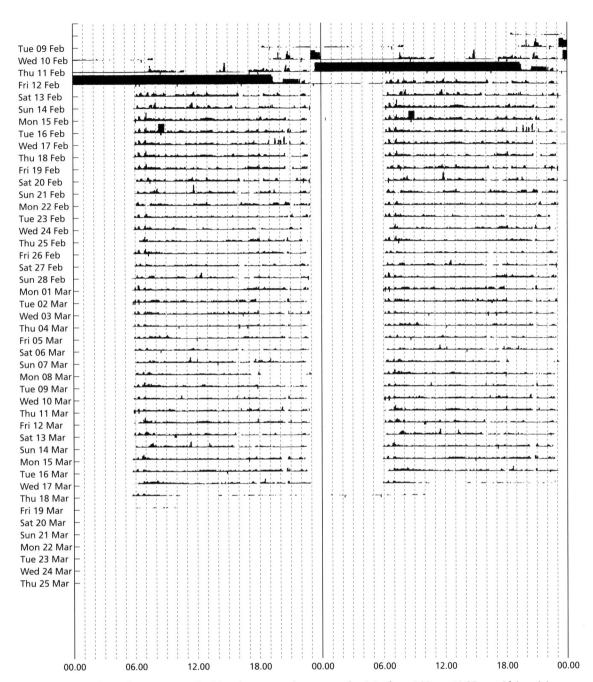

Fig. 5.2 Actigraphy readings in a normal subject shows a regular pattern of activity from 6.00 AM–11.30 PM with inactivity at night corresponding to sleep.

their environmental influences. In practice, there is considerable overlap between these three groups. Endogenous disorders may also modify the influence of the environmental factors on sleep and the latter may accentuate endogenous disorders.

Endogenous disorders

Endogenous disorders may affect either the timing or the amplitude of the circadian sleep rhythms. Organic abnormalities are uncommon, but may cause the sleep rhythms to become completely irregular with no discernible relationship to time, or light exposure. More commonly, however, there is a regular 24-h cycle which is set at a different point from normal. The onset of sleep and the natural waking time can both be delayed while the quality and duration of sleep remain normal, without any excessive sleepiness, if the patient is allowed to sleep as desired (delayed sleep phase syndrome, DSPS). In contrast, a pattern of early sleep onset and waking-up time, with a normal sleep quality and duration and no excessive sleepiness, can also develop (advanced sleep phase syndrome, ASPS).

Disorders of endogenous and exogenous linkage

These disorders lead to alterations in the timing of sleep so that there is a complaint of either insomnia or excessive sleepiness, or both. The sleep rhythm usually approximates to a free-running cycle of around 24.2 h which changes its relationship to the environment each day (non-24-h sleep–wake rhythm).

The connection between the endogenous circadian rhythms and time givers, particularly light, is reduced or absent. Insomnia and excessive sleepiness fluctuate from day to day according to the degree of mismatch of the endogenous cycle and environmental time. The failure to link the circadian rhythms to the external environment also leads to internal desynchronization of the sleep, temperature and endocrine rhythms which may contribute to the sleep disorder.

Exogenous disorders

The imposition of unusual or artificial changes in the environment induces physiological responses in the circadian rhythms which may cause symptoms, usually insomnia or excessive sleepiness, or both. These may be due to social factors, jet lag or shift work. The most important environmental factor is a change in the exposure to light, which often leads to alterations in sleeping times. A mismatch between the circadian time and environmental time develops, to which the circadian rhythms adjust slowly, and internal desynchronization of sleep, temperature and endocrine rhythms may arise. A DSPS, ASPS or irregular sleep–wake rhythm may be seen.

Delayed sleep phase syndrome (DSPS)

Pathogenesis

The delayed sleep phase syndrome can be caused by a circadian rhythm which is too long to be entrained to a 24-h cycle by light and other stimuli, or by an insensitivity to light as a sleep phase modifier, or by an asymmetry in the response to light, so that exposure in the evening causes a longer phase delay than the phase advance in response to early morning light. A high-amplitude circadian rhythm would also tend to delay the onset of sleep since it opposes the homeostatic drive to sleep more effectively in the evening.

Clinical features

This syndrome is characterized by a stable sleep rhythm in which sleep onset and time of awakening occur later than normal, but with a normal total sleep time and sleep architecture unless sleep is curtailed early in the morning. It causes difficulty in initiating sleep and in waking at conventional times. The latter in particular may be very disruptive and lead to recurrent episodes of lateness for school or work which may be interpreted as laziness or a lack of motivation. Sleepiness often continues through the morning, especially if the subject has been prematurely woken up, but excessive sleepiness later in the day is not a problem. Alertness is maximal later in the afternoon, evening and even after midnight, and sleep is often only initiated at around 3.00 AM. The natural waking time is usually 10–12 AM so it is predominantly REM rather than NREM sleep that is lost if the subject is woken prematurely (Fig. 5.3).

Delayed sleep phase syndrome is by definition characterized by an unusually late time of sleep onset and of waking. It may be worse in the winter, particularly in northern latitudes, when the intensity of light exposure is reduced in the mornings, compared to the summer when the earlier dawn promotes a phase advance.

The prevalence of DSPS depends on the conventional sleeping times of society. In warmer climates a late bedtime is common and DSPS is less frequently diagnosed than in northern climates where sleep onset is usually earlier and where individuals with this disorder are more conspicuous. In temperate climates a DSPS is seen in approximately 7% of adolescents and 1% of adults.

Causes

Normal adolescence

A mild DSPS is normal in adolescence from the age of around 16–18 years and into the early twenties. This tendency is often accentuated by social pressures, for instance late-night parties, or watching television or

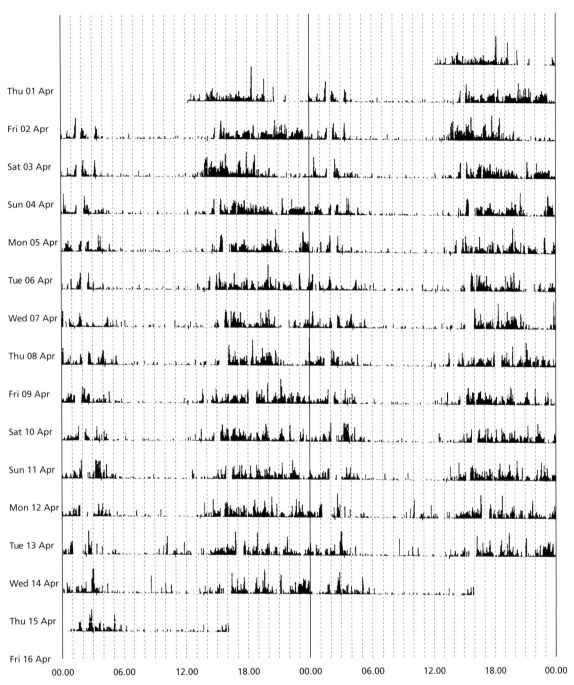

Fig. 5.3 Actigraphy readings in DSPS. The actigraphy tracing shows that inactivity starts around 3.00–4.00 AM and lasts until around midday, corresponding to the delayed sleep phase. The subject is then active later in the day and into the first part of the night.

videos. Students without fixed class times find it easier to adapt to their DSPS, but this situation may also encourage the maintenance of this sleep pattern.

Intrinsic delayed sleep phase syndrome

This disorder is familial. It may be due to a genetic abnormality but the exact mechanism has not been established. A short per 3 allele has been detected, but genetic influences are probably polymorphic.

Its onset is usually in childhood or adolescence and it usually worsens from the age of 16–18 for a few years. It may simply be an exaggeration of the normal changes in adolescence and merges into the 'owls' or 'evening types', who prefer to stay awake late, wake up late and are most alert in the evenings.

Extrinsic delayed sleep phase syndrome

This is due to psychosocial factors which promote the DSPS pattern. It often begins in childhood or as a teenager with staying up late on holidays, at weekends or on other special occasions, but may be triggered by a single major event. The habit of choosing to remain up late or being encouraged to do so then persists, and this may come to have secondary gains such as avoiding school on the following morning. Light exposure late in the evening tends to delay the sleep phase and perpetuate the DSPS.

The complaint usually comes from the parent rather than the child and this condition is unlikely to respond to treatment unless the priorities and motivation of both parents and child can be altered.

Seasonal affective disorder (SAD)

This is a seasonal circadian rhythm disorder which is four times more common in women than in men, is occasionally familial and is most frequent between the ages of 20 and 40 years. It is most prevalent in high latitudes where there is a greater seasonal change in the intensity and duration of exposure to light. Abnormalities of clock genes, for instance per 2, have been identified. They may change porphyrin metabolism which influences melatonin production.

The seasonal affective disorder develops during autumn and winter and remits in spring and summer, at which time there may even be mild hypomania. In the winter a DSPS pattern develops, associated with depression, an increase in appetite, particularly for carbohydrates, weight gain, fatigue and reduction in physical activity.

In the seasonal affective disorder there is slow elimination of circulating melatonin leading to a raised blood level in the mornings despite normal nocturnal secretion. The total sleep time increases, which is unlike other forms of depression, and the duration of both NREM and REM sleep increases, including stages 3 and 4 NREM sleep. The rhythm of cortisol secretion is phase delayed.

Seasonal affective disorder may be the extreme end of the normal range of seasonal variation in mood and behaviour. As winter approaches, the duration of the melatonin signal overnight lengthens and the abnormal elimination of melatonin initiates the DSPS.

Seasonal affective disorder responds to light therapy in up to 75% of patients, particularly if it is given on waking in the morning. Dawn simulation may be helpful and a combination of light therapy and exercise has been shown to be effective. Melatonin may help the depression slightly and this also responds transiently to sleep deprivation. Tricyclic and SSRI antidepressants are effective, but propranolol, which suppresses melatonin secretion, has no effect.

Brain and neck injuries

These may impair the secretion of melatonin from the pineal gland, or more commonly cause damage to its connections, especially the tortuous path between it and the suprachiasmatic nuclei through the cervical spinal cord. Cervical cord transection and whiplash injuries to the neck are particularly associated with DSPS.

Restless legs syndrome

The abnormal sensations in the limbs and repetitive arousals from sleep due to periodic limb movements early in the night often lead to difficulty in initiating sleep and the adoption of a delayed sleep phase pattern.

Diagnosis

The diagnosis of DSPS depends on the presence of the clinical features, especially a stable phase delay of the major sleep episode in relation to the desired time for sleep. This introduces a subjective element into the diagnosis, according to the patient's perception of the impact of the disorder, in addition to the difficulties in diagnosis due to the differing sleep times that are prevalent in individual societies. Delayed sleep phase syndrome should be distinguished from psychophysiological insomnia, and other causes of difficulty in initiating sleep, and other causes of excessive sleepiness, particularly idiopathic hypersomnia.

Polysomnography excludes other causes for the symptoms and reveals a normal sleep structure if it is

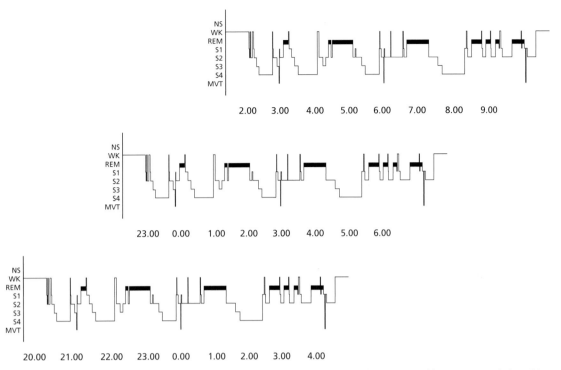

Fig. 5.4 Polysomnography in DSPS, normal subject and ASPS. The middle tracing shows a normal hypnogram with the subject asleep from around 11.00 PM–7.00 AM. In the top tracing the same normal hypnogram does not start until around 2.00 AM because of the delayed sleep phase syndrome (DSPS) and in the lower line the same sleep pattern is initiated at around 8.00 PM due to an advanced sleep phase syndrome (ASPS).

carried out at the subject's usual sleeping time (Fig. 5.4). If it is carried out at normal hours there may be a long sleep latency, low sleep efficiency, difficulty in waking the subject and a short duration of REM sleep which is truncated by the early time of ending the study in relation to the subject's usual sleep time. Sleep diaries and actigraphy recordings may confirm the sleep pattern of DSPS, and secretion of melatonin is delayed. The distinction between intrinsic and extrinsic DSPS can be difficult, but patients with the latter may assume more normal sleep times when removed from their usual environment if they are motivated to do so.

Treatment

The aims of treatment are to reset the sleep phase and to maintain this. This can be achieved by the following methods.

Sleep hygiene

Application of sleep hygiene principles may enable sleep to be initiated earlier and improve the sleep architecture. This is particularly important if early awakening from sleep is essential because of school or work attendance. These measures may need to be combined with the other treatments listed below in order to maintain resetting of the sleep phase. The success of this type of treatment depends very much on the motivation of the patient.

Chronotherapy

The aim of this, as with light therapy and melatonin, is to reset the circadian rhythm. Over a period of days or weeks the sleep–wake cycle is shifted by gradually introducing a phase delay and avoiding naps during the day. The time of sleep onset should be retarded in 3-h steps each night until it reaches the desired or socially acceptable sleep time. The sleep cycle is in effect lengthened to 27 h and kept constant until it has been realigned. Hypnotics may help to reduce sleep during the 'wake maintenance zone' and the changes should be supported by careful sleep hygiene. Once the new pattern has been established it is important to maintain a constant time of going to bed and of waking in the morning. Less than 1 h deviation from the intended time should be the aim, and this should be maintained at weekends as well as during weekdays. It is important to avoid naps during the day, and particularly during the 2 h preceding sleep. Sleeping late in the morning should be avoided, even after going to sleep late on the previous night.

These routines should be combined with other aspects of sleep hygiene, especially taking physical activity during the day, and, if necessary, with light therapy.

Light therapy (phototherapy, luminotherapy)
Exposure to bright light has an alerting effect and leads to sleep phase changes. These are influenced by the following.

Timing of light therapy
The effect of light on the sleep phase is determined by the phase response curve (page 31). This has an inflection point at around the time of the temperature nadir (3.00–5.00 AM). Light has more effect on changing the phase of sleep when it is applied close to the inflection point. Before this time it delays the onset of sleep and afterwards it causes a sleep phase advance. Light exposure during the middle of the day has virtually no effect on the sleep phase, but it does increase alertness.

The 'time of light exposure' is conventionally taken as the mid-point of the exposure to light. This is particularly important if it is applied close to the inflection point since the onset of light exposure may, for instance, be before the inflection point, despite the mid-point falling afterwards.

Light therapy is most effective in advancing the sleep phase if it is given between 6.00 and 10.00 AM. As the wake-up time becomes earlier so the timing of the light therapy can be moved earlier to further advance the phase shift. Once the circadian phase has been modified, light should be presented at a consistent time each day to maintain this change.

Light intensity
The sleep phase shift produced by light therapy is approximately proportional to the log of the light intensity. The maximum response is seen with around 1000 lux and 50% of this with around 100 lux, but even 25 lux can alter the sleep phase. Dawn stimulation, with a gradually increasing light intensity, may be particularly effective, even if the eyes are closed, because 5–10% of light reaches the retina through the eyelids. An intensity of 2500 lux is usually given for 2 h, or 5000 lux for 1 h or 10 000 lux for 30 min,

but high intensities of light exposure can cause eye damage.

Duration of light treatment
The phase shift is approximately proportional to the duration of light exposure up to around 3 h, but brief exposures for even around 1 min can have a significant effect.

Wavelength
The retinal ganglion cells which project to the suprachiasmatic nuclei have a peak sensitivity to light of wavelengths 445–475 nm, especially around 460 nm. This bluish light is most effective in shifting circadian rhythms and suppressing melatonin secretion. Ultraviolet light is not required and should be filtered out since it can cause cataracts and skin cancer.

Bright lights in the bathroom, bedroom and kitchen, and encouragement to walk to work may help, but sitting by a window and exposure to ordinary indoor electric light are insufficient. Light therapy is best delivered from a fluorescent light which is situated on a white or light-coloured surface to increase reflection, or from a visor or mask which can be worn on the head. Fluorescent bulbs are more energy-efficient and produce less heat, but are noisy and flicker. They have diffusers which enable the light to reach a wide area of the retina, in contrast to incandescent light bulbs which tend to give a point source, which stimulates a smaller area of the retina and has less effect. It is usual for the light source to be 1 m from the patient and at eye level. The light does not need to be directed along the line of gaze, and its projection onto the nasal side of the retina inferiorly may produce more melatonin suppression than other orientations.

Side-effects include headache and agitation. Hypomania may develop in bipolar disorders and there is a risk of eye damage with high intensities of light exposure.

Light therapy should be combined with sleep hygiene, particularly with regular sleep-onset and wake-up times, and can be used in conjunction with chronotherapy. It is particularly effective in seasonal affective disorder. Once the DSPS has been controlled, the maintenance dose of light may be reduced or the frequency of light therapy decreased to two to three times per week.

Melatonin
Melatonin is able to shift the circadian sleep rhythms and is also a sedative. It advances the sleep phase if it is

given in the evening and, rather less reliably, delays it if it is administered in the morning. The phase response curve for melatonin is therefore the opposite of that for light exposure, although its inflection point is probably the same as that for light exposure at around 3–5 AM. It is able to advance the onset of endogenous secretion and of sleep by 1.5 h per day. It does not alter sleep architecture [1].

Melatonin should be taken 1–2 h before the usual sleep onset time in DSPS and, as this becomes earlier, the timing of the melatonin dose is brought forward by intervals of 30 min. It acts in effect as an early night replacement treatment for endogenous melatonin, but its long-term efficacy is variable.

Advanced sleep phase syndrome (ASPS)

Pathogenesis

The advanced sleep phase pattern may be due to a circadian rhythm periodicity that is shorter than 24 h, or to asymmetry in response to light so that exposure in the evening causes less of a phase delay than the phase advancement in response to early morning light. A low-amplitude circadian rhythm would tend to bring forward the onset of sleep since it would fail to oppose the homeostatic drive to sleep sooner in the evening.

Clinical features

This syndrome is characterized by a stable sleep rhythm which is offset relative to normal, so that the sleep-onset and waking-up times occur earlier than is conventional and desired. Sleep often begins around 9.00 PM and ends between 3.00 and 5.00 AM. The total sleep time and sleep architecture are normal and daytime sleepiness is not a problem, unless going to sleep early in the evening is prevented.

Advanced sleep phase syndrome causes fewer problems than DSPS, although it is common for subjects to fall asleep in the evening and to have to be woken in order to go to bed. The early awakening time can disrupt the sleep of the partner and family, but occurs even if sleep onset is delayed, in which case sleepiness is worse during the day because of sleep restriction. Alertness is maximal in the mornings and sleepiness develops early in the evening.

Like DSPS, the criteria for the diagnosis depend on the normal sleep patterns within each society. Advanced sleep phase syndrome is more frequent and more troublesome when the conventional sleep times

are late, as in most warmer climates. It has probably become more prominent since the introduction of the electric light bulb because it was previously usual to fall asleep by around 9.00 PM or soon after sundown. The ASPS may be a biological adaptation to the natural light–dark cycles.

Causes

Old age

The amplitude of the circadian rhythm is reduced in the elderly and its timing may change so that it fails to combat the homeostatic drive to enter sleep early in the evening. This tendency is compounded by a variety of behavioural and other factors (Chapter 6).

Intrinsic advanced sleep phase syndrome

This syndrome is less common than intrinsic DSPS. It is often familial and it usually appears in late middle age or in the elderly. It may represent an exaggeration of the ASPS of the elderly and an extreme form of the 'lark' or 'morning types' who wake in the morning and are least alert in the evenings. It can be due to a genetic defect in the circadian sleep rhythms, or in the way in which they control the release of or respond to melatonin. An autosomal dominant mutation of per 2 gene has been demonstrated, but inheritance is probably usually polygenic.

Extrinsic advanced sleep phase syndrome

This syndrome may be socially induced, for instance by tiredness following early awakening for a morning shift or to commute to work, especially when this is associated with factors which promote sleep early in the evening, such as a large meal, dim lighting and watching unstimulating television. Early morning waking with exposure to light also leads to a sleep phase advance and this may perpetuate, and even in some people initiate, the ASPS.

Depression

This frequently causes an ASPS.

Diagnosis

Advanced sleep phase syndrome needs to be distinguished from other causes of excessive daytime sleepiness and early morning waking. Polysomnography carried out at the patient's normal sleep time shows a normal sleep architecture and duration, but if this is carried out at more conventional times, the duration of NREM sleep, particularly stages 3 and 4, is reduced

(Fig. 5.4). The pattern of sleep and wake can be confirmed by sleep diaries and actigraphy, and melatonin secretion occurs earlier than in normal subjects. Intrinsic ASPS may be difficult to distinguish from extrinsic ASPS unless modification of the factors responsible for the latter causes it to resolve.

Treatment

Sleep hygiene

This is as important as in DSPS. Sleep onset should be delayed, a regular wake-up time adopted, and naps avoided during the day.

Chronotherapy

A gradual delay in the sleep phase may realign it with environmental conditions, based on similar principles to the treatment of DSPS, but there is little evidence regarding its effectiveness.

Light therapy

The sleep phase can be delayed by exposure to bright light in the evening, but not within 1 h of the intended time of going to sleep. A bright light bulb used while eating, reading or watching television may be of some help, but formal light therapy with a light box or visor is preferable. The duration and intensity of the light therapy needed vary between individuals, but 1–3 h treatment is commonly given. Exposure to bright light early in the morning may cause a phase advance and should be avoided either by staying indoors or by wearing dark glasses in sunlight. The effects of light therapy may take 1–8 weeks to appear. Advanced sleep phase syndrome often relapses within a month of stopping treatment, which may need to be maintained in the long term to prevent relapses.

Melatonin

Exogenous melatonin taken in the morning delays endogenous melatonin secretion and may help to postpone the onset of sleep.

Non-24-h sleep–wake rhythm

Clinical features

This results from a failure of environmental factors to control the circadian sleep rhythm and melatonin secretion. The rhythm has an intrinsic cycle of around 24.2 h and if it becomes independent of the environment (free running) their relationship changes each day. At one point in the cycle the two are in phase, but the sleep rhythm then moves progressively forward, leading initially to what appears to be a DSPS, and then through sleep reversal with insomnia at night and sleepiness during the day to an ASPS, before returning temporarily to synchrony with the environment again. The rhythm may be partially entrained by cultural and social factors, depending on their intensity and the entrainability of the individual's circadian rhythm. The fluctuating insomnia and daytime sleepiness can be difficult to cope with, and while the same symptoms arise in partially entrained subjects as in those with free-running cycles, they are milder. Daytime naps tend to occur at the times of melatonin secretion.

Causes

Changes in ambient light

A reduction in the variation of light intensity, as experienced by cave dwellers, residents at polar latitudes, and space travellers, diminishes the influence of the environment on the circadian sleep rhythm and predisposes to a non-24-h sleep–wake rhythm. An extreme example is space travel, in which there is exposure to the sun rising and setting about 16 times in each 24-h period. The unusual pattern of activity and sleeping position in an environment with little gravitational force, and the imposed and restricted social interactions, all combine to alter circadian rhythms and sleep.

Blindness

A non-24-h sleep–wake rhythm is common if there is visual impairment [2]. It is most marked if there is no light perception, but it is also present in around 20% of those with unilateral blindness. It usually responds to 0.5 mg melatonin at around 9.00 PM. This not only entrains the circadian rhythms, but also has a soporific effect.

Damage to the retinohypothalamic tract and disorders of the hypothalamus
These are rare.

Idiopathic

An identical pattern can occur in otherwise normal subjects with no detectable visual or neurological abnormality, probably because of a functional defect in the suprachiasmatic nuclei or its connections which prevents the circadian sleep rhythm from being entrained by environmental factors.

Diagnosis

This requires a careful history and analysis of sleep diaries, supplemented by actigraphy to detect diurnal variations in movements which are an indirect marker of sleep and wakefulness.

Treatment

The symptoms of these partially or totally free-running circadian rhythms are often difficult to eliminate, but treatment comprises sleep hygiene advice, chronotherapy, light therapy, melatonin, or a combination of these. Melatonin is especially effective in blind people.

Irregular sleep–wake rhythm

Clinical features

The pattern of sleep may become irregular and fail to retain a constant relationship to the environmental time, or to light and darkness. The temperature and endocrine rhythmicity may also be lost or be dissociated from the sleep cycle. Insomnia, excessive daytime sleepiness or the need to nap during the day reflect the irregular sleep and wake patterns, but total sleep time is often normal.

Causes

Irregular sleep–wake rhythms may be due to the following.

Endogenous disorders

Structural neurological conditions causing endogenous circadian rhythm disorders are uncommon. They may involve the suprachiasmatic nuclei or the pathways leading to and from these in the hypothalamus and from the pineal gland. The most important examples are as follows.

Brain injuries

The irregular sleep–wake pattern may be either temporary or permanent and probably reflects damage to the circadian and other control mechanisms.

Degenerative disorders

The irregular sleep–wake pattern in these conditions reflects the extensive disorganization of sleep controlling mechanisms. It is a feature of Alzheimer's disease, fatal familial insomnia and African sleeping sickness.

Tumours

Tumours of the pinealocytes, but not the pineal glia, hypothalamic and pituitary tumours and craniopharyngiomas cause this type of disorder. These tumours are often associated with endocrine abnormalities and weight gain which may induce obstructive sleep apnoeas.

Social factors

The availability of artificial light, initially with the electric light bulb, and now from a variety of other sources, has both extended the time for which waking activities can be performed and also distorted the influence of light on the sleep–wake cycle. Previously this artificial light could only be provided by candles and fire and most members of society tended to wake up soon after dawn and go to bed soon after dusk. This pattern maximized the opportunities during daylight hours for farming, hunting and social activities. It not only minimized sleep restriction, except in polar regions during the summer, but also tended to maintain regular sleep–wake routines.

Exposure to light during the natural hours of darkness is often combined with less exposure to light during the day than in the past. Modern urbanized indoor life removes many people from sunlight for most of the day, particularly in the mornings. Work, recreation and other activities, including many sports and shopping, often entail remaining indoors for prolonged periods. Atmospheric pollution, particularly in the cities, reduces the amount of sunlight that reaches the eye, and climatic conditions such as rain, cold and the early onset of darkness in high latitudes increase indoor rather than outdoor activities. The intensity of light is significantly less with artificial lighting than in most outdoor environments (Table 2.3).

The irregularity of the timing of activities using artificial light also disturbs the circadian sleep rhythm by constantly altering the stimuli that regulate sleep and wakefulness. Artificial light has allowed the concept of a '24-hour' or '24/7' society to develop. Shift work, nocturnal entertainment and other activities previously confined to the daytime can now be carried out at night. Business activities involving contacts in other continents often require working at night. The increased noise level caused by these and other activities, such as driving, also hinders sleep, especially in urban societies. The development of the 24-hour society has also had an impact on other time givers for sleep, such as meals, exercise and social activities, so that the endogenous circadian rhythms increasingly conflict with the often rapidly changing external factors that control them. These effects are magnified by any pre-existing insomnia, excessive sleepiness and restriction of sleep duration.

Sleep patterns during the week are often very different from those at weekends. Sleeping for longer in the mornings at weekends to catch up with the sleep debt that has accumulated during the week may be equivalent to a time zone change of 1–3 h and this requires subsequent adjustments of the circadian and sleep control mechanisms.

Advice about sleep hygiene is important in order to minimize the impact on circadian rhythms of these sleep–wake patterns.

Time zone changes (jet lag)

Clinical features
Jet lag, which is the term used for the symptoms arising from time zone changes, is due to a failure of the circadian rhythms to synchronize with the new environment after a sudden time zone shift. Jet lag does not occur with travel from north to south or south to north, but only with transmeridian journeys. It is not due to sleep deprivation, but this may contribute to the problems that develop. Sleep may be lost because of the timing of the departure and arrival, and the poor quality of sleep during the journey. Reclining seats improve sleep quality.

Jet lag is characterized by insomnia and excessive daytime sleepiness, usually with a reduction in total sleep time and sleep efficiency and with frequent naps during the day. The first night's sleep after the journey is least affected because of prior sleep deprivation. The circadian sleep rhythm adjusts more quickly to the new environment than the temperature rhythm and most endocrine rhythms, leading to internal desynchronization. Travellers who make frequent time zone changes may develop a persistent combination of insomnia and excessive daytime sleepiness.

Causes
The severity of jet lag depends on the following factors.
1 Number of time zones crossed. Symptoms are usually significant if more than six time zones are crossed.
2 Individual susceptibility. This varies considerably and, in general, jet lag is more severe in the elderly.
3 Direction of travel. Eastward travel is more disruptive than travelling westward. Most long haul flights take place overnight. Adaptation to the new time occurs at a rate of around 1 h per day travelling

eastward and 1.5 h per day travelling westward. Eastward travel leads to an earlier night and therefore requires a sleep phase advance. This is more difficult to adapt to than a phase delay because the circadian sleep rhythm is longer than 24 h. The symptoms mimic the DSPS with a delay in sleep onset and difficulty in waking in the morning.

In contrast, travelling westward mimics the ASPS, and as the new environment is delayed relative to the old, sleep onset REM is common. Most long haul westward flights take place during the day.

Treatment
The treatment of jet lag depends on the duration and direction of travel. If transmeridian journeys are frequent, their need should be assessed. It may be preferable to travel less frequently, but stay abroad for longer, to reduce the problems of jet lag. If the stay abroad is less than around three days it is usually better to remain on 'home time' so as to avoid any need for adjusting to the new clock time while abroad and again after the journey home. Daytime activities such as social contacts, exercise, meals and exposure to light should all remain unchanged relative to home time.

The measures that should be taken for longer episodes depend largely on whether the journey is eastward or westward (Table 5.1). The new sleep-onset time is ahead of 'home' bedtime with eastward travel and occurs before the release of melatonin and often in the 'forbidden zone' when it is difficult to initiate sleep. Travelling westward, however, encourages sleep onset later than 'home time' so that sleep occurs readily on the first night. The sleep latency is short, sleep efficiency is high and there is a normal or increased duration of stages 3 and 4 NREM sleep. Awakening may occur early with loss of REM sleep which increases (rebounds) on the second night.

Short-acting hypnotics may be useful both during the flight and for a few nights after arrival if taken to establish sleep at the onset of night time at the destination.

Resetting of the circadian rhythms can be accelerated by carefully timed exercise and exposure to light. Excessive light in the morning leads to a phase advance and in the evening to a phase delay.

Exposure to light is useful in the early morning with eastward travel, even for a few days beforehand, since it advances the sleep phase, but it should be avoided in the evening by staying indoors or wearing sunglasses. Arrival after 3.00–5.00 AM on eastward journeys, but

Table 5.1 Jet lag prevention.

	Eastward travel	*Westward travel*
Before travel	Go to sleep and wake up early for 1–2 days Bright light exposure in morning for 1–2 days or melatonin on evening before journey	Go to sleep later for 1–2 days Bright light exposure in evening for 1–2 days Wear sunglasses in bright light in mornings for 1–2 days Melatonin early in morning before journey
During travel	Arrive between 5.00 AM and 9.00 PM Avoid hypnotics and alcohol except when travelling in the evening Avoid stimulants, e.g. caffeine, late in the journey	Arrive between 10.00 AM and 3.00 AM
After arrival	Adopt new time immediately Avoid naps on day of arrival Bright light exposure in morning for 1–2 days or melatonin on evening after flight	Adopt new time immediately Consider stimulants, e.g. caffeine, for 1–2 days Bright light exposure in the evening for 1–2 days or melatonin in morning after flight

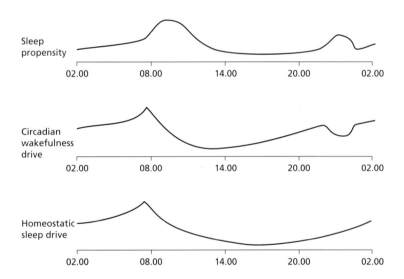

Fig. 5.5 Sleep–wake control immediately after 8 h eastward travel. The sleep propensity is the sum of the circadian and homeostatic drives.

before 9.00 PM, avoids any phase delay due to light exposure at the destination.

Conversely, when travelling westward, light should be avoided in the morning, but exposure obtained in the evening, even for a few days before travel, to hasten circadian adaptation. An arrival time from 10.00 AM to 3.00 AM is best, in order to avoid the phase advancing effect of light in the early morning.

Whether travelling east or west, loss of sleep is minimized with daytime flights, but if sleep is lost it will enhance sleepiness and increase the duration of stages

3 and 4 NREM sleep on the first night after arrival. It is best to go to bed progressively closer to the usual time of sleep at the destination each night after arrival.

The effects of melatonin are opposite to those of light. With eastward travel 2–5 mg of a fast release preparation should be taken 1 h before sleep onset at the new location, both for its hypnotic effect and to advance the sleep phase. With westward travel it should be taken at bedtime or if waking occurs during the night.

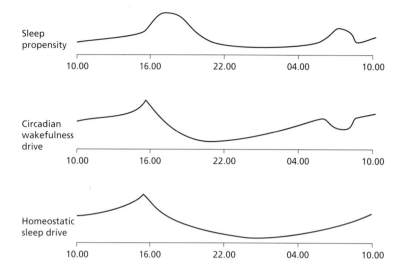

Sleep
propensity

10.00   16.00   22.00   04.00   10.00

Circadian
wakefulness
drive

10.00   16.00   22.00   04.00   10.00

Homeostatic
sleep drive

10.00   16.00   22.00   04.00   10.00

Fig. 5.6 Sleep–wake control immediately after 8 h westward travel. The sleep propensity is the sum of the circadian and homeostatic drives.

Shift work

In most developed societies 20–30% of the adult workforce carry out some form of shift work. This was introduced early in the twentieth century following the development of the assembly line, interchangeable parts, mass production and the idea of continuous use of production equipment. Henry Ford first applied this to the development of his Model T car which was produced in 1908. He was thereby able to reduce its price and make it available to large sections of society.

Public pressure in most developed societies has subsequently prioritized short-term productivity and artificial working practices above the need for the individual worker to obtain adequate sleep. This, and a lack of awareness of the importance of sleep, circadian rhythms and their disorders, has had wide-ranging detrimental effects.

Shift work entails working outside conventional daylight hours on a regular or intermittent basis. Shifts may be either fixed, with an unchanging pattern of work times, or rotating, in which the times change regularly [3]. At these times there is often a 7–10 h change in the timing of sleep, equivalent to a time zone shift of this degree.

Effects on sleep

Complete adaptation to shift work is very rare even after many years of such work, and, as a result, it causes both insomnia and excessive sleepiness at times when wakefulness is desired. The term 'shift work sleep disorder' is used if the symptoms are marked,

persist for more than 3 months and if there is no other cause. Subjects who have difficulty in coping with these problems often obtain alternative employment, but difficulty in initiating sleep and early morning waking insomnia may persist for months or years after shift work has ceased.

The effects on sleep are due to the following factors.
1 A mismatch between the circadian sleep rhythms and the external environment [4]. This is particularly important in rotating shifts in which the association between the circadian rhythms and external time changes frequently. During the first night at work it is difficult to stay awake, particularly at around 5.00 AM, and during the following day the circadian rhythms promote alertness and make it difficult to sleep. An 8-h shift change takes the circadian sleep rhythms around a week to adjust to and this may be further slowed by exposure to light during the day. Internal desynchronization of the circadian rhythms is common, particularly since, for instance, the temperature cycle takes longer than the sleep cycle to adapt to any external change.
2 Poor quality of sleep, not only because attempts to sleep are out of phase with circadian rhythms, but also because of noise, light and other disturbances during the day [5].
3 Sleep restriction. This is a common but not inevitable consequence of shift work. Sleep has to compete with family, social and recreational activities and the sleep pattern often becomes irregular. Most night shift workers sleep early during the day with the result that they are often awake for around 8 h before starting

work. In this they differ from people who work in the day who may only be awake for 2 h before going to work.

4 Sleep inertia. This is a problem particularly if naps are taken during work time, and is especially important for heavy goods vehicle (HGV) drivers if they begin to drive soon after taking a nap.

General effects

Increase in accidents and reduction in work performance. Work during the night shift takes place at the nadir of the circadian rhythm for alertness. Early morning shifts often cause subalertness because of the reduction in sleep quality and duration during the previous night, and because the shift takes place at a time when the circadian drive to sleep is still strong.

Both these shifts are associated with an increase in the frequency of accidents at work and a reduction in productivity. The number of errors in repetitive activities increases, particularly in those who are unable to develop coping strategies to handle their sleepiness. There is an increased risk of accidents between 2.00 and 4.00 PM and between 10.00 PM and 6.00 AM, especially around 3.00 AM. The decrement in performance is related to the extent of sleep deprivation, the time spent carrying out the task and the time of day, and the number of consecutive night shifts that have been worked.

Increased use of hypnotics and alcohol. These are often used to help re-establish an acceptable sleep pattern, but may lead to dependency and chronic disturbance of the sleep pattern.

Shortened life expectancy. This has been shown in several studies, but the cause is uncertain. It may be related to repetitive cycles of internal desynchronization of circadian rhythms, but other factors including increased alcohol consumption, and tobacco smoking may be relevant.

Social effects. Shift workers are often marginalized from family, social and recreational activities because they sleep for much of the day. This may lead to difficulties with relationships and with bonding to their children.

Metabolic effects. The metabolic effects in shift workers are similar to those seen in sleep deprivation and sleep fragmentation and include alterations in glucose and lipid metabolism (page 135).

Table 5.2 Factors determining effects of shift work.

Shift work	Fixed or rotating shifts
	Duration of shifts
	Direction of shifts
	Frequency of shifts
	Interval between changes
Individual	Age
	Previous sleep habits and quality
	Motivation to alter sleep habits

Physical effects. There is an increased incidence of heart disease and risk of peptic ulcer in shift workers, and frequently a change of bowel habit, particularly with rotating shifts. Irregular menstrual periods and an increased risk of spontaneous abortion, premature labour and low birthweight children occur in female shift workers, although there is no effect on fertility.

Psychological effects. Anxiety and depression are commoner in shift workers than in those who work during the day.

Shift work patterns and sleep
The degree of disruption to the sleep–wake cycle caused by shift work (Table 5.2) depends on the factors described below.

Whether the shift is fixed or rotating. The total sleep time of fixed-shift workers is less than that of regular daytime workers, but longer than that of rotating-shift workers.

Duration of shift. Shift lengths are usually 8–12 h. Longer shifts are often preferred because they fit in better with life outside work, but are probably no better at preventing sleep disturbances.

Number of hours shifted. It is common for shifts to last from around 6.00 AM to 2.00 PM, 2.00 to 10.00 PM and 10.00 PM to 6.00 AM. In the first of these the subject has to wake early and so it is best to go to bed earlier, although because of both social and circadian rhythm factors this may be difficult. The sleeping time is therefore shortened and there may be difficulty in waking and sleepiness later in the day due to sleep restriction. A 30–60 min nap in the afternoon after the end of the shift may be of help.

The 2.00 to 10.00 PM shift causes fewer problems, although many people find it difficult to mentally unwind after work and need time with their family and for social activities. This leads to a late onset of sleep with a reduction in time spent asleep unless the awakening time in the morning is delayed.

Most workers feel tired during the 10.00 PM to 6.00 AM shift and it is common to nap during this time. The first night shift often entails being awake for over 24 h so that sleepiness during this night shift is especially frequent. It is also common to feel sleepy after working a night shift, particularly at around 6.00–7.00 AM. This increases the risk of road traffic accidents while driving home at this time. Exposure to bright light early in the morning prevents a phase delay occurring which would adapt the subject better to the night shift, unless dark glasses are worn after work.

After the shift many people sleep until around midday, although this may be difficult because of external noise and light. After the morning sleep there is an interval of around 8–10 h of wakefulness before starting work. This is different from conventional daytime work which usually starts soon after waking. Tiredness during the next shift can be reduced by taking a 30–60 min nap in the evening, with the duration determined by the degree of loss of sleep during the main sleep episode. An alternative is to remain awake during the morning until around midday or 2.00 PM and then to obtain the main sleep episode. This has the advantage of utilizing the afternoon circadian tendency to fall asleep and also reduces the length of time awake before starting the next shift. Nevertheless, the total sleep time is often 2–4 h less than that of daytime workers because of the mismatch between the circadian rhythms and the opportunities for sleep.

Direction of shift. Adaptation is quicker and more complete if the shifts move forward rather than backwards. An early morning shift followed by a daytime shift and night-time shift is preferable to the opposite sequence.

Duration of rotation. Rapid shift changes cause the subject more difficulty in adapting to the environmental changes. The circadian rhythms fail to adapt to the constantly changing shift pattern, with the result that work is frequently carried out around the time of the temperature nadir when the circadian drive to enter sleep is strongest.

Slowly rotating shifts or fixed shift work reduce this problem, but the latter, in particular, do not give relief from sleepiness because of the restriction and poor quality of sleep that are inevitably associated with continual shift work. A compromise of five nights at work and two nights off may be best.

Interval between shift changes. A short interval between shifts, as with, for instance, working a 2.00–10.00 PM shift and then 6.00 AM–2.00 PM, leads to sleep restriction and hinders the adaptation that can take place to the new work pattern. An interval of 12–16 h, which usually in practice includes the main sleep period and one or more naps, is of help, but whole rest days between shifts are preferable.

Individual adaptability. The factors that determine this are poorly established but include the following.

Age. Younger subjects adapt more quickly and more completely to shift changes. Over the age of around 45 years, increasingly troublesome symptoms appear.

Previous sleep habits. Misalignment between the natural sleep tendencies and the hours of shift work magnifies its adverse affects. In practice workers tend to select jobs which fit their natural sleep patterns. 'Evening types', for instance, often work for some or all of the night, which fits their endogenous pattern of a late sleep-onset and wake-up time. Conversely, 'morning types' are better suited to work between 6.00 AM and 2.00 PM.

Subjects with relatively fixed circadian rhythms which are slow to entrain to environmental changes are likely to have more sleep problems with shift work. In other people there is a disproportionate decrement in performance following a slight loss of sleep (vulnerable sleepers).

Personality and motivation. The achievement of good quality sleep of an adequate duration has to compete with the desirability of social, recreational and other activities outside work. The degree of motivation to modify these, in order to obtain a reasonably quiet and dark sleep environment, and to prioritize an adequate sleep time outside work above other activities varies considerably. The temptation to stay awake and keep socially active during the time when sleep is best entered often leads to sleep restriction and sleep being taken at the least appropriate time in the circadian rhythm. These and other aspects of sleep hygiene

Table 5.3 Coping with night shift work.

To promote sleep during the day	To stay alert at night
Avoid bright light in the morning	Take a nap before going to work
Delay going to bed, ideally until 12.00 midday	Take caffeine, but not after 5.00 AM
Develop pre-sleep routines, e.g. hot bath	Keep work area brightly lit
Avoid caffeinated drinks before sleep	Avoid excessive overtime working
Keep bedroom at 18°C and dark	Avoid heavy meals before night shift
	Avoid alcohol or hypnotics

have a large impact on how successfully each individual copes with the potential disturbance of shift work on sleep–wake function.

Management
Both the employer and employee have responsibilities in managing problems associated with shift work. The employer has to balance the health of the employee, difficulty in obtaining cover if he or she is unable to work because of a shift work related illness and the risk of accidents due to sleepiness against the need for maximizing productivity. The employee with excessive daytime sleepiness and insomnia should be aware of how to minimize these symptoms, particularly through coping strategies and lifestyle changes.

The successful management of sleep–wake problems due to shift work (Table 5.3) entails the following counter-measures.
1 Optimization of shift schedules according to the principles described above.
2 Optimization of sleep environment to minimize awakenings due, for instance, to noise, light and temperature changes.
3 Adaptation of activities outside work so that a reasonable total sleep time is obtained. This may be most easily achieved as a single sleep episode, but division into a main sleep and one or more naps before starting the night shift often improves alertness at work at night [6].
4 Naps taken just before [7] or during work [8] can relieve excessive daytime sleepiness. In practice it may be difficult to take naps during work, both because facilities are not provided and because the employer expects the subject to be at work rather than sleeping. Naps during work may be followed by sleep inertia which can be dangerous if the subject is working with moving machinery or driving a motor vehicle.
5 Modification of circadian rhythms.

(a) Physical activity. Planning the timing of physical activity may assist adaptation of circadian rhythms.
(b) Light therapy. The timing of light exposure is determined by the details of the shifts that are being worked. Light exposure in the evening and at night will enhance alertness during the night shift [9]. Four hours light exposure at the start of the night shift, or even 5 min every 30 min during the shift, is effective in causing a phase delay, but may not be acceptable because all members of staff are exposed. Blue light is most effective, and while treatment with 100 lux has only half the phase-shifting effects of 1000 lux, it may be more practical to provide for the individual.

A phase delay prevents sleepiness developing until after the shift on subsequent nights. Light exposure after 3.00–5.00 AM may, however, cause a phase advance and light should be avoided in the morning, for instance by wearing sunglasses, e.g. welder's goggles.
(c) Melatonin may be used to alter the time of the main sleep episode in order to adapt to the changes in shift-working hours. It delays the next sleep phase if it is taken in the morning, but taken in the evening will advance the next sleep phase. Melatonin can also hasten adaptation of the circadian rhythms after a period of shift work, but in practice is often ineffective.
6 Hypnotics. These may be useful when taken intermittently, but only short-acting benzodiazepines, and drugs such as zaleplon, zopiclone and zolpidem, should be considered. Their main value is in initiating sleep, but since most of the hypnotics cause sleepiness after waking during the day, and some during the night shift as well, they have not proved popular.
7 Caffeine increases alertness when taken during the night shift, particularly in repeated small doses. It is probably less effective in the second half of the night and tolerance may develop.

8 Modafinil. 200 mg taken 30–60 min before the start of the night shift has been shown to improve alertness during the shift and to reduce sleepiness while driving home on the following morning. It is more effective than caffeine, but should be reserved for sleepiness which persists despite other counter-measures.

References

1 Nagtegaal JE, Kerkhof GA, Smits MG, Swart ACW, van der Meer YG. Delayed sleep phase syndrome: a placebo-controlled cross-over study on the effects of melatonin administered five hours before the individual dim light melatonin onset. *J Sleep Res* 1998; 7: 135–43.
2 Sack RL, Lewy AJ. Circadian rhythm sleep disorders: lessons from the blind. *Sleep Med Rev* 2001; 5(3): 189–206.
3 Akerstedt T. Shift work and disturbed sleep/wakefulness. *Sleep Med Rev* 1998; 2: 117–28.
4 Sallinen M, Harma M, Mutanen P, Ranta R, Virkkala J, Muller K. Sleep–wake rhythm in an irregular shift system. *J Sleep Res* 2003; 12: 103–12.
5 Weibel L, Spiegel K, Follenius M, Ehrhart J, Brandenberger G. Internal dissociation of the circadian markers of the cortisol rhythm in night workers. *Am J Physiol* 1996; 170: E608–13.
6 Sallinen M, Harma M, Akerstedt T, Rosa R, Lillqvist O. Promoting alertness with a short nap during a night shift. *J Sleep Res* 1998; 7: 240–7.
7 Garbarino S, Mascialino B, Penco MA, Squarcia S, Carlie F de, Nobili L, Beelke M, Cuomo G, Ferrillo F. Professional shift-work drivers who adopt prophylactic naps can reduce the risk of car accidents during night work. *Sleep* 2004; 27(7): 1295–302.
8 Purnell MT, Feyer A-M, Herbison GP. The impact of a nap opportunity during the night shift on the performance and alertness of 12-h shift workers. *J Sleep Res* 2002; 11: 219–27.
9 Burgess HJ, Sharkey KM, Eastman CI. Bright light, dark and melatonin can promote circadian adaptation in night shift workers. *Sleep Med Rev* 2002; 6(5): 407–20.

6 Excessive Daytime Sleepiness

Introduction

Sleepiness is a common and physiological event in certain circumstances such as while relaxing after a meal in the early afternoon. It can be difficult to differentiate a normal degree of sleepiness from a pathological degree of, or tendency towards, sleepiness or falling asleep. Excessive daytime sleepiness (EDS) is not a diagnosis, but only a symptom. Whether sleep occurs or wakefulness continues depends on the balance of the homeostatic and adaptive drives and the circadian rhythms. Each of these may be accentuated, diminished or modified in sleep disorders, but very often more than one of these aspects of sleep–wake control is disturbed.

The nature of sleepiness is probably similar whatever its cause. The subject is usually aware of feeling sleepy before sleep is entered, although subsequent recall of the degree of sleepiness varies considerably. Sleepiness can increase rapidly so that there is only a brief warning before sleep onset. 'Sleep attacks' of this type may occur in narcolepsy and Parkinsonism, particularly when this is treated by dopamine receptor agonist drugs.

Definitions

Subalertness

Consciousness is the awareness of oneself and the environment but its level ranges from extreme vigilance and alertness to the state of barely perceiving any stimulation. Subalertness is a state of diminished arousal rather than true sleepiness. It varies according to the phase of the circadian rhythm and the duration and quality of the previous sleep episode.

Hypersomnolence

This is an excessive sensation of sleepiness or drowsiness during the day but does not necessarily lead to sleep. It is similar to excessive daytime sleepiness. The term excessive sleepiness is preferable in some situations, since shift workers in particular need to be alert at night rather than during the day, which is when sleepiness is desired.

Sleep propensity

This is the ease with which sleep can be entered. It may be due to pathological sleepiness, but some subjects have a physiological sleepiness trait whereby they are able to fall asleep readily [1]. They have a short multiple sleep latency test on objective testing, and a normal level of alertness, and can resist sleep when this is not desired. This state may have a genetic basis, but can also be the result of training as in, for instance, soldiers who need to be able to sleep for short periods when they can.

Microsleeps

These are brief episodes of sleep, lasting only a few seconds. The subject may not have any recollection of falling asleep, but is usually aware of having been sleepy and of waking suddenly at the end of the microsleep.

Hypersomnia

This implies an increase in duration of sleep during each 24-h cycle. The patient may wake up late or go to sleep early in the evening and there may be frequent naps or a single main daytime sleep episode, usually in the afternoon. The sensation of sleepiness is usually but not invariably prominent, and sleep is easily entered.

Fatigue

Sleepiness should be distinguished from tiredness and fatigue. Tiredness may be either physical or mental and is also used to describe sleepiness. Tiredness is the state the subject feels that he or she is in, whereas fatigue is the inability to sustain an effort which may be emotional, mental or physical. Fatigue either leads to an increased effort or an aversion to continuing with the activity. Sleep does not necessarily improve fatigue, but normally relieves sleepiness.

Both tiredness and fatigue are subjective and difficult to quantify. Fatigue may be 'central' if it is due

Table 6.1 Causes of central and peripheral fatigue.

Central	Head injuries
	Parkinsonism
	Multiple sclerosis
	Cancer
	HIV
	Depression
	Chronic fatigue syndrome
Peripheral	Myasthenia gravis
Both	Post poliomyelitis syndrome

to abnormalities within the central nervous system, or 'peripheral' when it is the neuromuscular junction that is abnormal (Table 6.1). Central fatigue appears to be the result of abnormal relationships between the cerebral cortex and basal ganglia. The latter are involved not only with coordination and anticipation of movements, but also with processing sensory information. Lack of drive from the cerebral cortex to the basal ganglia or a failure of these to respond to cortical input probably leads to the sensation of excessive and increasing effort being required to carry out activities [2]. Abnormalities of dopamine and opioid (endorphin) transmitter systems may be involved. In the chronic fatigue syndrome the adrenal glands are small (in contrast to depression where they are hyperplastic) due to a reduction in ACTH production.

There are often psychological reactions to this fatigue if it persists. These include acceptance, particularly in the elderly, preoccupation, often leading to depression, or rationalization of the fatigue as a biological dysfunction due to an external agent.

The drug treatment of fatigue is unsatisfactory but modafinil 100–200 mg daily, amantadine, methylphenidate, dexamphetamine and antidepressants, especially amitriptyline, have been used.

Prevalence

Population surveys have indicated that EDS is associated with sleep deprivation, snoring and hypnotic use, and is commonest in young adults, shift workers and the elderly. Excessive daytime sleepiness has been documented to occur in around 5% of the adult population in developed countries, but the prevalence varies according to its definition.

Excessive daytime sleepiness forms a spectrum which merges with normality on the one hand and an inability to remain awake at all during the day at the other extreme. The usual duration of sleep is longer in infants and young children than in adults, but even in adult life some otherwise normal people have normal sleep architecture but require a long sleep duration to feel refreshed (long sleepers). They may fall into the conventional definition of hypersomnia because of the increase in their sleep requirements during each 24-h cycle. The degree of alertness or sleepiness also varies between individuals. Those who are habitually subalert may become significantly drowsy or fall asleep in response to minor events or changes in lifestyle that would not affect other people.

The methods for assessing the severity of daytime sleepiness have been described in Chapter 3, but many of the tests do not assess the subjective component of the symptom. The complaint of sleepiness is related to the expectations and requirements of each individual. In the elderly, who may be confined to their home, a degree of sleepiness during the day may not elicit a complaint of sleepiness, but in, for instance, a professional vehicle driver a similar degree of sleepiness would be intolerable. Patients also vary considerably in their ability to cope with a certain level of sleepiness. A complaint of EDS without any objective change in the quality or duration of sleep may be precipitated by stress within the family, or with friends or at work.

Effects of sleepiness

Neurophysiological effects

Sleepiness has widespread effects on the central nervous system, but most of the psychological and behavioural features reflect changes in the function of the prefrontal cortex. This integrates sensory information from multiple modalities and has close connections with the hippocampus and amygdala, which are concerned with memory and reward-seeking behaviour, as well as with the hypothalamus, which controls the autonomic nervous system. The prefrontal cortex is involved specifically with attention and perception, abstract thought, creative problem solving, executive function and temporal sequencing of behaviours. Its primary function is goal-directed behaviour, and lesions lead to a failure to integrate environmental and internal stimuli [3].

The dorsolateral region of the prefrontal cortex is completely inactivated during both stages 3 and 4 NREM and REM sleep, and it is likely that this area is also under-active during the state of sleepiness. The dorsolateral region has a greater sensory input than the orbitomedial prefrontal cortex. Its under-activity

Table 6.2 Consequences of excessive daytime sleepiness.

Psychological	Reduced alertness and attention
	Mood swings, irritability
	Loss of mental flexibility
	Hallucinations
Motor	Automatic behaviour
	Impaired physical performance
Social	Poor school and work performance
	Hyperactivity in children
	Impaired social interactions
	Accidents (travel, home, occupational)

leads to an inability to maintain attention, loss of cognitive function and of the ability to think abstractly. There is a reduction in motivation and verbal fluency, apathy and a reduction in physical activity, although social functioning is maintained. In contrast, underactivity of the orbitomedial prefrontal cortex, which receives input from the limbic system and projects particularly to the basal ganglia, leads to euphoria, hyperactivity, antisocial behaviour and disinhibition, for instance of the sexual drive.

Neuropsychological effects

The level of alertness falls, concentration deteriorates, and attention for prolonged monotonous tasks shortens (Table 6.2). The subject is usually distractible and mood changes, particularly irritability, are common. These deficits can be partially offset by an increased effort and by caffeine and other wakefulness promoting drugs.

Stereotyped behaviours with a loss of innovative responses to stimuli, a more limited vocabulary [4], and a loss of mental creativity and of flexibility of thought processes develop [5]. Working memory is reduced, probably because of active suppression in order to attempt to protect executive functioning. Word fluency is reduced with shorter sentences and preservation and repetition of statements is common. These changes probably involve active inhibition and suppression as well as a failure to generate recall of the appropriate words. There is a reduction in the ability to think abstractly and of verbal creativity. Planning and executive functions are impaired, thoughts are disorganized and there is a perception that it is difficult to think clearly. There may also be disinhibition of mood control, often with a loss of empathy, irritability and a feeling of suspicion. Psychosis is not a feature of sleepiness.

Hallucinations due to altered perceptions of reality or to intrusion of REM sleep into wakefulness may appear and there is a deterioration in short-term memory. Illusions are usually visual, but not auditory. There is also a reduction in the visual field and the ability to search the visual field for important features.

Presleep behaviour

Severe sleepiness requires an increased mental effort to maintain wakefulness, keep alert, concentrate and maintain attention. Intermittent restlessness, which may be a mechanism of increasing alertness, alternates with a vacant expression with little eye movement, infrequent blinking, drooping of the eyelids, head nodding, yawning and rubbing of the eyes. Simple motor tasks such as walking or driving may continue, but the response time to changes in environmental situations is prolonged with an increased risk of errors and accidents. The automatic behaviour of acute sleepiness is similar to that seen on waking from sleep (confusional arousals) and there is often poor or fragmented recollection with distorted perceptions of this presleep phase.

Microsleeps are brief episodes of sleep lasting 1–10 s. They are common and identifiable by a fixed gaze, absence of blinking and a blank facial expression. The subject may not have any recollection of falling asleep, but is usually aware of having been sleepy and of waking suddenly at the end of the microsleep.

Motor effects of sleepiness

Motor dysfunction includes a deterioration in physical performance, particularly for long or monotonous tasks, a sense of fatigue, lack of energy, weariness and episodes of automatic behaviour in which purposeful but inappropriate actions are performed in association with diminished vigilance and with subsequent amnesia (Table 6.2). Automatic behaviour of this type includes inappropriate actions such as putting sugar into a kettle, writing nonsense and missing motorway exits while driving. Speech becomes flat and monotonous with less intonation than usual.

When sleepiness is severe, dysarthria, tremor, ptosis, nystagmus and epileptic seizures may develop. The respiratory drive and probably respiratory muscle strength and endurance are reduced.

There are large inter-individual differences in the effects of sleep deprivation on performance. Complete lack of sleep is unsustainable, but many people can manage everyday activities with around 5 h sleep each night as long as they are motivated. An increased 'vulnerability' to sleep deprivation may be specific to certain types of performance [6]. It is uncertain whether 'vulnerability' is related to a lack of resilience and difficulty in coping with other types of stress.

There is a progressive performance decrement of around 25% if wakefulness is maintained continuously for 24 h, but 10% of this can be reversed by a 30-min nap. Deficits in attention and motivation can be improved by effort, caffeine and amphetamines. A loss of creative activity and word fluency cannot be compensated for in these ways, but may be at least partially reversed by modafinil [7].

Social and educational effects

Excessive daytime sleepiness can have a serious impact on family and social life, particularly if the patient's relatives and friends do not understand the sleep problem. Recreational activities may have to be curtailed or may become dangerous if the subject is excessively sleepy.

Children with excessive daytime sleepiness have difficulty in learning and often perform poorly at school and in examinations. They may develop secondary psychological responses such as hyperactivity or aggression which cause additional problems. Accidents in the home and during recreational activities are common, and these can be wide ranging if, for instance, they involve cooking or electrical appliances.

Occupational effects

Excessive daytime sleepiness causes difficulties with employment, since it may be interpreted as laziness, poor motivation or even drunkenness. The psychological and motor consequences of chronic excessive daytime sleepiness impair work performance, particularly at night or during shift work. Productivity may fall and decision making becomes slower with an increased number of errors. A study of Swedish gas meter readings showed that the greatest number of errors were made when they were read between 2.00 and 4.00 AM, and a second smaller peak was noted between 2.00 and 4.00 PM.

Sleepiness also contributes to occupational accidents [8] and working with heavy or moving machinery should be avoided. Accidents with milling machinery have been documented to increase by 25% during night shifts compared to an early morning shift, and doctors who have been working long hours or shifts tend to operate more slowly and may be prone to

errors. The extent to which this occurs depends on the personality of the individual and their ability to develop coping strategies, as well as on the degree of sleep deprivation.

The combination of poor productivity and accidents at work frequently leads to loss of employment or failure to be promoted and thereby to financial difficulties and depression.

Individual sleep-related accidents can have a major impact on society. In the Chernobyl nuclear plant incident, at 00.28 AM on 26 April 1986 the water circulation around the plant failed because of a stuck valve. This led to over-heating of the plant, but the staff were slow to become alert to the problem and to respond appropriately because of the long shifts that they had been working. The nuclear plant was close to meltdown before the fault was corrected. The population of eastern Europe was exposed to considerable radiation and the mean lifespan of men in the Ukraine fell from 74.5 to 63.4 years over the 5 years after this incident. A similar episode occurred at 4.00 AM in the Three Mile Island nuclear plant, in Pennsylvania, on 28 March 1989, and the failure to act appropriately was again associated with excessive daytime sleepiness due to shift work.

It is important that employers are aware of the risks of sleepiness and of the problems due to sleep deprivation. They have a duty of care to protect employees against foreseeable risks to their health and safety at work, due for instance to long working hours and shift work, and to take reasonable care with regard to these. This may involve increasing the flexibility of the workforce to cope with needs such as continuous running of processes and provision of services or on-call cover while maximizing utilization of machinery.

Counter-measures which may improve sleepiness at work and reduce the risk of problems developing include:

1 Reducing the workload and in particular the number of hours worked, and reviewing the timing of work.

2 Reviewing shift work patterns [9] and the need to travel, which may cause jet lag.

3 Reviewing work conditions, providing appropriate lighting, and ensuring that there is less noise and fewer distractions at work.

4 Changes in working patterns, such as working in teams of two or more to provide more supervision between 4.00 and 8.00 AM when sleepiness is most likely to be severe and to lead to errors or accidents.

5 Provision of facilities for napping at work [10, 11]. 'Nap rooms' are increasingly becoming available in the USA.

6 Provision of stress coping strategies and counselling.

7 Travel. Employers also have a duty of care to ensure that employees are able to travel home safely. Provision of facilities for sleeping after work or to transport employees home may be needed.

Sleepiness and transportation

Motor vehicle accidents

Size of the problem

The importance of motor vehicles has increased steadily during the last 100 years with the increasing emphasis on mobility both for work and social reasons. Comfort and speed of the vehicles have been the priorities and the safety of driving has been relatively neglected. In one survey, 25% of New York State drivers admitted to having fallen asleep at the wheel, particularly during long journeys at night after a lack of sleep. It is estimated that 1–3% of all road traffic accidents are due to driver drowsiness and perhaps 10% of serious accidents, and 20% of motorway accidents. The number of near misses is probably much greater. In the UK there are now more fatal accidents related to driver sleepiness than to driving with a blood alcohol concentration above the legal limit.

These accidents particularly involve males under the age of 30 who are driving alone, who appear to be poor at recognizing their degree of sleepiness. They are often involved in single-vehicle accidents and 40% are driving a commercial vehicle. Ninety per cent of sleep-related accidents at all ages involve male drivers [12].

Types of accident

It can be difficult to be certain whether an accident is due to drowsiness or not. Drowsiness is, however, likely to be at least a contributory factor in single-vehicle accidents occurring at night, particularly between 2.00 and 6.00 AM, since at this time there is least traffic on the roads, and between 2.00 and 4.00 PM (Fig. 6.1). These accidents are often fatal and 40% of them occur on motorways or on dual carriageways.

Pre-accident behaviour

The first observable sign of a sleepy driver is a change in speed due to intermittent loss of muscle activity in the leg controlling the accelerator. Shunting accidents

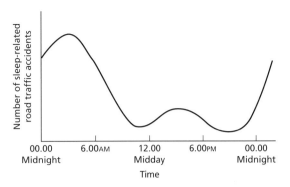

Fig. 6.1 Biphasic timing of accidents due to EDS.

at traffic lights or roundabouts are frequent, and it is common to weave or change lanes. If the driver veers off the road the vehicle may collide with an oncoming car or a static object. Articulated lorries may jackknife if the driver suddenly regains alertness after a lapse of concentration or a microsleep and over-reacts by making a sudden corrective steering action. This type of accident is most common on motorways early in the morning.

It is possible to drive for several miles while extremely drowsy or even lightly asleep. This type of automatic behaviour is characterized by a glazed expression, absence of blinking, reduced responsiveness to external stimuli and a loss of peripheral vision. Drivers are occasionally drawn towards lights or other features, for instance the rear of other vehicles, leading to fatal accidents. Microsleeps are common and awakening may occur without any recollection of having fallen asleep or of changing lanes before the accident, although awareness of being sleepy before the incident is usually retained.

Causes of accidents

Those who are chronically, mildly sleep deprived or have an undiagnosed sleep disorder are more vulnerable to additional acute episodes of sleep loss. Accidents are more common after working long hours before driving, and in those who drive frequently when they are drowsy [13]. There is also an increased risk while driving after working night shifts, which often end at around 7.00 AM. This is particularly important after the first night of shift work when the subject may have been awake for more than 24 h before attempting to drive home. The longer 12-h overnight shifts are more of a risk than shorter 8-h shifts. Employers have a duty of care to ensure that the employee is safe to drive home from work. A charge of corporate manslaughter may be brought if there is gross management negligence in this respect.

Commercial drivers are particularly at risk of sleep-related accidents [14] – 50% of accidents involving sleepiness are work related. In order to meet deadlines or make emergency deliveries journeys often occur at night, or involve shift work and long driving times. The comfortable cabs and power steering of modern large goods and passenger carrying vehicles make driving easier and less stimulating. Alertness falls after around 60 min driving and the mean duration of driving before a sleep-related accident is around 4 h. Many commercial drivers are obese due to the ready availability of junk food during their journeys and the sedentary nature of their job. This obesity predisposes to obstructive sleep apnoeas and increases the risk of sleep-related accidents.

The tachographs in heavy goods vehicles detect vehicle movement and give an indication of how long the vehicle has been driven. Nevertheless the driver may be awake at times between vehicle movements with the result that there may be severe sleep restriction and an increased risk of an accident. European Union regulations indicate that heavy goods vehicle (HGV) and bus drivers should not drive for more than 9 h continuously without a rest period in any 24 h, and for not more than 56 h each week. In general, HGV drivers cover 7–10 times the mileage of domestic drivers and often drive through the night when the risk of accidents is greatest. There are no regulations concerning taxi drivers' hours of work.

Medical causes of excessive daytime sleepiness are less frequent than social factors, but the presence of frequent obstructive sleep apnoeas increases the risk of motor vehicle accidents about sixfold [15, 16]. The risk increases as sleep fragmentation worsens. The accident rate in those with narcolepsy is lower, probably because they are well aware of their limitations and of the possibility of sleepiness while driving.

Drug-induced sleepiness

Some drugs help to reduce accident rates, for instance anticonvulsants for epilepsy, treatment for diabetes and antidepressants in certain situations.

Sedative drugs and alcohol accentuate sleepiness following sleep restriction and irregular sleeping patterns [17], particularly if they are taken when the circadian rhythms facilitate sleep (2.00–6.00 AM and 2.00–4.00 PM). The effect of one drink of alcohol at these times may be equivalent to two or three taken at 10.00 AM [18]. The risk of a sleep-related driving accid-

ent is three times greater in those taking hypnotics, such as benzodiazepines, and it is also increased with sedating tricyclic antidepressants. The effects of these drugs may exceed that of consumption of alcohol which is sufficient to raise the blood concentration above the legal limit of 0.8 g/l (80 mg/100 ml). Sedative drugs may impair vigilance, vision, coordination, cognitive function, the perception of risk and important aspects of memory such as anticipation of exits from motorways. Driving performance can be altered without drowsiness being apparent.

The effects of sedative medication on driving vary according to the specific drug, its timing and half-life, sleep-related factors, such as previous shift work or sleep deprivation, individual vulnerability, age and in some situations gender. The most important individual drugs are as follows.

1 *Benzodiazepines*. The main effect is sedation, but they can occasionally cause disinhibition and aggression. They impair cognitive function, reduce the appreciation of changes in conditions, and increase muscle relaxation. Benzodiazepines also interact with antidepressants, alcohol and antihistamines. Women appear to be more sensitive to the effects of benzodiazepines on driving performance than men, but the newer shorter-acting drugs related to benzodiazepines have less effect on driving. Zaleplon taken 10 h previously does not affect driving, although zopiclone may impair driving slightly in this situation.

2 *Barbiturates*. These cause sedation and occasionally aggression.

3 *Antidepressants*. The serotonin re-uptake inhibitor and related antidepressants have little or no sedative effect, except for trazodone, which has an antihistaminic action. Some of the tricyclic antidepressants can, however, cause sedation, including clomipramine.

4 *Opiates*, e.g. codeine. These cause sleepiness and often euphoria.

5 *Antihistamines*. These are present in a wide variety of medications, including many cough suppressants, and can cause prolonged sedation.

6 *Dopamine receptor agonists*. These have been reported to cause sudden 'sleep attacks', particularly in Parkinsonism. This may be a class effect, but pramipexole and ropinirole appear to cause this most frequently. The sleepiness is probably dose related and has only been reported in those with Parkinsonism, suggesting that it is at least partly due to the underlying disorder.

7 *Progesterone*. This is a constituent of the oral contraceptive pill and can have a hypnotic effect.

8 *Alcohol.* This leads to disinhibition as well as to sedation in higher doses.

9 *Cannabis.* This has a rapid onset of action which lasts for 2–6 h. It reduces attention, causes disinhibition, and impairs concentration and the perception of the environment. The driver may appear drunk as in alcoholic intoxication.

It is estimated that in France at present there are 45 million who drink alcohol, 2.2 million who take cannabis and 0.3 million who use opiates. Addiction to any of these drugs adds extra risks, since the driver is unable to control his or her consumption and remains at risk until the addiction is effectively treated. Withdrawal effects, which may be acute or last for several weeks or months, also impair driving.

The only drug for which a roadside test is available is alcohol, but various tests have been proposed to assess a driver's ability to drive safely. These include driving simulators [19], vigilance tests, divided attention tests, tracking tests, cognitive and perception tests, and reaction times, both simple and complex. None has proved satisfactory.

Despite wide-scale recognition of the problem there are very few prosecutions for driving with impaired performance because of drugs other than alcohol. Surveys have shown that between 10 and 20% of drivers test positive for alcohol, cannabis or other sedative drugs. The precautions indicated in the summary of product characteristics by the pharmaceutical industry often fail to adequately address the risks and the physician has a duty to inform the patient if there is a significant risk that the prescribed drug may impair driving and lead to an accident.

Accident prevention

Counter-measures to reduce the risk of a motor vehicle accident [20] due to sleepiness include:

1 Avoiding sleep deprivation and, if possible, shift work before driving, together with encouraging good sleep hygiene practices and a greater awareness of the problems of driving while sleepy.

2 Treat any underlying sleep disorder. Effective treatment of obstructive sleep apnoeas with nasal continuous positive airway pressure (CPAP) treatment reduces the risk of road traffic accidents [21].

3 If driving after sleep deprivation is unavoidable, it is best to nap for 15–30 min before starting driving and to take 50–100 mg caffeine [22]. This has a stimulant effect within 15–30 min. Activities such as keeping the car windows open and playing music may have a brief beneficial stimulant action, but can encourage sleepiness in some people.

4 It is essential to stop driving before sleepiness becomes marked and it is probably those drivers who ignore this warning symptom who are most likely to be involved in fatal accidents.

5 Road design. The design of roads has a large influence on the frequency of sleep-related accidents. Accident blackspots on motorways are usually due to a combination of a previous monotonous stretch of driving, coupled with a complex junction or slip road system. Warning signs on motorways alerting drivers to be aware of sleepiness and the provision of laybys on major roads, so that drivers can stop to sleep, should be encouraged. Ridged surfaces (rumble strips) are effective in alerting drivers to a lane change and have significantly reduced accident rates.

6 Detection of driver's sleepiness. Equipment to detect the driver's blink rate or eye closure, which then alerts the driver, has been introduced, but is unlikely to be effective since accidents frequently occur before these signs develop. It is preferable to stop driving at the onset of sleepiness rather than to wait until this late stage before attempting to detect it.

7 Increase public awareness. Prevention of sleep-related motor vehicle accidents involves increasing public awareness and altering public policies regarding roads and driving.

8 Medical care. The physician has a role in educating patients about the risks of driving while sleepy, in diagnosing any underlying sleep disorder, in giving sleep hygiene advice, especially for shift workers, and in assessing whether or not the patient is fit to drive. This decision is influenced not only by the degree of sleepiness, but also by the presence of any underlying sleep disorder and the distance that is usually driven and the time of day. The doctor has a duty to inform the patient that he or she should notify the Driver and Vehicle Licensing Agency (DVLA) and the driver's insurance company of any sleep disorder that may impair the ability to drive. It is not the doctor's role to make these notifications except in exceptional circumstances when the duty to society as a whole may outweigh the duty of confidentiality to the individual patient because of a substantial risk from an accident and the patient's unwillingness or inability to notify the authorities.

9 Driver licensing. Legislation has to balance the costs to society of the dangers while driving against the loss of individual liberty, including for instance the loss of employment if driving is prevented. There

are wide international variations in the regulations and criteria for revoking driving licences.

The DVLA are responsible for identifying drivers with sleep disorders who are likely to be a source of danger while driving. 'Likely' in this sense is interpreted as 'more than a bare possibility'. The DVLA do not require notification of EDS due to poor sleep hygiene, sleep deprivation, shift work or sedative medication. The patient has a legal duty to report narcolepsy, irrespective of the extent of any perceived difficulty with driving. Approximately 2500 patients with obstructive sleep apnoeas and 300 with narcolepsy are identified each year in the UK. This is probably considerably fewer than the total number that are diagnosed with these conditions.

Medical disorders which affect the ability to drive may require a report from the doctor caring for the patient before a licence is issued, whether it is for a restricted period, such as 1–3 years before being reviewed, or for a longer period. In general, the licence is usually retained in those with obstructive sleep apnoeas if these are satisfactorily controlled with nasal continuous positive airway pressure (CPAP) for around 3 months and if there is satisfactory compliance with treatment.

The DVLA do not continue to supervise drivers with obstructive sleep apnoeas who have Group 1 licences (vehicles less than 3.5 tonnes), but those with Group 2 licences (vehicles weighing more than 3.5 tonnes or with more than eight passenger seats) require annual assessment for at least 2 years to establish whether improvement with CPAP has been maintained. Treatment of excessive daytime sleepiness and cataplexy in narcolepsy usually enables the licence to be retained for a limited period.

Falling asleep while driving is not a defence in law by itself and is regarded as evidence of a lack of due care and attention. The act of falling asleep is in effect a self-induced automatism (page 197) for which the subject is considered guilty. The driver has a duty of care not to drive while sleepy, whatever the cause of the sleepiness may be.

The law assumes that there is adequate warning of sufficient sleepiness that might cause lapses of attention or sleep to be entered. The ability to recall the sleepiness before the accident is often denied, particularly by younger drivers, but is not a defence since it is felt that sleepiness would have been recognizable at the time, even if it is not later recalled. Driving while under the influence of sedative medication, even if it is medically prescribed, is not a defence.

Driving while sleepy is well documented in arousal disorders, such as sleep walking, but the defendant has to demonstrate that the episode involved an automatism, which is distinct from simply feeling sleepy or having microsleeps while driving. Driving without any awareness of the surroundings is normal if the mind is preoccupied, and is distinct from driving while sleepy or during an automatism.

Sea and rail travel accidents

The combination of shift work, comfortable cabins or similar areas for controlling the mode of transport, and the reduction in the number of staff on each shift have all contributed to the increased risk of accidents. The Exxon Valdez disaster on 25 March 1989, in which the oil tanker hit a reef off the Alaska coast and released 240 000 barrels of oil, was related to the captain being asleep and a third mate being left to navigate difficult waters. His long shift at night caused his tiredness which contributed to the accident in the early hours. Similarly, in the Sante Fe rail accident in 1990, all the crew were asleep at the time of the accident and $4.4 million of damages were paid.

Aviation accidents

Awareness of the risks of flying while tired surfaced after Charles Lindbergh's flight from New York to Paris in 1927 which involved him being awake for 24 h beforehand and 33.5 h during the flight. Investigation into the crash of flight US2860 at 02.38 AM on 18 December 1977 near Salt Lake City revealed that this was due to flight-crew fatigue, coupled with inadequate advice from an air traffic controller who was also sleep deprived. The pilot's reliance on automatic controls, which makes flying more monotonous, and the possibility of jet lag and sleep deprivation all contribute to the risk of this type of accident. Surveys in the past have indicated that 75% of pilots have fallen asleep briefly in the cockpit, but aviation authorities now take pilot sleepiness into consideration when planning long-haul flights.

Long-haul flights often cross time zones and lead to sleep deprivation, particularly when flying at night, and from west to east. Short-haul flights occur during the day and have little time zone effect. Flight schedules should be designed to maximize the amount of flying time occurring while the circadian rhythm is promoting wakefulness rather than sleep, and should allow for sleep deprivation after a series of long-haul flights. Brief naps may be taken during the flight while the co-pilot is awake in order to avoid sleepiness and to minimize the risk of sleep inertia.

Time zone changes are less easily adapted to by older pilots. Hypnotics are not allowed during flight, but are often taken before and after flights because of difficulty in sleeping in the new environment against the tendency of the circadian rhythms.

Space travel accidents

Frequent brief naps may partially offset the erratic sleep schedules and sleep restriction of space travel, but it was sleep deprivation of the managers at National Aeronautics and Space Administration (NASA) which appears to have led to the error in the timing of the launch of the Challenger space shuttle that contributed to its explosion.

Causes of excessive daytime sleepiness

There are many individual causes of excessive daytime sleepiness, but they can be grouped into three main categories.

Insufficient duration of sleep (sleep deprivation, restriction)

Sleep deprivation is the commonest cause of sleepiness and is usually due to social or work pressures arising from the conflict between the need to complete various activities and to obtain sufficient sleep. There is pressure in westernized societies to carry out an increasing variety of activities during wakefulness, and the expectation that these can be achieved tends to push sleep into the background. Sleep can seem a semi-expendable commodity which is to be fitted around apparently more important events. Increasing social and recreational activities, shopping outside normal daylight hours, the need to work shifts, and to communicate across time zones for business purposes, computer and internet activities, travel related to, for instance, employment in transportation, and the need to continuously provide emergency and medical services have all contributed to the development of a '24 hour' or '24/7' society. The possibility of carrying out many of these activities at any time has enabled them to take priority over obtaining sufficient sleep.

The timing as well as the duration of duties at work also impact on the ability to obtain sufficient sleep. Shift work, for instance, leads to considerable disruption of sleep–wake patterns. Cultural influences have a similar effect. In cold climates it is usual to go to sleep earlier and to wake up later than in hotter areas. In some Mediterranean countries an afternoon siesta is taken, which coincides with the normal 2.00–4.00 PM phase of increased drowsiness. In these societies it is usual to stay awake until later at night. This pattern makes difficulty initiating sleep less apparent than in colder climates, but conversely the advanced sleep phase syndrome would be more obvious than in colder climates where an earlier sleep onset is usual.

The development of artificial light sources has enabled the 24-h society to develop. The increased noise level caused by activities at night, such as driving, also hinders sleep, particularly in urban societies. The 24-h society has also had an impact on other time givers for sleep, such as meals, exercise and social activities, so that the endogenous circadian rhythms increasingly conflict with the often rapidly changing external factors that control sleep. These effects are magnified by any pre-existing insomnia, excessive daytime sleepiness or restriction of sleep duration.

A careful history should elicit the nature and extent of sleep deprivation and the reasons for this. It is important to discuss methods of altering the balance between daytime activities and sleep in favour of the latter. Constraints, such as fixed working hours, may be difficult to change, but advice about regularity of sleep times and earlier onset of sleep, planning of naps during the day to compensate for sleep restriction at night, improving the sleep environment in order to maximize the quality of sleep, avoiding stimulant drugs such as caffeine in the evening, and other aspects of sleep hygiene, such as taking exercise during the day to increase alertness, may all be of value. It is ultimately the responsibility of each individual to select his or her own combination of sleep and wakefulness by choosing between the opportunities that present themselves every day.

Impaired quality of sleep (sleep fragmentation)

This is the failure to sustain sleep or a stage of sleep because of frequent transitions to a lighter stage of sleep or to wakefulness. The time spent in bed and the duration from the start to the end of the sleep period may be normal, but continuity of sleep is broken. Fragmentation of stages 2–4 NREM sleep appears to be particularly important in leading to EDS, but it is not known how much this is influenced by the duration of each arousal or whether there is a minimum length of sleep between arousals which is required to retain the refreshing function of sleep.

Sleep fragmentation may be due to one or more of the following factors.

1 External factors. These may be a noisy, light, hot or cold sleep environment, or an uncomfortable bed. These problems should be corrected.

2 Conditions which only appear during sleep. This important group of disorders includes obstructive and central sleep apnoeas (see Chapters 10 and 11), periodic limb movements in sleep (see Chapter 9) and occasionally other motor disorders during sleep if they occur frequently. The history and examination may need to be supplemented by blood gas analysis and a sleep study, usually polysomnography, to confirm the diagnosis and to assess the severity of these disorders.

3 Medical disorders which are exacerbated by sleep. These include gastro-oesophageal reflux, nocturnal angina and asthma (see Chapter 12). Patients often present with the primary symptom of the disorder, but EDS can be significant. The history should be supplemented by relevant investigations.

4 Symptoms that are largely unrelated to sleep. These include pain and discomfort due to rheumatoid arthritis or other types of arthritis and neurological diseases such as Parkinsonism and multiple sclerosis. These symptoms require appropriate investigation and treatment of their cause, together with analgesic and other symptomatic treatment and modification of the sleep environment and sleeping position.

5 Drugs may fragment sleep through several different mechanisms. Stimulant drugs such as caffeine and amphetamines cause frequent sleep-stage shifts and arousals. Tricyclic antidepressants may increase the frequency of periodic limb movements, and drugs such as dopamine agonists may cause awakening due to vivid dreams. Alcohol and short-acting hypnotics cause rebound insomnia at the end of the night, and other drugs cause side-effects which may develop during sleep leading to frequent arousals and awakenings.

Hypersomnias

Hypersomnias are characterized by unrefreshing sleep at night leading to a prolonged nocturnal sleep episode or the need to sleep during the day. They are the result of intrinsic abnormalities of sleep–wake function. The most typical example is idiopathic hypersomnia. Narcolepsy is usually included in this group because of the unrefreshing nature of nocturnal sleep and the need to nap during the day, but unlike true hypersomnias the total sleep time during each 24-h period is hardly increased because the time spent awake at night almost matches the time spent asleep during the day.

Narcolepsy is primarily a REM sleep disorder but most of the other hypersomnias lead to an increase in NREM sleep. Little is known about the mechanisms underlying the need to sleep for prolonged periods, but they probably involve primarily the homeostatic sleep drive, and this may lead to secondary changes in the adaptive drive to sleep.

A wide range of disorders can cause hypersomnias (Fig. 6.2), but a similar clinical picture can result from drug administration and withdrawal (Table 6.3). A careful drug history should always be taken. Blood and urine tests are indicated if there is doubt about whether the drug has been taken or if a combination of drugs may be contributing to EDS. The need for each drug should be reassessed and if necessary the drug should be changed to a non-sedating alternative.

Drug-induced anaesthesia has some similarities to sleep in that the sleep debt appears to dissipate during a general anaesthetic, and similar regions of the brain are influenced by the drugs and sleep [23]. Anaesthesia is not, however, spontaneous or reversible with external stimuli and no distinct electroencephalogram stages are apparent. The duration and depth of the anaesthetic are proportional to the dose and type of the drug and not related to the influence of the sleep–wake control systems. Anaesthetic agents probably act on multiple neurotransmitters, particularly to facilitate GABA and adenosine activity.

Table 6.3 Sedative drugs which cause excessive daytime sleepiness.

Hypnotics
Antipsychotics
Antidepressants, especially MAOIs and tricyclics
Anticonvulsants
Alpha-agonists, e.g. clonidine, methyldopa
Alpha-blockers, e.g. prazosin, indoramim
Antihistamines (older drugs, e.g. chlorpheniramine)
Melatonin (slight effect)
Withdrawal of amphetamines and related drugs

MAOIs, monoamine oxidase inhibitors.

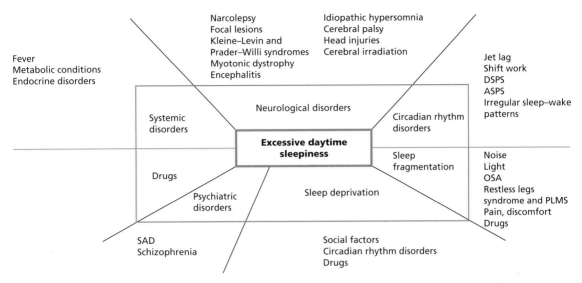

Fig. 6.2 Causes of excessive daytime sleepiness (EDS). ASPS, advanced sleep phase syndrome; DSPS, delayed sleep phase syndrome; OSA, obstructive sleep apnoeas; PLMS, periodic limb movements in sleep; SAD, seasonal affective disorder.

Effects of sleep deprivation and sleep fragmentation

Effects on sleep

Intermittent sleep deprivation leads to a short sleep latency, increased total sleep time and rebound increase in NREM sleep, particularly stages 3 and 4, on the next night and a subsequent rebound increase in the duration of REM sleep on the following night. If sleep deprivation is chronic and only around 3 h sleep is achieved each night the duration of stages 3 and 4 NREM sleep is maintained at approximately normal levels with a reduction in stages 1 and 2 NREM and REM sleep to around 50% of normal. Sleep deprivation increases the frequency of theta and alpha waves, particularly in the frontal region, and reduces sleep spindle frequency. It increases slow-wave activity, especially in the frontal region, but also in the central and parietal regions, but has little effect on occipital slow waves.

Selective NREM or REM sleep deprivation is very difficult to achieve even under experimental conditions because of rebound of whichever state of sleep is restricted. In general, however, REM sleep deprivation occurs particularly with an early wake-up time since REM sleep is concentrated towards the end of the night. NREM sleep restriction can be induced either by a later sleep onset time or a reduction in total sleep time.

NREM sleep restriction leads predominantly to defects of attention, although simple psychomotor tasks and actions may be maintained. REM sleep deprivation probably causes more disorganization of thoughts and impairment of memory. REM sleep disruption may increase appetite and REM sleep deprivation improves depression, leads to mania and in animals may increase sexual activity. Chronic sleep restriction is an effective treatment for primary insomnia.

Autonomic effects

Sleep deprivation increases the sympathetic activity during wakefulness. This raises the heart rate, reduces the inter-beat variability and raises the blood pressure, probably through causing systemic vasoconstriction [24]. This, together with the metabolic and endocrine consequences of sleep deprivation, may be responsible for the reduced life expectancy and possible increase in myocardial infarction associated with a short sleep duration.

Metabolic and endocrine effects

Both acute and chronic sleep deprivation impair glucose tolerance during wakefulness. Sleep deprivation alters glucose uptake in the cell membrane and cytoplasm. It also reduces the initial insulin response to glucose, probably because of increased sympathetic activity which regulates pancreatic beta cell function and insulin release. There may also be effects on the later increase in plasma insulin because of impaired synthesis of insulin in response to a raised blood glucose level.

Impaired glucose tolerance is also due to other endocrine responses to sleep deprivation. First the hypothalamic pituitary adrenal axis is activated with a rise in cortisol secretion early in the night, as is seen in depression and with ageing. There is a reduction in prolactin secretion and a loss of the circadian rhythm and quantity secreted of TSH. Sleep fragmentation reduces growth hormone secretion during the initial NREM sleep cycle, although there is some compensatory increase in secretion during wakefulness. This effect on growth hormone and the autonomic abnormalities both reduce lipolysis.

The peak level of leptin, which is produced by fat cells, is normally seen at around 9.00 PM. In sleep deprivation less leptin is secreted. There is a smaller diurnal amplitude in its secretion, particularly in those who are obese and have a high initial leptin level. The findings are similar to those seen in the elderly. Ghrelin, released by the stomach, has opposite effects to leptin, and its secretion increases by around 25% in sleep deprivation.

The lack of leptin and increase in ghrelin reduce the sensation of satiety and increase hunger and appetite, with an increase particularly for carbohydrate and fatty foods. Sleep deprivation in effect leads to an internal misperception of body fat and other energy stores, leading to increased energy intake coupled with an impaired ability to utilize the absorbed carbohydrates and fats. The insulin resistance due to sleep deprivation further increases the risk of diabetes and is associated with an increased triglyceride level and reduced high-density lipoproteins (HDL). These features, together with hypertension, constitute the 'metabolic syndrome'.

Immunological effects

Acute sleep restriction reduces antibody production, for instance in response to influenza immunization, but also increases inflammatory mediators such as cytokines, including IL-6 and C reactive protein (CRP), which is a predictor of cardiovascular morbidity. Sleep deprivation increases the white blood count, reduces the production of interferon and increases the natural killer (NK) lymphocyte activity [25] and phagocytic activity. It may increase the frequency of infections. Sleep deprivation also affects melatonin secretion which influences immunological function.

Excessive daytime sleepiness in children

Excessive daytime sleepiness in children is usually manifested not by a tendency to sleep, but by 'paradoxical' hyperactivity, impulsiveness and lack of concentration. It leads to emotional lability, frustration and disinhibition, shown by aggression and cognitive impairment, such as changes in mood and inattention. Failure to cope with school work and to develop friendships is common. Sleep deprivation also leads to failure to thrive with lack of growth.

The causes of excessive daytime sleepiness in children (Table 6.4) include narcolepsy, restless legs syndrome, and periodic limb movements in sleep, circadian rhythm disorders, sleep apnoeas, medical and psychiatric disorders, especially depression, drug abuse, the Kleine–Levin syndrome and sleep deprivation.

Excessive daytime sleepiness in the elderly

This may be due to sleep deprivation, but sleep fragmentation due to age-related sleep disorders is particularly important. These include:

1 Restless legs syndrome and periodic limb movements in sleep.
2 Obstructive sleep apnoeas. These are less closely related to the presence of obesity than in younger subjects, and while the familial tendency persists in old age, the male to female ratio falls to approximately 1.5 : 1. The impact of obstructive sleep apnoeas in the elderly may be less than in younger subjects and is difficult to assess because of the presence of other comorbidities, but they can lead to neuropsychological consequences.
3 Central sleep apnoeas. These are more common in the elderly because of the increased prevalence of cardiovascular and central nervous system disorders.
4 Sedative medication. Sedation with, for instance, benzodiazepines is more common than in younger subjects, but other drugs such as olanzapine and sedating antidepressants are also important.

Assessment

The most important points to establish when assessing excessive daytime sleepiness are whether the sleepiness is physiological or pathological, its severity, its impact on the patient's lifestyle and its cause. These issues may be difficult to evaluate because of the normal changes in sleepiness with age and environmental factors that may promote sleep or wakefulness. The cause of excessive daytime sleepiness is often multifactorial and if it fails to improve with treatment the process of assessment should be reconsidered.

History

A careful history is essential in assessing excessive daytime sleepiness accurately (Table 6.5; see Chapter 3). The following issues should be considered.

Table 6.4 Age and excessive daytime sleepiness.
ASPS, advanced sleep phase syndrome; CNS, central nervous system; DSPS, delayed sleep phase syndrome; OSA, obstructive sleep apnoeas; PLMS, periodic limb movements in sleep.

Childhood	Adolescence	Young and middle-aged adults	Old age
		Sleep deprivation	
	Drugs		
			ASPS
	DSPS		
		Shift work	
		OSA	
			PLMS
			Pain and discomfort
		Narcolepsy	
		Idiopathic hypersomnia	
		Focal CNS lesions	
	Kleine–Levin syndrome		
	Prader–Willi syndrome		
	Myotonic dystrophy		
Cerebral palsy			
		Head injury	
	Encephalitis		
		Cerebral irradiation	
	Psychiatric disorders		
	Metabolic and endocrine disorders		

Nature of excessive daytime sleepiness

Drowsiness and subalertness should be distinguished from similar symptoms such as fatigue. It should be established whether the subject is sleeping for more than the normal length of time during each 24-h cycle and the distribution of sleep during the day and night. Microsleeps during the day are characteristic of sleep deprivation, whereas refreshing naps of 5–30 min are usual in narcolepsy, and longer, less refreshing naps are characteristic of idiopathic hypersomnia.

Severity of excessive daytime sleepiness and its impact on lifestyle

This can be gauged by whether sleep occurs in situations in which a passive role is adopted or whether it extends into more active situations such as holding a conversation. Drowsiness, microsleeps or sleepiness while driving and deteriorating concentration with mood lability and irritability should be enquired about. Automatic behaviour is a feature of severe excessive daytime sleepiness.

The effects of excessive daytime sleepiness on the patient and his or her family, friends and colleagues at work, any accidents it has caused with moving machinery or while driving, and its influence on performance at school and work should be ascertained.

Causes of excessive daytime sleepiness

Questions should be asked regarding:
1 Sleep hygiene, especially the duration and regularity of sleep times.
2 Drugs, such as sedatives, analgesics or antidepressants.
3 Causes of sleep fragmentation, such as obstructive sleep apnoeas, periodic limb movements in sleep, asthma, pain or discomfort at night.
4 REM sleep-related symptoms might indicate narcolepsy or a similar disorder.

Table 6.5 Differential diagnosis of sleepiness.

	Characteristics	Causes
Physical tiredness	Sensation of fatigue or weariness	Organic illness and, less prominently with sleep deprivation, insomnia, and chronic fatigue syndrome or prolonged or intense exertion
Mental fatigue	Lack of attention	Depression
	Short concentration span	Chronic fatigue syndrome
	Difficulty in assimilating information	Sleep deprivation
Boredom	Loss of interest in immediate surroundings which lowers the threshold for sleep	Sleepiness predisposes but is not the cause
Automatic behaviour	Subalertness with poor motor control (ataxia) and complex but inappropriate actions	Any cause of sleepiness with entry into stages 1 and 2 NREM sleep
Confusional arousal (sleep drunkenness)	As for automatic behaviour, often with mental slowness and confusion	Partial arousal from sleep especially stages 3 and 4 NREM sleep
Hypnosis	A state of increased suggestibility	Occurs with EEG features of wakefulness not sleep
Meditation	A state of altered awareness	Dissociation of level of consciousness from reflex control
Fugue states	Amnesia with episodes of wandering	Psychogenic (hysterical), often precipitated by stress or depression
		Epilepsy, brief episodes often with other complex motor activities
Catalepsy	Prolonged maintenance of unusual postures	Hysteria: apparent unrousability but with EEG features of wakefulness
		Catatonia
Catatonia	Catalepsy with increased muscle tone and purposeless motor activity	Affective disorders, schizophrenia, metabolic disorders, drugs
		Organic brain damage
Confusion	Alertness with disorientation for time, place or person	Diffuse cerebral disorders, e.g. dementia
		Infection
		Metabolic disorders
		Drug effects and withdrawal
Delirium (toxic confusional state)	Confusion with restlessness and over-activity	As for confusion
Stupor	Unconsciousness and physical inactivity, but rousable to make brief verbal responses	As for coma
	Merges into coma	
Coma	Unconsciousness, not readily reversible	Diffuse bilateral cerebral cortical damage, e.g. encephalitis, head injury
	Responds reflexly but not with speech	Upper brainstem lesions
	Regular EEG slow-wave activity, but not influenced by external stimuli	Metabolic disorders
		Drugs
Persistent vegetative state (PVS)	Unresponsive and unaware of surroundings	Extensive cerebral cortical damage
	No communication	
	A few simple movements	
Akinetic mutism	Involuntary movements, except of eyes	Extensive brain damage, especially to reticular activating system
	Some sleep–wake rhythms detectable	
Locked-in syndrome	Conscious and aware of surroundings	Pontine lesions with intact midbrain and cerebral cortex
	Able to see and hear but paralysed except for vertical eye movements and blinking	
	NREM and REM sleep alternate with wakefulness	
General anaesthesia	Reduced awareness and, to a variable extent, memory, pain and movements	Chemical agents with widespread CNS effects, in some cases affecting sleep control mechanisms
	Arousability brief and incomplete	

CNS, central nervous system; EEG, electroencephalogram; NREM, non-rapid eye movement; REM, rapid eye movement.

Table 6.6 Role of investigations in diagnosis of excessive daytime sleepiness.

Diagnosis	Investigation
Sleep deprivation	Sleep diary, PSG Actigraphy
Sleep fragmentation	Respiratory monitoring for OSA Arterial blood gases for ventilatory failure Polysomnography for PLMS or occasionally for other causes
Circadian rhythm disorders	Sleep diary Actigraphy 24-h temperature monitoring Diurnal cortisol secretion Melatonin profile
Neurological disorders	Narcolepsy: HLA type, PSG, MSLTs Idiopathic hypersomnia, PSG to exclude other causes Focal lesions – head MRI or CT scan Prader–Willi syndrome: respiratory sleep study
Psychiatric disorders	Nil
Systemic disorders	Metabolic and endocrine investigations
Drugs	Blood and urine drug levels

CT, computerized tomography; HLA, human leucocyte antigen; MSLTs, multiple sleep latency tests; MRI, magnetic resonance imaging; OSA, obstructive sleep apnoeas; PLMS, periodic limb movements in sleep; PSG, polysomnography.

5 Neurological problems such as a previous head injury or encephalitis and current neurological symptoms that might indicate a focal lesion.
6 Systemic disorders, e.g. hypothyroidism.

Physical examination

Physical examination is often unrewarding, but an impression of the subject's mental state and level of alertness is important. Abnormalities of the upper airway and obesity which might be related to obstructive sleep apnoeas should be sought. Examination of the nervous system is only indicated if a neurological cause is being considered.

Investigations

Further investigation is not required if the history and examination provide sufficient information for the cause and severity of the excessive daytime sleepiness to be established, and for treatment to be initiated. Disorders of sleep hygiene, including a suboptimal sleep environment, drug-related problems and systemic disorders such as hypothyroidism, can usually be managed without referral to a specialist centre, but in most other situations this is required for further investigations to be carried out (Table 6.6). These are discussed below.

Sleep study

The complexity of the sleep study varies according to the suspected diagnosis. If obstructive sleep apnoea is most likely, an oximetry study may be sufficient on its own, or combined with measurement of airflow and abdominal and rib cage movement. In most other situations polysomnography is needed to give information about sleep architecture, arousals, sleep-onset REM, and the cause of arousals from sleep, such as periodic limb movements in sleep, central sleep apnoeas or gastro-oesophageal reflux. Serial sleep studies may be required to monitor progress with treatment.

Assessment of severity of excessive daytime sleepiness

This can be carried out with the tests described in Chapter 3, including the Epworth Sleepiness Scale and multiple sleep latency tests, which also demonstrate the sleep-onset REM Sleep characteristic of narcolepsy.

Investigation of the cause of excessive daytime sleepiness

1 Imaging techniques, e.g. computerized tomography (CT) and magnetic resonance imaging (MRI) scans of the brain to detect organic neurological disorders.
2 Human leucocyte antigen (HLA) typing, which is of use in narcolepsy.
3 Arterial blood gases, to assess ventilatory failure.
4 Cerebrospinal fluid hypocretin concentration to diagnose narcolepsy.

Principles of treatment

The aims of treatment (Fig. 6.3) are described below.

Assist adaptation

The nature of the disorder should be explained and advice should be given about lifestyle modifications to assist in managing any residual excessive daytime sleepiness despite optimal treatment. This may include coping strategies, and advice about when to take naps and how to plan activities around episodes of sleepiness and driving. Explanation and reassurance about the nature of the condition to family, friends, school teachers, employers and colleagues at work may be helpful.

Optimize sleep hygiene

This is almost invariably an important aspect of the management of excessive daytime sleepiness. It entails:
1 altering the sleep environment so that the bed is comfortable and the bedroom warm, dark and quiet;
2 improving sleep–wake patterns, increasing physical activity, and light exposure during the day, regularizing sleep and wake times and avoiding daytime naps.

Treat the underlying cause

Disorders such as obstructive sleep apnoea, periodic limb movements in sleep, hypothyroidism, gastro-oesophageal reflux and nocturnal asthma may all be amenable to treatment. Treatment of circadian rhythm disorders is described in Chapter 5.

Optimize drug treatment

Hypnotics

It is important to avoid sedatives and hypnotics such as alcohol, benzodiazepines and opiate analgesics if possible.

Central nervous system stimulants and wakefulness promoting drugs

These should be considered once all the above measures have been implemented and if any residual excessive daytime sleepiness is sufficiently severe to have a significant impact on the subject's life, for instance by interfering with the ability to cope with interpersonal relationships, family responsibilities, driving or at work. The issues that should be addressed when choosing a stimulant preparation are as follows.
1 Effectiveness. The ability to convert sleepiness to wakefulness and the level of alertness that can be achieved vary.
2 Duration of action. Short-acting drugs are less likely to cause insomnia, unless they are taken late in the day, but are more likely to cause the level of alertness to fluctuate.
3 Specificity for sleep–wake actions. Stimulant preparations, such as dexamphetamine, may affect mental function, changing the ability to perform complex mental tasks and causing emotional changes with

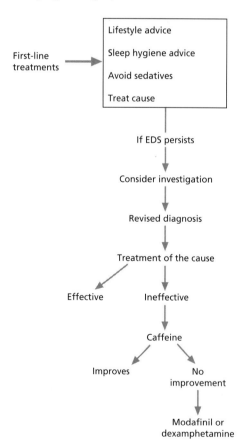

Fig. 6.3 Management of excessive daytime sleepiness.

euphoria, irritability or occasionally a psychosis. Motor hyperactivity, muscle tremor, autonomic effects such as sweating and palpitations, and sensory changes, including hallucinations, may appear.

4 Side-effects. These and the toxic : therapeutic ratio vary between individual stimulant drugs.

5 Drug interactions.

6 Potential for dependency.

7 Tolerance to therapeutic effects.

Caffeine is the usual first-line mild stimulant for excessive daytime sleepiness, and is often taken in tea, coffee, cola or 'energy' drinks, or as caffeine tablets. Nicotine is a stimulant in high doses and has a useful alerting effect. If excessive daytime sleepiness is more severe, modafinil should be considered before amphetamines and related drugs. It has a more specific sleep-promoting action with fewer central or peripheral nervous system stimulant effects. Side-effects and drug interactions are uncommon and it has little potential for dependency. It has a more gradual onset and a longer duration of action than dexamphetamine, but lacks the 'lift' that amphetamines give. It is as effective as dexamphetamine as a wakefulness promoting drug, but should not be taken late in the day since its long duration of action may lead to insomnia.

Amphetamines and related drugs should be reserved for those in whom modafinil is ineffective or for occasional patients who develop side-effects with modafinil. Those who have been established on dexamphetamine or similar drugs, but who have side-effects or who have developed other management problems, should be considered for transfer to modafinil, but this is not required for those who are effectively treated with amphetamines and do not have problems with them. The combination of modafinil and dexamphetamine may be required and can provide the peaks of alertness due to the amphetamine on the background of wakefulness due to the modafinil.

Circadian rhythm disorders

These may cause either EDS or insomnia, or both (see Chapter 5).

Narcolepsy (narcoleptic syndrome)

Overview

The term narcolepsy was for many years used almost synonymously with the symptom of EDS, but it now implies a specific disorder of REM sleep which has various manifestations both during sleep and during wakefulness. Sleep–wake control is destabilized so that there are frequent awakenings at night and episodes of sleep during the day. Loss of muscle tone, which is a feature of REM sleep, occurs during wakefulness as sleep paralysis or cataplexy. Abnormally vivid dreams occur during sleep and the same processes are responsible for visual, auditory and other types of sensory hallucinations during drowsiness or falling asleep after waking up, and occasionally while fully awake.

Occurrence

The prevalence of narcolepsy is around one in 2000–3000 people in most societies, with an annual incidence of one in 70 000. It is least frequent in Israeli Jews and most common in Japanese, although the clinical features and disease severity appear to be similar in all populations. In the UK there are an estimated 20 000 people with narcolepsy of whom 80% are currently untreated and most of these are undiagnosed.

Narcolepsy is equally common in males and females. It occasionally appears before the age of 5 years, develops before the age of 10 years in around 10%, and in one-third the first symptom is present before the age of 15 years. The most frequent age of onset is 20–40 years and it is unusual for it to appear after the age of 55.

Patients with narcolepsy often give a family history of EDS, but in only around 10% is there a relative with narcolepsy. The chance of this being a first-degree relative is increased 20 to 40 times to 1–2%. The risk of a child of a narcoleptic having the disease is around 1%. Twin studies have been inconclusive, but there is a concordance of 30% with identical twins. The familial tendency to narcolepsy probably has a polygenic basis [26].

Narcolepsy may appear during pregnancy, but usually persists after the birth of the child.

Pathogenesis

Sleep control

Narcolepsy is primarily a disorder of the control and structure of REM sleep, but NREM sleep and wakefulness may also be abnormal. It can be regarded as a tendency to a mixed sleep–wake state or as a sleep state boundary control disorder in which REM sleep intrudes into NREM sleep and wakefulness. A characteristic feature is, however, that only fragments of REM sleep appear. The reduced awareness of external stimuli which is characteristic of sleep may become separated from dreams and from the motor inhibition of REM sleep and any one or a combination of these three components may be present at any one time. Each component is also less stable than normal. It is uncertain whether REM sleep in narcolepsy is as effective in promoting mental associations as in normal subjects. The deeper stages of NREM sleep are shortened and, perhaps because the lighter stages are more prevalent, there are more arousals to wakefulness during sleep.

Cataplexy and sleep paralysis probably represent waking manifestations of the normal inhibition of muscle tone and activity during REM sleep. The cholinergic LDT/PPT and its surrounding area project to the medial medulla which inhibit the alpha motor neurones in the spinal cord and cranial nerve nuclei. The association between loss of muscle tone in cataplexy and emotion may be due to the links between the amygdala, which is activated during emotional states, and the LDT/PPT and nearby regions.

Genetic factors

There is an abnormality in the short arm of chromosome 6 which is closely associated with the HLA type DR2 and subtype DR15 and more particularly with the subtype DQB1*0602 (Table 6.7). Human leucocyte antigen is a protein which is present in cell membranes and is linked to the susceptibility to autoimmune diseases.

There is a close association between HLA type and classical idiopathic narcolepsy. This association with the HLA type is the strongest of any disease [27], but only around 50% of those with familial narcolepsy have this HLA association. Its presence does not invariably lead to narcolepsy since HLA DQB1*0602 is present in around 25% of the normal Caucasian population. The expression of the genetic tendency requires other factors which may act through altering the immune state. HLA DR2 is positive in 50–60% of those with multiple sclerosis and 85% of patients with Goodpasture's syndrome, but neither of these is associated with narcolepsy.

Neurochemistry

The features of narcolepsy probably involve an increase in cholinergic activity relative to that mediated by noradrenaline and dopamine. These abnormalities appear to be mainly located in the pons and medulla, and at least in part are related to abnormalities in hypocretin (orexin) secretion from the perifornical area in the postero-lateral hypothalamus.

In idiopathic narcolepsy less than 15% of the normal number of cells in this area are functioning, possibly because they are inactivated or because too few were present at birth, because of a developmental abnormality, but more probably because of cell damage and death later in life. This may have an autoimmune basis, particularly in view of the HLA association, but little evidence for this has been detected histologically. Auto-antibodies are no more frequent than in the general population and there is no evidence for any organ-specific autoimmunity. Narcolepsy is no more frequent in women than in men, unlike other autoimmune diseases, and there is no association with any other autoimmune diseases. Humoral immunity appears to be normal and inflammatory markers, such as C reactive protein, are normal.

Hypocretins are almost invariably absent or markedly reduced (less than 40 pg/ml) in the cerebrospinal fluid (CSF) in those with idiopathic narcolepsy, even at the time of presentation. Deficiency of hypocretin 1 may be more closely associated with cataplexy and sleep-onset REM sleep on polysomnography, and deficiency of hypocretin 2 with EDS and REM sleep episodes during wakefulness.

Table 6.7 Human leucocyte antigen type and narcolepsy.

HLA type	African-American		Caucasian		Japanese	
Population (% positive)	Narcolepsy	Normal	Narcolepsy	Normal	Narcolepsy	Normal
DQ1	95–100	75	90–100	67	100	75
DQB1*0602	90–95	35	95–100	25	100	12
DR2						
DR15	65–75	30	90–100	25	100	35
DRB1*1501	10–20	7	95–100	25	100	12

Aetiology

Idiopathic narcolepsy

This is by far the commonest type and is usually associated with HLA DQB1*0602 and hypocretin deficiency. Environmental factors are, however, probably twice as important as genetic factors in determining the onset of this condition. It often follows a febrile illness and it may represent an abnormal immune reaction to a streptococcal infection. Physical and emotional stress frequently precede the onset of narcolepsy.

Narcolepsy has also been associated with physical trauma, particularly head injuries. Loss of consciousness at the time of the injury is usual, but not invariable, and narcolepsy may follow injuries to any part of the head. It usually appears immediately afterwards or within a few weeks or months of the injury. HLA DQB1*0602 is present in only around half of those with post-traumatic narcolepsy. This may be triggered by damage to the blood–brain barrier or by direct damage to structures controlling REM sleep, but more probably the injury initiates changes in neurotransmitters or an inflammatory response, which lead to symptoms of narcolepsy.

Narcolepsy is most common in those born in March and least common when the birth date is in September [28]. This suggests that either prenatal or early postnatal experiences predispose to or protect against the subsequent development of narcolepsy.

Secondary (symptomatic) narcolepsy

This is due to an organic abnormality in the hypothalamus, midbrain or pons. Secondary narcolepsy should be suspected if symptoms develop before the age of 5 years, since idiopathic narcolepsy is unusual at this age. Sudden sleep attacks may be present and it is usual for the subject to sleep for an abnormally long time during each 24 h, unlike idiopathic narcolepsy.

Cranial nerve abnormalities, such as conjugate gaze defects, are usually present and there may be other features of a hypothalamic disorder such as changes in appetite and temperature control. Lesions affecting the rostrocentral midbrain tegmentum cause a combination of EDS, intense colourful visual hallucinations (peduncular hallucinosis) and a vertical gaze palsy. Lesions confined to the pontine tegmentum may reduce or alter the nature of both NREM sleep and REM sleep, and if they are severe enough to cause

the locked-in syndrome there may be no recognizable NREM or REM sleep.

Secondary narcolepsy may also be due to the following.

1 Tumours of the hypothalamus and related lesions. These include an astrocytoma, lymphoma, craniopharyngioma, meningioma, pineal tumour or a colloid cyst of the third ventricle.
2 Hypothalamic stroke. This may be caused by a vascular malformation or vasculitis, in which case the features of narcolepsy are usually preceded by an acute episode of loss of consciousness.
3 Hypothalamic inflammation. This may be due to sarcoidosis or tuberculosis.
4 Anti-Ma2 paraneoplastic encephalitis. This is usually associated with a germ cell tumour of the testis or a bronchial carcinoma.
5 Encephalitis lethargica. Excessive daytime sleepiness was associated with this infection, particularly when it involved the lateral and posterior hypothalamus.

Genetic syndromes

EDS with cataplexy-like attacks is recognized in the Prader–Willi syndrome, Niemann–Pick disease type C, Norrie and Moebius syndromes and autosomal dominant deafness with ataxia. The exact nature of the cataplexy-like attacks in these conditions is poorly documented.

Clinical features

The most common symptoms of narcolepsy in children are prolongation of the main sleep episode with EDS, but the tiredness that is experienced can lead to paradoxical hyperactivity. This may be incorrectly diagnosed as the attention deficit hyperactivity disorder.

In adults the onset is sudden in around 15%, particularly in older subjects in whom the various manifestations tend to arise almost simultaneously and often in a severe form. In younger adults EDS usually appears before cataplexy. This is often seen within the next 2 years, but may be delayed for up to 30 years, and other symptoms subsequently develop. Complete remissions are uncommon, although the symptoms may fluctuate in severity, probably due to a change in the intrinsic severity of the disorder, to external factors, or to the patient's lifestyle and ability to cope with the problems that arise [29]. Sleep paralysis, cataplexy and vivid dreams are more likely to spontaneously improve than EDS.

The specific effects of narcolepsy are as follows (Table 6.8).

Feature of sleep		Abnormality
Changes in sleep	*Night*	Short sleep latency
		Insomnia
	Day	Sleep attacks
		Subalertness
Dreams		Vivid
		Occur while going to sleep, asleep, waking up and occasionally while awake
Motor control		Sleep paralysis
		Cataplexy
		Other behavioural disorders, e.g. PLMS, REM sleep behaviour disorder

Table 6.8 Features of REM sleep related effects of narcolepsy.

PLMS, periodic limb movements in sleep; REM, rapid eye movement.

Disorders of sleep

Insomnia

It is usual for those with narcolepsy to fall asleep within 5 min of going to bed, but the sleep pattern is then unstable. Awakenings from sleep or shifts from deeper to lighter stages of NREM sleep are frequent. The total duration of sleep during the night is only slightly reduced, and episodes of REM sleep are shorter than in normal subjects. Most narcoleptics feel unrefreshed when they wake in the morning, but this does not correlate with the number or frequency of awakenings during the night.

Excessive daytime sleepiness

The total sleep time during each 24 h is normal or only slightly increased because the loss of sleep time at night is only just outweighed by the time spent asleep during the day. There are two components to daytime sleepiness.

Daytime naps. These are usually of 5–30 min duration and rarely last for more than 1 h. They are temporarily refreshing and there is usually a refractory period of over an hour before the next nap is taken, often at a time corresponding to the 90 min ultradian REM sleep cycle. Sleep-onset REM sleep is common during the naps. The naps may occur in situations where sleep might be anticipated, such as while sitting as a car passenger, but sleep 'attacks' may be sudden and irresistible and occur in such situations as while talking, walking or during sexual intercourse.

Subalertness. This is probably due to a disorder of wakefulness rather than of sleep, although sleep fragmentation and poor quality of NREM sleep may contribute. Cognitive function is normal, but attention and concentration span are reduced and reaction times prolonged. Poor memory is often reported, but this is probably due to low self-esteem, subalertness and the anterograde amnesia of microsleeps rather than a true memory defect.

Automatic behaviour is closely related to subalertness during the day and consists of semi-purposeful behaviour in which familiar and often complex tasks are carried out without any subsequent recollection. They include inappropriate actions, such as stacking dishes in a refrigerator, and may lead to accidents. Automatic behaviour should be distinguished from the stereotyped behaviour of epilepsy and fugue states.

Disorders of dreams

Dreams during sleep

These are vivid and there is usually good recall. The dream theme may continue even after interruption by a period of wakefulness. Dreams occur at sleep onset and the perception of dreaming all night is common. The most intense emotional experience during dreams is in the first REM sleep episode during the night, which contrasts with the experience of normal subjects in which dreams much later in the night are the most emotionally charged [30]. Dreams may be in colour with vivid sounds as well as taste, smell and pain. A sensation of levitation, such as flying or swooping, or being pushed up or pressed down, is common, probably representing fluctuations in the inhibition of muscle spindle activity. The dreams are often sufficiently unpleasant and realistic to become nightmares.

Dreams during wakefulness

Dreams often occur shortly before sleep (hypnagogic hallucinations) or shortly after waking (hypnopompic hallucinations), but can occur during wakefulness; 60% of those with narcolepsy and cataplexy have these types of dreams and 30% of those without cataplexy. They represent partial REM sleep intrusion into wakefulness or the intrusion of consciousness into partially formed REM sleep at the end of a sleep episode.

These dreams merge into wakefulness and are usually vivid and sufficiently realistic for the subject to be unsure whether they represent reality or not. Awareness of semi-formed images, the presence of people, or animals such as insects is common, and a feeling of levitation (and even 'out of body' experiences), with a visual and auditory content such as hearing voices, is usual. The subject is sufficiently awake to be able to think and talk during the dream. This temporary loss of contact with reality can be embarrassing and the dream images may lead to vague but intense emotions, particularly fear.

Sensory disturbances due to migraines are common in narcolepsy, but they can usually be readily distinguished from dream disorders.

Disorders of motor control

Motor disorders during sleep

Narcolepsy is associated with a variety of parasomnias due to fluctuations in the degree of motor inhibition in REM sleep. Sleep terrors, sleep talking and walking are common, and irregular jerking movements and periodic limb movements may be seen during REM sleep because of a failure of motor inhibition. This also underlies the appearance of REM sleep behaviour disorder. Obstructive sleep apnoeas are more common than in normal subjects, probably because of an alteration in the inhibition of the activity of the dilator muscles of the upper airway and also because of obesity.

Sleep paralysis

This is a motor disorder which has been particularly associated with narcolepsy. Over 60% of those with narcolepsy and cataplexy have sleep paralysis. It is present in only around 10% of those without cataplexy. It is the inability to move while consciousness is retained, either at the onset of sleep or, less commonly, when waking up. The respiratory muscles, or more probably only the diaphragm, retain activity but speech is impossible. The episodes usually last for less than 2 min but can occasionally persist for up to 30 min. The intense relaxation may be pleasurable, but much more commonly it is perceived as frightening because of the inability to move, the loss of control, and the occasional association with vivid dreams.

Sleep paralysis episodes are less common in the upright position and can be terminated by an intense effort to move or by a touch from the partner, who may be alerted to the situation by a change in the pattern of breathing or faint sounds that may be uttered.

Cataplexy

This is the sudden onset of muscle weakness during wakefulness. It usually appears within 2 years of the development of excessive daytime sleepiness, although it precedes this in around 10% of narcoleptics. Excessive daytime sleepiness is usually more severe in those with cataplexy. Cataplexy is present in at least 75% of those with narcolepsy.

It may follow an abnormal sensation around the mouth or face, which is succeeded by twitching of the lower face, and occasionally the upper limbs, and rapid eye movements due to an intermittent loss of muscle tone. This usually leads to symmetrical muscle weakness which may remain localized or become generalized. Mild episodes may simply cause drooping of the face, double vision, dysarthria or nodding of the head. The weakness may spread to cause loss of strength in the arms, trunk muscles and legs, causing the knees to buckle and the subject to fall to the ground, occasionally with persisting twitching of the limbs. Consciousness and memory of the episode are retained, although paralysis may be complete apart from the respiratory and extra-ocular muscles. Incontinence and tongue biting are not features of cataplexy.

Recovery from an episode of cataplexy is usually sudden and complete. Cataplexy attacks usually last for a few seconds or up to 2 min, but can occur repetitively for up to 20–60 min (status cataplecticus) and are then usually followed by REM sleep.

Cataplexy in narcolepsy is almost invariably triggered by a sudden intense emotion. There is no disorder of emotional control, but laughter or anger, or the anticipation of these emotions, or surprise are usually the triggers. It may also occur during or after sexual intercourse, or while being tickled. It varies considerably in frequency and severity, but is more common and more severe if the subject is tired, mentally relaxed and in the company of familiar people.

Situations in which sudden or intense emotions may be felt tend to be avoided and techniques of controlling the emotions and a flattened affect are often developed to avoid cataplexy. The attacks can sometimes be prevented by tensing the muscles at the onset of an attack, for instance by clenching the fists. Injuries and accidents including drowning may occur because of cataplexy.

Other conditions

Narcolepsy is also associated with several conditions apparently unrelated to sleep.

1 Migraines. These occur in around 75% of subjects.

2 Obesity. An increase in weight and appetite is an early and often the initial symptom of narcolepsy, particularly in children. It is associated with a reduction in hypocretin production which stimulates appetite, and a reduction in leptin which is an appetite suppressant. Initially there is an increase in appetite, particularly for carbohydrates, but later in the natural history food intake appears to be reduced, although some subjects retain a craving for carbohydrate food during the night. The fall in serum leptin is probably due to a reduction in sympathetic activity and there is also a loss of the nocturnal increase in leptin. In general, carbohydrates appear to have a tendency to promote sleep in narcolepsy.

3 Type 2 diabetes mellitus.

4 Thyroid disorders.

5 Hypotension. There is a relative increase in parasympathetic compared to sympathetic activity in narcolepsy, with a tendency towards a lower blood pressure, body temperature and metabolic rate, which contrasts with conditions in which there is sleep fragmentation in which there is increased sympathetic activity.

Investigations

Self-reported rating scales

The severity of narcolepsy can be estimated using the Ullanlinna Narcolepsy Scale (Appendix 8).

Human leucocyte antigen (HLA) typing

Absence of the HLA DQB*0602 is useful in excluding narcolepsy if the clinical picture and physiological investigations are equivocal. It is of little value in confirming the diagnosis since the subtype is present in a significant percentage of normal subjects in most populations (Table 6.8).

Polysomnography

This may help to establish the diagnosis of narcolepsy, exclude other diagnoses and assess the presence of complications, such as insomnia, periodic limb movements in sleep, obstructive sleep apnoeas, or REM sleep behaviour disorder. It characteristically shows a short sleep latency, usually less than 5 min, without an increase in the total sleep time at night, although the total sleep time during each 24-h cycle is slightly greater than normal because of the daytime naps (Fig. 3.4). Sleep-onset REM (defined as the appearance of REM sleep within 20 min of onset of sleep) is present in around 50% of subjects and REM sleep episodes are often shorter in duration and have more variable muscle tone than normal. There is no increase in the duration of REM sleep episodes later in the night, as in normal subjects, but REM density is increased. The duration of stage 1 NREM sleep is increased, and stages 3 and 4 are shortened. Sleep efficiency is decreased, particularly in older subjects.

Multiple sleep latency tests (MSLTs)

These should be carried out after a period of withdrawal from drugs such as amphetamines and anticataplectic agents, which may affect the results. MSLTs are not suitable for children under the age of around 6 years. They show a short sleep latency with a mean of less than 5 min in 80% of narcoleptics. Sleep-onset REM sleep in two or more of the four or five MSLTs is present in over 75% of narcoleptics, but may also be seen in depression, REM sleep deprivation due to sleep restriction or fragmentation due, for instance, to obstructive sleep apnoeas, and in REM suppressant drug and alcohol withdrawal.

Maintenance of wakefulness test

This is usually reduced to around 10 min. This finding is not specific to narcolepsy and 15% of those with narcolepsy remain awake for 20 min.

CSF hypocretins (orexins)

A concentration of less than 110 pg/ml is seen in over 95% of subjects with narcolepsy and cataplexy and it is usually less than 40 pg/ml (normal > 200 pg/ml) [31, 32]. The hypocretin level is occasionally normal in the presence of EDS and cataplexy, but in the absence of the characteristic HLA type. If there is no cataplexy, either a low or a normal hypocretin level may be found. It is reduced in only 2% of subjects with other neurological disorders, particularly Guillain–Barre syndrome, Hashimoto's encephalopathy and myotonic dystrophy. It is raised in periodic limb movements in sleep and Lewy body disease.

Low hypocretin levels can also be seen in secondary narcolepsy due, for instance, to the paraneoplastic syndrome associated with Ma2 antibodies and tumours causing narcolepsy. CSF hypocretin is normal in Niemann–Pick disease type C, and probably in the Prader–Willi syndrome.

The hypocretin level is inversely related to body weight and fluctuates by around 40% in a diurnal pattern. It may double after exercise, is higher in wakefulness than in NREM sleep, lowest in REM sleep and is not affected by drugs, such as antidepressants and stimulant and wakefulness promoting agents.

Estimation of CSF hypocretin levels may be useful in the following situations.

1 The clinical features are suggestive of narcolepsy, but there is no cataplexy or a doubtful history.
2 There is difficulty in interpreting polysomnography or MSLT findings because of the presence of other sleep disorders or the effects of medication.
3 In younger subjects who have not yet developed the characteristic polysomnography or MSLT abnormalities, but in whom it is important to establish a definite diagnosis.
4 There is an atypical presentation, such as onset of symptoms in later life.

Differential diagnosis

A prolonged delay in the diagnosis of narcolepsy is common. Surveys have shown mean delays of around 3–6 years and patients often see several doctors from different specialties before the correct diagnosis is made. A delay in diagnosis is particularly likely if cataplexy is not present, since this is virtually pathognomonic of narcolepsy.

Before the widespread use of polysomnography and HLA typing, narcolepsy was often confused with or misdiagnosed as schizophrenia. The combination of an unusual affect and auditory and visual hallucinations led to this error, and the overlap of the symptoms of these two conditions led to the theory that schizophrenia was a REM sleep disorder. The two conditions are, however, unrelated [33]. The individual symptoms of narcolepsy can be confused with other disorders.

Excessive daytime sleepiness

The characteristic features are the sudden onset of an irresistible need to sleep (sleep attacks), episodes of sleep which are often brief but refreshing, and dreams which occur even during naps during the daytime, indicating that REM sleep has been entered.

Cataplexy

This may arise as an isolated familial disorder, but needs to be distinguished from epilepsy, especially if this is triggered by laughter (gelastic epilepsy). Gelastic syncope is related to the physical intensity of laughter, whereas in cataplexy it is the emotional intensity which acts as the trigger. Cataplexy may also be confused with atonic epileptic seizures although depression of the level of consciousness is usual in epilepsy (Table 6.9).

In cataplexy there is a similar but more intense loss of muscle tone than is seen transiently with laughter and exercise in normal subjects. This response is no more common in those with narcolepsy and is not accompanied by twitching of the face or jerking of the limbs. Weakness of the head and neck is common with cataplexy, but rare with laughter or exercise.

Cataplexy may also be misdiagnosed as a cardiac dysrhythmia or as a sleep attack, although consciousness is retained throughout episodes of cataplexy. It can be confused with an exaggerated startle response and psychogenic pseudo-epilepsy.

Sleep paralysis

This occurs occasionally in around 50% of normal subjects and frequently in around 6%, usually in adolescents and the elderly, especially with REM sleep rebound following sleep deprivation and jet lag following east–west travel which induces sleep-onset REM sleep. There is also a familial tendency to sleep paralysis.

Table 6.9 Differential diagnosis of cataplexy.

Sleep 'attack'
Epilepsy, especially gelastic and atonic
Vertebro-basilar insufficiency
Cardiac dysrhythmias
Drop attacks
Myasthenia gravis
Periodic paralysis
Faints
Gelastic syncope
Hysteria

Table 6.10 Differential diagnosis of vivid dreams in narcolepsy.

Schizophrenia
Epilepsy
Alcohol and benzodiazepine withdrawal
Hallucinogenic drugs
Parkinsonism
Occipital lobe lesions
Nocturnal visual hallucinations

Sleep paralysis should be distinguished from the generalized fatigue on waking which is common in the chronic fatigue syndrome and depression and is due to a lack of motivation rather than true paralysis. This lasts longer than sleep paralysis and small movements, for instance of the fingers, are possible. Sleep paralysis may also be confused with atonic seizures, transient cerebrovascular attacks and psychogenic disorders.

Hypnagogic and the hypnopompic hallucinations and vivid dreams

The characteristic features are the realistic nature of the hallucination while drowsy and the often intense emotions and perceived activities, often including flying, in the nocturnal dreams. Dreams may occur during brief naps during the day. The hallucinations of epilepsy are much more stereotyped than the dreams of narcolepsy (Table 6.10).

The diagnosis of narcolepsy is highly likely if there is a combination of EDS and well documented or observed cataplexy [34]. The probability of this being present is only slightly increased by positive polysomnography or MSLT findings. The likelihood is increased if other clinical features are present, including a short sleep latency, nocturnal insomnia, vivid dreams, both during wakefulness and during sleep, and sleep paralysis. The last two of these only occur in around 60% of those with narcolepsy.

When some of these features are absent the diagnosis may be in doubt. Some examples of situations that may arise are as follows.

EDS is the only symptom. If the HLA type is appropriate and polysomnography and MSLT findings are typical of narcolepsy or if CSF hypocretins are absent, narcolepsy is likely. If, on the other hand, the polysomnography or MSLT findings are atypical for

narcolepsy, the diagnosis is likely to be incorrect unless it is early in the natural history of the condition or unless CSF hypocretin is absent.

EDS without cataplexy, but with dreams during wakefulness and sleep paralysis. This may represent an early or mild form of narcolepsy which can be diagnosed if the polysomnography, MSLT and CSF hypocretin findings are typical. If they are not, the diagnosis may only become clear at a later stage when cataplexy develops.

Subjects with typical features of narcolepsy such as dreams during wakefulness and sleep paralysis, but in whom cataplexy never develops, probably form a homogeneous group which is distinct from those with the classical form of idiopathic narcolepsy with cataplexy. This form has been termed variant narcolepsy. Sleepiness is usually less severe than in classical narcolepsy with cataplexy, but the presence of symptoms such as dreams during wakefulness and sleep paralysis distinguishes these patients from those with idiopathic hypersomnia. The HLA DQB1*0602 is positive in only around 45% of subjects and CSF hypocretin is absent in only around 15%.

Cataplexy without EDS. This is unusual since EDS usually precedes rather than follows cataplexy, but in around 10% of subjects cataplexy is delayed for over 1 year after the onset of EDS. One view is that narcolepsy cannot be diagnosed in this situation since EDS is considered to be a prerequisite, but if the HLA type is appropriate and polysomnography and MSLT findings are typical of narcolepsy, this is likely to be the correct diagnosis.

REM sleep behaviour disorder. Narcolepsy should be suspected in this condition if there is excessive daytime sleepiness.

Restless legs syndrome and periodic limb movement in sleep. Narcolepsy should be suspected if periodic limb movements occur predominantly during REM sleep.

Social effects

The impact of narcolepsy on the quality of life varies according to its severity, the combination of symptoms, age of onset and the patient's understanding and ability to cope with the symptoms, as well as the availability of support from those around the patient [35]. The impact is, in general, comparable to that of epilepsy or multiple sclerosis.

Narcolepsy particularly affects interpersonal relationships. Social activities are avoided because of the risk of falling asleep or of cataplexy during any excitement, and alcohol may precipitate an irresistible sleep attack. Problems may arise during marriage, particularly if the partner does not have a full understanding of the difficulties arising from the condition. Failure to adapt to this often causes confusion and anger, and separation or divorce is frequently attributed to their disorder by those with narcolepsy.

The children of those with narcolepsy may be exposed to danger if the parent falls asleep or during a cataplexy episode. Accidents to children may occur, for instance, if the parent is carrying the child and has a cataplectic episode or if the children are alone with the parent who has an irresistible sleep attack which leaves the children unsupervised. Parental anxiety about whether the children may also develop narcolepsy, and guilt about the restrictions that this condition imposes on how they care for their children, may be intense.

Intelligence is normal in narcolepsy, but the poor concentration and attention span reduces educational achievements. Falling asleep in class and during examinations is common. An inability to take part in many sports often leads to a feeling of being different from other children, and after leaving school there may be problems in employment. Monotonous work may precipitate sleep and computer and desk jobs and jobs involving frequent meetings are particularly difficult to cope with. Working at heights or with moving machinery may be unsafe, and frequent job changes are common, as well as limitations on which types of employment are suitable.

Recreational opportunities are also restricted, both because of the risk of accidents, and because any emotional response may cause cataplexy which is usually embarrassing. Accidents occur at home or at work, but particularly during driving, although the exact risk of this is uncertain. There is usually sufficient warning of sleepiness to be able to pull over to the side of the road. Cataplexy is infrequent while driving.

As a result of these difficulties secondary psychological problems are common. Emotional development may be retarded if narcolepsy appears in childhood, and a low self-esteem, little confidence and anxiety are common. Awareness of being underachievers, depression, embarrassment about their symptoms, and weight gain, due to the metabolic effects of narcolepsy, a craving for carbohydrates and a lack of physical activity, are common. These aspects are especially important in adolescence when the individual's pattern of interpersonal relationships is becoming established.

The only influence of narcolepsy on lifespan is through increasing the risk of accidents, such as road traffic accidents and those related to drowning and fire.

Treatment

Treatment of narcolepsy is often delayed for many years because of a failure to make the diagnosis early in its natural history. During this time important psychological responses to the problems of narcolepsy develop and these may be only partially reversible once they have become established. The most important aspects of treatment are discussed below.

Advice

Understanding of narcolepsy
Explanation and reassurance about the nature of the symptoms and the outcomes of narcolepsy are important, not only for the patient but also for the parent, partner, school teachers and employers, where appropriate. Those with narcolepsy are often thought to be depressed or lazy, or to have a mental disorder, and their sleep and cataplexy attacks often generate resentment, anger or occasionally guilt, all of which can harm interpersonal relationships.

Sleep hygiene
The nocturnal sleep episode should not be shortened, and regular sleep–wake routines should be adopted. These may be difficult to achieve, particularly in adolescence. Other aspects of sleep hygiene which are detailed in Chapter 1 are also important.

Modification of daytime activities
Alertness can be increased by exercise and exposure to bright light, but exercise should be avoided in situations where falling asleep or cataplexy might be dangerous, e.g. boxing, mountaineering, or while swimming alone. Alcohol and large meals, particularly those containing carbohydrates, are likely to induce sleep and should be avoided.

Naps during the day should be planned either to coincide with the circadian rhythms, so that they are taken between 2.00 and 4.00 PM, or around essential activities. Naps should be taken before events for which it is important to be particularly alert, but equally, the timing of these events should be coordinated with the optimal time for naps.

Coping strategies

It is important to accept that narcolepsy is a lifelong condition which has to be managed and integrated into the everyday lifestyle. Coping strategies, including cognitive techniques, may help.

School activities

An understanding of narcolepsy by teachers and others at school is important. Narcolepsy does not affect the intelligence or memory, but concentration and attention span are often reduced. Careful planning of study schedules should be adopted. Examinations should be arranged for the mornings or at whatever time of day alertness is greatest. The length of the examination may need to be extended in order to take into account the periods of sleep that are needed. Individualized careers advice should be offered.

Employment

An awareness and understanding of narcolepsy by the employer is important so that planned short naps, and regular breaks from tasks involving immobility or prolonged concentration, can be taken. The work area should be well lit.

The most suitable work for those with narcolepsy involves exercise and contact with other people, together with a stimulating environment, e.g. shop assistant, hairdresser, porter. Shift work, particularly rotating shifts, should be avoided, and part-time work should be timed for when alertness is greatest, which is usually in the morning. Occupations where continuous concentration is required, e.g. air traffic controller, and those involving confrontation or situations which might induce cataplexy, such as a policeman or traffic warden, should be avoided. Work involving moving heavy machinery could be dangerous because of cataplexy, and jobs involving water, such as a swimming pool attendant, are unsuitable because of the risk of drowning due to cataplexy or a sudden sleep attack. Work with computers may be satisfactory if there is a particular interest in this, but if not, episodes of sleep are likely and these may increase the chance of dismissal.

Driving

Narcoleptics need to be aware that driving while drowsy is dangerous because the reaction time is increased, peripheral vision is reduced and judgement is impaired. Once narcolepsy has been diagnosed, the individual has a duty to notify the DVLA and their own insurance company. The DVLA usually seeks a medical report regarding the fitness to drive, and a licence is granted initially for 1–3 years if this is satisfactory, before the situation is reviewed.

Awareness of the times of day when sleepiness is most likely enables these to be avoided for driving. Taking a nap before driving, and timing stimulant medication so that alertness is optimized at the time of driving, may help. Driving for any longer than has previously been found to lead to drowsiness should be avoided. Cataplexy is rarely a problem during driving. Situations which could lead to sudden or intense emotions, such as anger or laughter, and which might trigger this should be avoided, but there remains a small risk of sudden unexpected events involving other cars or pedestrians which might cause cataplexy.

Drugs

Hypocretin replacement treatment is not yet feasible in humans and has only led to transient benefits in dogs. Hypocretin-containing neurones have been grafted into the pons of rats [36], but the potential role of this treatment in humans is uncertain.

The link between febrile illnesses and the onset of narcolepsy and the possibility of an autoimmune cause for the loss of function of the hypocretin-secreting cells in the perifornical region of the lateral hypothalamus have prompted the use of anti-inflammatory agents, particularly early in the natural history of narcolepsy. Prednisolone has not been found to be effective, but three administrations of intravenous immunoglubulin 2 gm/kg at monthly intervals can significantly improve both excessive daytime sleepiness and cataplexy and lead to weight loss. This treatment does not alter the hypocretin level in the CSF.

Drug treatment (Table 6.11) may also be indicated for the following conditions.

Excessive daytime sleepiness

Both subalertness during wakefulness, and episodes of sleep, respond to CNS stimulants and wakefulness promoting drugs. The timing of the dose of treatment needs careful consideration so that the level of alertness can be raised to cope with planned activity, and so that the effect wears off before the desired nocturnal sleep time in order to minimize the risk of insomnia.

Large quantities of caffeinated drinks are often taken, but are usually ineffective. The amphetamines and related drugs have been the mainstay of stimulant treatment for many years, together with drugs such as

Table 6.11 Drugs commonly used in narcolepsy.

Indication	EDS	Cataplexy	Other REM sleep symptoms	Insomnia
Drugs	Modafinil Dexamphetamine Methylphenidate Sodium oxybate	Trycyclic antidepressants SSRIs Venlafaxine Sodium oxybate Dexamphetamine	Antidepressants Sodium oxybate	Sodium oxybate Benzodiazepines and related drugs

selegiline and mazindol which are chemically unrelated, but which have similar effects. Dexamphetamine is the most commonly prescribed drug in this group [37], but has important drawbacks (Chapter 4). These usually limit the dose that can be prescribed so that EDS is often undertreated. The residual sleepiness commonly causes secondary effects such as loss of self-esteem, depression and unemployment which are potentially avoidable.

Modafinil is as effective as amphetamines and improves alertness in around 75% of patients [38, 39]. It has been shown to improve the quality of life and reduce the number of daytime naps. It has fewer unwanted central nervous system actions and side-effects [40]. It is preferable to dexamphetamine as initial treatment for EDS in narcolepsy. Patients who have developed side-effects with amphetamines, and those at risk of side-effects of amphetamines because of, for instance, ischaemic heart disease, should be transferred to modafinil instead.

Dexamphetamine is indicated in patients who have already been established on it with improvement in EDS and without side-effects, and in those who either fail to improve with modafinil or fall into the small group who develop troublesome side-effects. Modafinil can be combined with dexamphetamine so that it provides the background improvement in EDS, with dexamphetamine taken shortly before activities for which alertness is particularly important.

Sodium oxybate improves daytime alertness and also relieves cataplexy and improves continuity of sleep at night [41, 42]. It may be useful as monotherapy for treating these symptoms, but can also be used in conjunction with amphetamines or modafinil to relieve daytime sleepiness.

Cataplexy

Cataplexy is suppressed by drugs that increase dopamine, 5HT and noradrenergic activity, and is worsened by antagonists of these neurotransmitters, such as prazosin, an alpha 1 antagonist, and by cholinergic agents.

Amphetamines, and to a lesser extent mazindol and selegiline, have an anticataplectic action which may be related to their noradrenergic effects. Modafinil, which has a similar effect on alertness, does not have this action but may increase the blood level of anticataplectic drugs such as clomipramine.

Antidepressants have been widely used to treat cataplexy, although there is little data about their effectiveness. Their mechanism of action is probably different from their antidepressant action since the anticataplectic effect is apparent within one day, whereas relief of depression often takes around 2 weeks. The efficacy of the tricyclic antidepressants relates to their noradrenergic and anticholinergic activity, but the 5HT promoting effect of the selective serotonin re-uptake inhibitors and similar drugs may be important.

Each antidepressant has a different profile of activity at noradrenaline and 5HT synapses and of anticholinergic activity. Monoamine oxidase inhibitors are rarely used because of their drug interactions, but phenelzine is highly effective in cataplexy. Tricyclic antidepressants are probably slightly more effective than selective serotonin re-uptake inhibitors and related drugs, but have more side-effects, and in particular often cause weight gain and may exacerbate EDS. Clomipramine 10–150 mg nocte may be the most effective, is relatively selective for blocking 5HT uptake and is the most effective tricyclic antidepressant in suppressing REM sleep. The action of selective serotonin re-uptake inhibitors is limited to 5HT synapses and this may be responsible for their slightly lower efficacy compared to tricyclic antidepressants, but new drugs which also block the uptake of noradrenaline appear to be more effective. These include venlafaxine 37.5–375 mg daily, reboxetine 1–4 mg bd [43], and viloxazine and sibutramine may also be useful. Bupropion is a noradrenaline and dopamine re-uptake blocker which is useful if REM sleep behaviour disorder or periodic limb movements are present, since it is the only antidepressant which does not exacerbate these problems.

Sodium oxybate is chemically unrelated to the antidepressants, but is effective in relieving cataplexy as well as improving daytime sleepiness and continuity of sleep in a dose of 1.5–4.5 gm taken before sleep and 2.5–4 hours later [41]. It also leads to gradual weight loss, counteracting the tendency of those with narcolepsy to gain weight, particularly on tricyclic antidepressants. Withdrawal of sodium oxybate does not lead to a rebound worsening of cataplexy which is a problem with antidepressants.

Clonazepam 1–4 mg nocte and clonidine 150–300 μg daily also have some anticataplectic effect. Propranolol and carbamazepine have also been reported to be effective.

Hallucinations, dreams and nightmares
Antidepressants and sodium oxybate reduce the frequency and duration of these events through their action in reducing the duration of REM sleep.

Insomnia
This responds best to sodium oxybate, but also to hypnotics such as zopiclone 7.5 mg nocte, benzodiazepines, e.g. temazepam 10 mg nocte, or sedating tricyclic antidepressants such as imipramine. Sleep hygiene advice may also be helpful.

Motor disorders during sleep
Obstructive sleep apnoeas, REM sleep behaviour disorder and periodic limb movements all require specific treatment.

Depression
This is a frequent response to the problems of narcolepsy and may require a tricyclic or selective serotonin re-uptake inhibitor antidepressant. Bupropion is the only antidepressant that does not worsen REM sleep behaviour disorder or periodic limb movements during sleep.

Idiopathic hypersomnia

Occurrence
This is an uncommon condition, but its true incidence is uncertain because of the variable criteria which have been used to make the diagnosis. The term is often used when no definite diagnosis for EDS has

been established. Patients diagnosed as having idiopathic hypersomnia therefore form a heterogeneous group unless a comprehensive clinical and investigative evaluation has been undertaken to exclude other conditions.

Idiopathic hypersomnia is probably less common than narcolepsy. It is equally frequent in males and females. It usually appears before the age of 25 and in 25% of subjects is present before the age of 13. It is usually sporadic, but is occasionally familial, and may then be associated with autonomic disorders such as migraines, postural hypotension, faints and cold hands and feet.

Pathogenesis
Idiopathic hypersomnia is thought to be due to an increase in the intensity or amplitude of the homeostatic drive to sleep. This overcomes the circadian and adaptive drives more readily during the day, leading to EDS, and at night causes prolonged sleep. A similar syndrome has been produced in mice by damage to the locus coeruleus, thereby reducing the noradrenergic drive to wakefulness. No abnormality of neurotransmitters has been identified in humans.

Clinical features
Idiopathic hypersomnia tends to progress steadily over the weeks or months after its appearance and then persists throughout life with little change, although occasionally it improves spontaneously. It may cause secondary psychological reactions, particularly depression, loss of educational opportunities or employment and an inability to take part in recreational activities.

There are two clinical patterns of idiopathic hypersomnia [44].

Monosymptomatic
Excessive daytime sleepiness is the sole symptom. Nocturnal sleep is not prolonged and there is no difficulty in waking in the morning. Naps, often prolonged, are taken during the day and may be refreshing. They are not associated with dreams.

This group is probably heterogeneous. Some may have monosymptomatic narcolepsy or other undiagnosed causes for their excessive daytime sleepiness (see differential diagnosis below).

Polysymptomatic
This group is excessively sleepy during the day, but also has a prolonged sleep episode at night and difficulty in waking in the morning. They may sleep

for around 15 h at night and, unlike narcolepsy, there are few arousals or awakenings and dream recall is infrequent. It is difficult to rouse the subject from sleep, either during the night or during naps, and in the morning several alarms may be required. The subject characteristically remains confused for some time after wakening, probably due to a severe form of sleep inertia, and automatic behaviour with confusion and inappropriate actions, which are often aggressive, is characteristic.

Naps during the day are unrefreshing and often last for 30–120 min. There may be a sensation of sub-alertness between naps.

This is a more homogeneous group and autonomic problems such as migraines, postural hypotension, faints and cold hands may be associated.

Investigations

Clinical evaluation is insufficient to exclude other causes of EDS and polysomnography is required, often with MSLTs.

Polysomnography reveals a short sleep latency with a long total sleep time, high sleep efficiency and few arousals (Fig. 3.4). Sleep architecture is normal, except that the NREM sleep episodes may not shorten in duration during the night as in normal subjects and the duration of stages 3 and 4 NREM sleep may be increased. There is no sleep-onset REM, but there is often high spindle activity at the start and end of sleep.

Multiple sleep latency tests confirm a short sleep latency, usually 5–10 min, but with no sleep-onset REM sleep.

There are no associations with any HLA type and CSF hypocretin levels are normal or slightly reduced. CT and MRI scans of the brain are normal.

Differential diagnosis

1 Narcolepsy. Idiopathic hypersomnia can be distinguished from narcolepsy, as shown in Table 6.12, although secondary depression may shorten REM sleep latency.
2 Upper airway resistance syndrome.

Table 6.12 Narcolepsy and idiopathic hypersomnia.

Characteristic	Idiopathic hypersomnia	Narcolepsy
Age of onset (years)	15–30	15–30
Gender	M = F	M = F
Family history	Occasional	Occasional
EDS	Yes	Yes
Insomnia	No	Yes
REM sleep features		
Cataplexy	Nil	Prominent
Sleep paralysis	Nil	Common
Dreams	No	Prominent
Naps		
Duration	30–120 min	5–30 min
Refreshing	No	Yes
Night time sleep episode	Prolonged	Slightly shortened
Arousability on waking	Difficult	Variable
Natural history	Lifelong	Lifelong
Polysomnography	↓	↓↓
Sleep latency		
SOREM	No	Common
NREM sleep	Consolidated	Fragmented
MSLT	Short	Very short
HLA	No association	DQB1*0602 almost invariable

EDS, excessive daytime sleepiness; F, female; HLA, human leucocyte antigen; M, male; MSLT, multiple sleep latency test; NREM, non-REM; SOREM, sleep-onset REM.

3 Delayed sleep phase syndrome. Patients may have extreme difficulty in waking in the morning. They go to sleep late at night, but if they can obtain enough sleep they are not sleepy during the day.

4 Sleep deprivation. A history of sleep restriction at night is characteristic. The polysomnography findings may be similar to those of idiopathic hypersomnia, but EDS improves with an increase in time spent asleep.

5 Sedative drugs.

6 Post-traumatic hypersomnia.

7 Hypersomnia following infection, e.g. encephalitis. This is usually identifiable from the history.

8 Long sleepers. These subjects require more sleep at night than is normal, and if this is not obtained are sleepy during the day. If, however, they are allowed to sleep for as long as they need, their EDS disappears, unlike in idiopathic hypersomnia.

Treatment

The principles of treatment are similar to those for relieving EDS in narcolepsy. Counselling, lifestyle and sleep hygiene advice are important and the response to modafinil and central nervous system stimulants is at least as good as in narcolepsy. Modafinil has fewer side-effects than dexamphetamine and related drugs which are best reserved for patients who fail to improve with modafinil.

Disorders of the medulla

These cause sleepiness if they lead to either obstructive or central sleep apnoeas (see Chapters 10 and 11).

Disorders of the pons and midbrain

These can cause abnormalities of REM sleep such as narcolepsy and REM sleep behaviour disorder, but more commonly affect the ascending reticular activating system and predispose to an increase in NREM sleep, as in Parkinson's disease. There may be focal neurological signs which help to identify these lesions.

Disorders of the hypothalamus

These may be focal lesions, as in multiple sclerosis, tumours, or trauma, following surgery and the effects of radiotherapy. Excessive daytime sleepiness is associated with lesions of the posterior hypothalamus which increase the homeostatic sleep drive, but circadian rhythm disorders develop if the suprachiasmatic nuclei in the anterior hypothalamus are damaged. Hypothalamic lesions are often associated with endocrine and autonomic abnormalities and may also cause secondary narcolepsy.

There are several syndromes in which it is thought that diffuse hypothalamic abnormalities are the cause of excessive daytime sleepiness. The most important are described below.

Kleine–Levin syndrome (recurrent hypersomnia)

Occurrence

This rare syndrome is three times more common in males than in females. The onset is usually in adolescence or early adult life and, while it may gradually improve later in life, it rarely resolves completely.

Pathogenesis

The cause is usually uncertain but it occasionally follows a head injury, or more frequently a febrile illness, suggesting that it can be a post-encephalitic syndrome which runs a relapsing and remitting course. There is no abnormality of the circadian rhythms. It is thought to result from an instability of hypothalamic control of sleep, feeding, mood and sexual activity [45]. Abnormalities of the prefrontal cortex have also been detected. There is little direct evidence for any neurotransmitter abnormality, but a reduction in dopamine availability during exacerbations and an increase in 5HT have been proposed.

Clinical features

The three specific features of the syndrome are excessive daytime sleepiness, overeating and sexual disinhibition. An impaired memory, mood changes and other behavioural abnormalities are also common and fluctuate in parallel with the other symptoms. These symptoms characteristically occur in episodes lasting between two days and three weeks (usually less than one week), and occurring 2–12 times per year, although there is considerable variability both between patients and over time for individual subjects. They alternate with periods of apparent complete normality or partial remission of symptoms. Secondary psychiatric problems and social isolation are common.

Excessive daytime sleepiness
This may appear suddenly or develop over a few days and up to 20 h sleep per day may be obtained. The

subject may be very difficult to wake and between the sleep episodes may be confused, depressed and agitated, but able to eat, micturate and defaecate.

Overeating

A voracious appetite ('megaphagia'), equivalent to compulsive eating without satiety, is present in around 50% of subjects. There is no preference for any particular type of food, such as carbohydrates, and considerable weight may be gained during the attacks.

Sexual disinhibition

About 25% of patients make inappropriate sexual advances or repeatedly masturbate, and behaviour may be aggressive.

Psychological features

These include anxiety, depression, confusion, hallucinations, automatic behaviour associated with irritability, and often aggression. There is often amnesia for the episode and euphoria as the attack resolves.

Investigations

The main value of polysomnography is to exclude other causes of EDS since sleep is normal between attacks. During episodes it shows an increased duration of stage 2 NREM sleep with a raised arousal index, with a normal or reduced sleep efficiency, as well as an increased total sleep time.

CT and MRI scans of the brain are normal.

Differential diagnosis

1 Early stages of narcolepsy.
2 Depression with EDS in adolescence.
3 Bipolar mood disorder.
4 Psychogenic hypersomnia.

Treatment

Treatment is usually unsatisfactory. Lithium, carbamazepine and sodium valproate have been used to reduce the frequency and severity of attacks and modafinil may lessen the severity of sleepiness.

Prader–Willi syndrome

Pathogenesis

This multisystem disorder is associated with absence of part of chromosome 15. This impairs the development of the hypothalamus which leads to a loss of the sensation of satiety, leading to continual overeating and gross obesity.

Clinical features

Subalertness during the day is common and daytime naps are frequent. The excessive daytime sleepiness is usually due to sleep fragmentation caused by obstructive sleep apnoeas, but there may also be a hypothalamic abnormality causing EDS. The obesity and narrow upper airway contribute to the obstructive sleep apnoeas. The reduced respiratory drive and generalized respiratory muscle weakness also predispose to central sleep apnoeas. Episodes similar to cataplexy have been reported but are not well documented.

Investigations

Polysomnography shows an increase in the total sleep time with an increase in the duration of stages 3 and 4 NREM sleep, a short REM sleep latency, an increase in the number of REM sleep episodes, and a reduction of the inter-REM sleep interval. There is no association with HLA DQB1*0602.

Treatment

Treatment of obstructive sleep apnoeas with nasal continuous positive airway pressure or bilevel pressure support ventilation is effective, although compliance may be difficult to achieve and sustained weight loss is uncommon.

Disorders of the thalamus

Thalamic lesions more frequently cause insomnia than EDS, but this is occasionally seen with, for instance, thalamic infarcts, trauma or after bilateral thalamotomy for Parkinson's disease.

Diffuse organic neurological disorders

Cerebral palsy

This is usually due to birth trauma and the extent of the brain damage correlates with the degree of sleep disturbance. Excessive daytime sleepiness is common and may be due to obstructive sleep apnoeas and an abnormality of sleep control, but also to drugs, especially anticonvulsants, and to poor sleep hygiene.

Polysomnography is hard to interpret because of the poor definition of NREM and REM sleep, particularly in those who are severely affected. The number of arousals is increased, there are few spindles or K-complexes and the duration of stages 3 and 4 NREM and REM sleep appears to be reduced.

Myotonic dystrophy (dystrophia myotonica)

Excessive daytime sleepiness is commonly due to hypoventilation at night associated with frequent respiratory related arousals from sleep causing sleep fragmentation. Nocturnal hypoventilation is due both to weakness of respiratory muscles and to a disorder of the respiratory drive. It can also be due to disturbance of the sleep controlling mechanisms, independently of any respiratory abnormality [46]. This may be associated with damage to the dorsomedial thalamic nuclei. There is some evidence that circadian rhythms can be disorganized, possibly because time givers, such as light exposure, are less effective than in normal subjects.

Polysomnography may confirm the diagnosis of central sleep apnoeas and occasionally reveal obstructive apnoeas or periodic limb movements in sleep. The sleep latency is shortened and sleep-onset REM sleep is common. The cerebrospinal fluid hypocretin concentration may be low and many subjects with EDS are also HLA DQB1*0602-positive, raising the pos-sibility that there may be an overlap with narcolepsy.

Brain injuries

Head trauma causes both primary brain injuries, such as haematomas and diffuse axonal injury, and secondary effects due, for instance, to hypotension, hypoxia, raised intracranial pressure and release of free radicals. Both fatigue and sleep disorders commonly follow closed head injuries. Obstructive sleep apnoeas are common in those who have had head injuries, but whether they are related in any way to the injuries is uncertain. Periodic limb movements have also been associated with head injuries, and a delayed sleep phase syndrome may develop, although more characteristically it follows neck injuries with disruption of the tract between the suprachiasmatic nuclei and the pineal gland. Deterioration in vision after head injuries may lead to a non-24-h sleep–wake rhythm, and drugs to treat for instance epilepsy or psychiatric disorders following the head injury may also cause sedation.

The initial coma after head injuries is usually due to either diffuse cerebral cortical damage due to intracerebral haemorrhage or cerebral oedema, or malfunction of the brainstem. It is often followed by a phase of continuous sleepiness, usually with a reduction in REM sleep, which is punctuated by increasingly frequent awakenings. A gradual increase in the duration of REM sleep has been correlated with an improvement in cognitive function after the injury, but there is often poor dream recall.

In the recovery phase the poor differentiation of NREM and REM sleep may prevent accurate sleep staging. Excessive daytime sleepiness may improve for up to around a year, but recovery is often incomplete, so that there is a prolonged nocturnal sleep episode with frequent and prolonged naps during the day, and subalertness between these. The clinical features of this post-traumatic hypersomnia are similar to those of idiopathic hypersomnia.

Head injuries may also trigger narcolepsy and occasionally the Kleine–Levin syndrome.

Encephalitis

The acute phase of encephalitis characteristically causes a deterioration in the level of consciousness and even coma. There may be a full recovery of consciousness, but EDS can be a permanent result. This is usually due to inflammation in the midbrain and posterior hypothalamus which alters both the homeostatic sleep drive and circadian rhythms. Persistent EDS may also be due to central or obstructive sleep apnoeas which cause sleep fragmentation, and occasionally to carbon dioxide narcosis when hypoventilation due to damage to the medullary respiratory centres is severe.

The most important examples of EDS due to encephalitis are as follows.

Infectious mononucleosis

This infection with the Epstein–Barr virus (EBV) may be followed by EDS which can persist for several years. This may be difficult to distinguish from the chronic fatigue syndrome that is often caused by an EBV infection.

Human immunodeficiency virus infection (HIV)

A variety of sleep disorders occur with HIV infection. Patients who are HIV positive without features of the acquired immunodeficiency syndrome (AIDS) have an increased duration of stages 3 and 4 NREM sleep with reduction in REM sleep in the second half of the night so that REM sleep is more evenly distributed. As it advances, there is a decrease in sleep efficiency, an increase in the number of arousals, and a reduction in stages 3 and 4 NREM sleep which correlates with the fall in the CD4 lymphocyte count. Complaints of insomnia, daytime fatigue, drowsiness, poor concentration and memory are common.

These changes in sleep structure may be due to cytokines and other mediators of the immune response and changes in growth hormone secretion which initially promote NREM sleep. The later changes occur when the immune response is failing and may be partly due to neuronal death or dysfunction caused by direct effects of the HIV, or to changes in production or release of neurotransmitters.

African sleeping sickness (African trypanosomiasis)

This is due to a protozoan, *Trypanosoma brucei*, which is transmitted to humans by the tsetse fly from wild animals. It occurs in a wide belt of Africa between latitudes 22° north and south. The initial febrile illness is followed by a meningoencephalitis with demyelination, especially in the periaqueductal region of the midbrain but also in the pons, medulla, hypothalamus and frontal lobes. The mechanisms controlling sleep become severely disorganized due to both the destructive nature of the inflammation and the release of cytokines.

Sleepiness usually appears weeks or even years after the acute infection, is linked to the severity of the illness, and is often associated with fits, ataxia and tremor. Excessive daytime sleepiness is progressive and death usually occurs within around a year without antitrypanosomal drug treatment [47].

The total sleep time remains approximately normal, but the circadian rhythms of sleep, temperature and hormone secretion are lost, leading to a polyphasic sleep pattern. Nocturnal insomnia with severe sleep fragmentation is associated with EDS (sleep reversal) and the concentration of PGD2 is raised in the cerebrospinal fluid. Sleep episodes during the day often last 3–4 h, but become shorter as the disease progresses. Polysomnography shows loss of definition of NREM sleep, with absence of spindles and K-complexes, but the proportions of NREM and REM sleep are unaffected. The normal features of REM sleep are retained and sleep-onset REM sleep is common [48].

Treatment with trypanosomicidal drugs such as melarsoprol can reverse the loss of circadian function and lead to longer sleep episodes with more cycles of stages 3 and 4 NREM sleep and less sleep-onset REM sleep.

Encephalitis lethargica

This has caused several large epidemics of which the last was between around 1915 and 1927. Cocksackie and Echo viruses have been isolated from some subsequent sporadic cases. Cerebral damage is extensive, but sleep disorders are most prominent when the inflammation involves the midbrain and hypothalamus.

The manifestations include EDS, which appears to have similar features to narcolepsy, and sleep 'inversion', which probably represents a delayed sleep phase syndrome with an onset of sleep at around 3.00 AM. Occasionally patients remain awake all night, especially shortly after the acute phase of the illness, and the encephalitis also causes central alveolar hypoventilation due to damage to medullary respiratory centres.

Poliomyelitis

This can cause both central and obstructive sleep apnoeas associated with EDS due to damage to the medullary respiratory centres and weakness of the upper airway and chest wall muscles. Nocturnal hypoventilation may be severe enough to lead to carbon dioxide narcosis (Chapter 11).

Western equine encephalitis

This can damage the medullary respiratory centres and cause central alveolar hypoventilation. This may present with EDS due to respiratory-induced arousals from sleep and carbon dioxide narcosis.

General paresis

This form of neurosyphilis can cause EDS.

Multiple sclerosis

Physical fatigue related to muscle weakness is present in around 75% of those with multiple sclerosis but this should be distinguished from mental fatigue and from EDS. The latter is usually due to sleep fragmentation caused by immobility, discomfort, muscle spasms, nocturia and occasionally central or obstructive sleep apnoeas. Periodic limb movements in sleep have also been reported as being common in multiple sclerosis, and depression may have an important impact on sleep. Polysomnography may show an increased sleep latency and duration of time awake after sleep onset, and early morning awakening. The HLA DR2 type is present in 50–60% of those with multiple sclerosis, but narcolepsy, which shares this HLA type, is not commoner in multiple sclerosis than in the general population.

The fatigue of multiple sclerosis may respond to modafinil 200 mg daily.

Cerebral irradiation

Excessive daytime sleepiness often occurs within 6 weeks of radiotherapy to the brain. It may be due to a direct effect of the radiotherapy, possibly acting through cytokines and other inflammatory mediators, but occasionally the symptoms may be due to a raised intracranial pressure due to worsening of the tumour for which the radiotherapy was given.

Excessive daytime sleepiness is common when a large volume of brain is irradiated, for instance with prophylactic treatment for leukaemia or small cell carcinomas of the bronchus, whereas localized radiotherapy even close to the hypothalamus for pituitary tumours causes less EDS. Excessive daytime sleepiness following cranial irradiation should be distinguished from the physical fatigue that follows radiotherapy to areas outside the brain.

Parkinson's disease (idiopathic Parkinsonism)

Parkinson's disease (page 226) frequently causes excessive daytime sleepiness [49]. This is reported in around 40% of subjects and polysomnography reveals a reduced sleep efficiency proportional to the disease severity, and often markedly shortened MSLTs. There is a reduction in stages 3 and 4 NREM sleep and REM sleep, but sleep-onset REM sleep is common. The cerebrospinal fluid hypocretin concentration may be reduced in advanced disease, but there is no association with HLA DQB1*0602, unlike in narcolepsy. There are several causes for these abnormalities.

Poor sleep hygiene

This is associated with the physical limitations imposed by the motor and other disabilities.

Periodic limb movements

These cause sleep fragmentation and lead to excessive daytime sleepiness. They are rarely apparent in subjects treated with L-dopa or dopamine receptor agonists, but are common in untreated patients and often associated with symptoms of the restless legs syndrome. A low serum ferritin is common and symptoms may respond to iron supplementation as well as dopaminergic agents.

Obstructive sleep apnoeas

These may be slightly more frequent in Parkinsonism than in normal subjects.

Degeneration of sleep controlling mechanisms

The severity of excessive daytime sleepiness is related to both the extent and duration of the disease, probably due to degeneration of sleep controlling mechanisms in the brainstem.

Drugs

Sudden 'sleep attacks' have been documented in those with Parkinsonism treated with dopamine receptor agonists. This has been seen particularly with pramipexole and ropinirole, but may occur occasionally with other drugs, suggesting that it may be a class effect. It is dose related and may be specific to the combination of these drugs and the abnormalities of the sleep regulating systems due to the Parkinsonian degeneration. The attacks can be avoided by reducing the dose of the drug, changing to a different drug or, alternatively, adding a wakefulness promoting drug such as modafinil.

Surgical treatment

Thalamic damage from bilateral thalamotomy may cause excessive daytime sleepiness.

Psychiatric disorders

Excessive daytime sleepiness is much less frequently caused by psychiatric problems than is insomnia [50]. It may develop as a protective psychological reaction to circumstances which are difficult to cope with. If it persists it may be difficult to distinguish from idiopathic hypersomnia but MSLTs are usually normal.

Excessive daytime sleepiness is common in younger subjects with depression, whereas later in life this more frequently causes insomnia. EDS may persist despite adequate treatment of low mood by antidepressants and may even be worsened by sedative antidepressants. EDS in depression is usually associated with weight gain whereas depression and weight loss often lead to insomnia. EDS is also a feature of the seasonal affective disorder, which is associated with weight gain.

The daytime sleepiness seen in schizophrenia is occasionally due to the disorder itself, but more commonly to sedative medication.

Systemic disorders

These characteristically increase the duration of sleep during each 24-h period, often with a long nocturnal sleep episode. These sleep abnormalities have a wide range of mechanisms, some of which involve alterations in sleep factors, such as cytokines.

Premenstrual sleepiness

This usually occurs in adolescence for a few days before the onset of each menstrual period. A long sleep at night is associated with naps during the day and occasionally with an increased appetite. Polysomnography may be required to exclude other possible causes, including premenstrual exacerbation of periodic limb movements in sleep, but is normal in this condition. Multiple sleep latency tests are shortened.

Premenstrual sleepiness is related to the increase in progesterone secretion and can be treated by suppression of ovulation with oestrogens.

Pregnancy sleepiness
This usually occurs during the first trimester with an increase in total sleep time and in the number of daytime naps.

Metabolic disorders
These rarely cause EDS, but may alter the state of consciousness as in, for instance, hypoglycaemia, carbon monoxide poisoning and lead encephalopathy. Hepatic encephalopathy causes EDS, with difficulty in initiating sleep and a delay in the onset of melatonin secretion, similar to the delayed sleep phase syndrome.

Hypothyroidism
Excessive daytime sleepiness, apathy, stupor and coma may develop, either due to the metabolic abnormality or to obstructive sleep apnoeas caused by obesity. The duration of stages 3 and 4 NREM sleep is reduced but this and the EDS return to normal with thyroxine treatment.

References

1 Harrison Y, Horne JA. 'High sleepability without sleepiness'. The ability to fall asleep rapidly without other signs of sleepiness. *Neurophysiol Clin* 1996; 26: 15–20.

2 Chaudhuri A, Behan PO. Fatigue and basal ganglia. *J Neurol Sci* 2000; 179: 34–42.

3 Jones K, Harrison Y. Frontal lobe function, sleep loss and fragmented sleep. *Sleep Med Rev* 2001; 5(6): 463–75.

4 Harrison Y, Horne JA. Sleep loss impairs short and novel language tasks having a prefrontal focus. *J Sleep Res* 1998; 7: 95–100.

5 Fulda S, Schulz H. Cognitive dysfunction in sleep disorders. *Sleep Med Rev* 2001; 5(6): 423–45.

6 Van Dongen HPA, Baynard MD, Maislin G, Dinges DF. Systematic interindividual differences in neurobehavioral impairment from sleep loss: evidence of trait-like differential vulnerability. *Sleep* 2004; 27(3): 423–32.

7 Buguet A, Montmayeur A, Pigeau R, Naitoh P. Modafinil, d-amphetamine and placebo during 64 hours of sustained mental work. II. Effects on two nights of recovery sleep. *J Sleep Res* 1995; 4: 229–41.

8 Melamed S, Oksenberg A. Excessive daytime sleepiness and risk of occupational injuries in non-shift daytime workers. *Sleep* 2002; 25(3): 315–22.

9 Harma M, Sallinen M, Ranta R, Mutanen P, Muller K. The effect of an irregular shift system on sleepiness at work in train drivers and railway traffic controllers. *J Sleep Res* 2002; 11: 141–51.

10 Takahashi M. The role of prescribed napping in sleep medicine. *Sleep Med Rev* 2003; 7(3): 227–35.

11 Tietzel AJ, Lack LC. The short-term benefits of brief and long naps following nocturnal sleep restriction. *Sleep* 2001; 24(3): 293–300.

12 Akerstedt T, Kecklund G. Age, gender and early morning highway accidents. *J Sleep Res* 2001; 10: 105–10.

13 Suratt PM, Findley LJ. Driving with sleep apnea. *N Engl J Med* 1999; 340: 881–3.

14 Mitler MM, Miller JC, Lipsitz JJ, Walsh JK, Wylie CD. The sleep of long-haul truck drivers. *N Engl J Med* 1997; 337: 755–61.

15 Findley LJ, Unverzagt MR, Suratt PM. Automobile accidents involving patients with obstructive sleep apnea. *Am Rev Respir Dis* 1988; 138: 337–40.

16 Horstmann S, Hess CW, Bassetti C, Gugger M, Mathis J. Sleepiness-related accidents in sleep apnea patients. *Sleep* 2000; 23(3): 383–9.

17 Verster JC, Veldhuijzen DS, Volkerts ER. Residual effects of sleep medication on driving ability. *Sleep Med Rev* 2004; 8: 309–25.

18 Falleti MG, Maruff P, Collie A, Darby DG, McStephen M. Qualitative similarities in cognitive impairment associated with 24 h of sustained wakefulness and a blood alcohol concentration of 0.05%. *J Sleep Res* 2003; 12: 265–74.

19 George CFP. Driving simulators in clinical practice. *Sleep Med Rev* 2003; 7(4): 311–20.

20 MacLean AW, Davies DRT, Thiele K. The hazards and prevention of driving while sleepy. *Sleep Med Rev* 2003; 7(6): 507–21.

21 Sassani A, Findley LJ, Kryger M, Goldlust E, George C, Davidson TM. Reducing motor-vehicle collisions, costs, and fatalities by treating obstructive sleep apnea syndrome. *Sleep* 2004; 27(3): 453–8.

22 Valck E de, Cluiydts R. Slow-release caffeine as a countermeasure to driver sleepiness induced by partial sleep deprivation. *J Sleep Res* 2001; 10: 203–9.

23 Tung A, Mendleson WB. Anesthesia and sleep. *Sleep Med Rev* 2004; 8: 213–25.

24 Ogawa Y, Kanbayashi T, Saito Y, Takahashi Y, Kitajima T, Takahashi K, Hishikawa Y, Shimizu T. Total sleep deprivation elevates blood pressure through arterial baroreflex resetting: a study with microneurographic technique. *Sleep* 2003; 26(8): 986–9.

25 Matsumoto Y, Mishima K, Satoh K, Tozawa T, Mishima Y, Shimizu T, Hishikawa Y. Total sleep deprivation induces an acute and transient increase in NK cell activity in healthy young volunteers. *Sleep* 2001; 24(7): 804–9.

26 Chabas D, Taheri S, Renier C, Mignot E. The genetics of narcolepsy. *Annu Rev Genomics Hum Genet* 2003; 4: 459–83.

27 Mignot E. Genetic and familial aspects of narcolepsy. *Neurology* 1998; 50(Suppl. 1): S16–S22.

28 Picchioni D, Mignot EJ, Harsh JR. The month-of-birth pattern in narcolepsy is moderated by cataplexy severity and may be independent of HLA-DQB1*0602. *Sleep* 2004; 27(8): 1471–5.

29 Parkes JD, Chen SY, Clift SJ, Dahlitz MJ, Dunn G. The clinical diagnosis of the narcoleptic syndrome. *J Sleep Res* 1998; 7: 41–52.

30 Fosse R, Sitckgold R, Hobson JA. Emotional experience during rapid-eye-movement sleep in narcolepsy. *Sleep* 2002; 25(7): 724–730.

31 Krahn LE, Pankratz VS, Oliver L, Boeve BF, Silber MH. Hypocretin (orexin) levels in cerebrospinal fluid of patients with narcolepsy: relationship to cataplexy and HLA DQB1*0602 status. *Sleep* 2002; 25(7): 733–6.

32 Hungs M, Mignot E. Hypocretin/orexin, sleep and narcolepsy. *BioEssays* 2001; 23: 397–408.

33 Vourdas A, Shneerson JM, Gregory CA, Smith IE, King MA, Morrish E, McKenna PJ. Narcolepsy and psychopathology: is there an association? *Sleep Med* 2002; 3: 353–60.

34 Thorpy M. Current concepts in the etiology, diagnosis and treatment of narcolepsy. *Sleep Med* 2001; 2: 5–17.

35 Daniels M, King MA, Smith IE, Shneerson JM. Health-related quality of life in narcolepsy. *J Sleep Res* 2001; 10: 75–81.

36 Arias-Carrion O, Murillo-Rodriguez E, Xu M, Blanco-Centurion C, Drucker-Colin R, Shiromani PJ. Transplantation of hypocretin neurones into the pontine reticular formation: preliminary results. *Sleep* 2004; 27(8): 1465–70.

37 Mitler MM, Aldrich MS, Koob GF, Zarcone VP. Narcolepsy and its treatment with stimulants. *Sleep* 1994; 17: 352–71.

38 Schwartz JRL, Schwartz ER, Veit CA, Blakely EA. Modafinil for the treatment of excessive day-time sleepiness associated with narcolepsy. *Today's Therapeutic Trends* 1998; 16: 287–308.

39 US Modafinil in Narcolepsy Multicenter Study Group. Randomized trial of modafinil for the treatment of pathological somnolence in narcolepsy. *Ann Neurol* 1998; 43: 88–97.

40 Pigeua R, Naithoh P, Buguet A *et al.* Modafinil, d-amphetamine and placebo during 64 hours of sustained mental work. I. Effects on mood, fatigue, cognitive performance and body temperature. *J Sleep Res* 1995; 4: 212–28.

41 The US Xyrem^R Multicenter Study Group. A randomized, double blind, placebo-controlled multicenter trial comparing the effects of three doses of orally administered sodium oxybate with placebo for the treatment of narcolepsy. *Sleep* 2002; 25(1): 42–8.

42 Mamelak M, Black J, Montplaisir J, Ristanovic R. A pilot study on the effects of sodium oxybate on sleep architecture and daytime alertness in narcolepsy. *Sleep* 2004; 27: 1327–34.

43 Larrosa O, Llave Y de la, Barrio S, Granizo JJ, Garcia-Borreguero D. Stimulant and anticataplectic effects of reboxetine in patients with narcolepsy: a pilot study. *Sleep* 2001; 24(3): 282–5.

44 Billiard M, Dauvilliers Y. Idiopathic hypersomnia. *Sleep Med Rev* 2001; 5(5): 351–60.

45 Merriam AE. Kleine–Levin syndrome following acute viral encephalitis. *Biol Psychiatry* 1986; 21: 1301–4.

46 Gibbs JW III, Ciafaloni E, Radtke RA. Excessive daytime somnolence and increased rapid eye movement pressure in myotonic dystrophy. *Sleep* 2002; 25(6): 672–5.

47 Buguet A, Bourdon L, Bouteille B, Cespuglio R, Vincendeau P, Radomski MW, Dumas M. The duality of sleeping sickness: focusing on sleep. *Sleep Med Rev* 2001; 5(2): 139–53.

48 Buguet A, Gati R, Sevre JP, Develoux M, Bogui P, Lonsdorfer J. 24 hour polysomnographic evaluation in a patient with sleeping sickness. *Electroencephalogr Clin Neurophysiology* 1989; 72: 471–8.

49 Garcia-Borreguero D, Larrosa O, Bravo M. Parkinson's disease and sleep. *Sleep Med Rev* 2003; 7(2): 115–29.

50 Ohayon MM, Caulet M, Philip P, Guilleminault C, Priest RG. How sleep and mental disorders are related to complaints of daytime sleepiness. *Arch Intern Med* 1997; 157: 2645–52.

7 Insomnia

Introduction

Insomnia (agrypnia) is not a diagnosis, but a symptom, or more usually a symptom complex or syndrome. It is commonly defined as a perception of insufficient or poor quality sleep, despite an adequate opportunity for sleep, leading to a feeling of being unrefreshed on waking, during wakefulness, or in both of these situations. The relative importance of the two components of the syndrome, poor sleep at night and tiredness during the day, varies considerably. Most insomniacs find it difficult to fall asleep during the day despite feeling tired, and therefore do not have true excessive daytime sleepiness, although 'sleep reversal' is characterized by severe insomnia at night with prominent episodes of sleep during the day. It usually indicates severe disorganization of the sleep controlling mechanisms, as in Alzheimer's disease, African sleeping sickness and after encephalitis lethargica, but may occur in depression and schizophrenia. Insomniacs can be distinguished from short sleepers in that the latter, although they may sleep for no longer, wake feeling refreshed, function normally during the day, and do not complain about their sleep at night.

The large number of physiological factors that influence sleep often combine to cause a poor night's sleep. This is usually recognized as a natural response to the circumstances. A mild degree of insomnia merges into normality on the one hand, and into what can be a severe disability on the other, but the complaint of insomnia depends very much on the subject's expectations of the quality and length of sleep and of daytime tiredness. The correlation between the subjective reporting of sleep quality and objective findings at polysomnography is poor, although as a group those with insomnia tend to sleep less and wake more frequently than the general population.

Anxiety and frustration may lead to the degree of wakefulness during the night being overestimated. The extreme form of this is sleep state misperception, where the subject complains of insomnia, but has completely normal sleep as assessed at polysomnography. The mood, degree of boredom and medical disorders, both physical and psychological, also influence how severe insomnia is perceived to be. It therefore represents the degree of dissatisfaction with sleep or the mismatch between the expectation and reality rather than reflecting an absolute degree of sleep disturbance. It is less frequently due to organic disease than excessive daytime sleepiness, but, like this, its origin is often multifactorial.

Prevalence

Insomnia is the commonest sleep complaint. Almost every adult suffers from it at some stage in their life. Surveys have indicated that around one-third of adults in developed societies have some degree of insomnia each year, and 10–15% of the population have insomnia at any one time. At the age of 30 about 5% of males and 15% of females have insomnia, but by the age of 70 years 15% of males and 25% of females have this problem [1]. Difficulty in initiating sleep is twice as common in women as in men, but there is less gender difference in difficulty in maintaining sleep, and early morning awakening is equally common in men and women.

The high prevalence figures need to be interpreted cautiously because of the subjective nature of the complaint and differences in the definitions of insomnia. Its commonness may reflect the pressure in developed societies to function effectively during the day, particularly at work, while restricting sleeping time because of social activities and leisure opportunities, and combined with an increasing preoccupation with medical problems.

The complaint of insomnia is commoner in those who are anxious or depressed, those with chronic physical illnesses, and those who drink excessive quantities of alcohol or take drugs which affect the quality of sleep. In about half of these it is felt to be severe enough to require medical care, although this

Table 7.1 Causes of patterns of insomnia.

Difficulty in initiating sleep	Difficulty in maintaining sleep	Early morning waking
Poor sleep hygiene	Pain, discomfort	Old age
Poor sleep environment	Poor sleep environment	Poor sleep environment
Drugs	Drugs	Drugs
Anxiety	Medical problem, e.g. asthma, nocturia	Depression
Psychophysiological insomnia	RLS & PLMS	Mania
RLS	OSA, CSA, CSR	ASPS
DSPS	Dementia	
	Psychophysiological insomnia	

ASPS, advanced sleep phase syndrome; CSA, central sleep apnoeas; CSR, Cheyne–Stokes respiration; DSPS, delayed sleep phase syndrome; OSA, obstructive sleep apnoeas; RLS, restless legs syndrome; PLMS, periodic limb movements in sleep.

is surprisingly often not obtained. The reasons for this are uncertain, but the lack of attention directed to insomnia by the medical profession, the failure to develop coherent management plans and the perception that there is a lack of effective treatments probably all contribute.

Patterns of insomnia

Insomnia can be separated into the following three patterns (Table 7.1).

Difficulty in initiating sleep (DIS, sleep onset insomnia)

This is defined as a sleep latency of greater than 30 min and is often due to a high level of arousal associated with anxiety, and other factors.

Difficulty in maintaining sleep (DMS, sleep maintenance insomnia)

Waking may occur irregularly during the night, or at specific times as in cluster headaches occurring during REM sleep and the 90-min cycles of REM sleep behaviour disorder episodes.

Early morning waking without further sleep (EMW)

This is common in the elderly and in most of the conditions listed in Table 7.2.

Time course of insomnia

Insomnia may be a temporary phase, it may fluctuate or it may be a long-term problem. The causes and perpetuation of these three patterns are different.

Table 7.2 Common causes of secondary insomnia.

Medical disorders and physical disability
Dementia
Parkinsonism
Restless legs syndrome
Circadian rhythm disorders
Depression
Menopausal symptoms
Shift work
Drugs

Transient insomnia (adjustment sleep disorder, acute insomnia)

The diagnosis of transient insomnia can only be firmly made retrospectively after it has been relieved. It is usually defined as insomnia that lasts for less than three weeks, and very often has a close temporal association to an event which is clearly recognized by the patient and is often stressful. It is equally common in males and females and is more likely if there is a history of previous poor sleep, or if there is a low threshold for emotional arousal. Recurrent episodes of transient insomnia are also common.

Transient insomnia is usually triggered by one of the following factors.

Changes in sleep environment

These may be physical stimuli such as noise or bright lights, or movements or noises, such as snoring, made by the bed partner. Sleeping in unfamiliar environments such as a hotel or in hospital, including a sleep laboratory, may also impair sleep.

High arousal states

These may be due to emotional events which increase the level of alertness and physiological arousal. They include bereavement, apprehension before an examination, excitement before a holiday, anxiety about job insecurity, and brief illnesses or pain.

Poor sleep hygiene

Transient insomnia may result from temporary adoption of an irregular sleep–wake cycle. Drinking excess coffee or alcohol in the evenings, or other central nervous system stimulants or drugs which can impair sleep, either while being taken or during the withdrawal phase, may be responsible.

Short-term circadian rhythm disorders induced particularly by jet lag and rotating shift work

This type of transient insomnia may be severe, but resolves once the trigger factor is removed or the patient adjusts to the new circumstances. It may evolve into chronic insomnia if this adjustment fails to take place.

Cyclical insomnia (recurrent insomnia)

Cyclical insomnia is less common than transient insomnia and implies an unstable balance between the sleep and wake drives. This instability may be temporary or lifelong. The insomnia may recur in phase with physiological changes as in circadian rhythm disorders and premenstrual insomnia, with psychological changes such as manic depression and anorexia nervosa, or with recurring behavioural changes such as in drug addicts and alcoholics who binge drink.

Chronic insomnia (persistent insomnia)

Chronic insomnia represents a heterogeneous group of conditions that have been investigated less than most other sleep disorders. They fall into two main groups.

Primary insomnia

This type of insomnia is not due to a primary sleep disorder, psychiatric condition, or medical or neurological problem, or related to drug use or withdrawal. It is due to a hyperarousal state, possibly due to excessive activity of the ascending reticular activating system, which persists during wakefulness as well as sleep.

Secondary insomnia

This is the result of a primary sleep or circadian rhythm disorder, or a psychiatric, neurological or medical condition, or related to drug use or withdrawal (Fig. 7.1). It is often multifactorial, and is particularly common in the elderly who have more medical problems and in whom sleep is more easily disrupted.

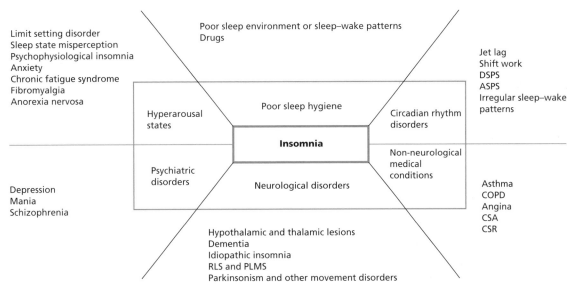

Fig. 7.1 Causes of insomnia. ASPS, advanced sleep phase syndrome; COPD, chronic obstructive pulmonary disease; CSA, central sleep apnoea; CSR, Cheyne–Stokes respiration; DSPS, delayed sleep phase syndrome; RLS, restless legs syndrome; PLMS, periodic limb movements in sleep.

Effects of insomnia

Physiological effects

The electroencephalogram shows lower delta power and increased beta activity than normal during sleep in primary insomnia, suggesting that there may be a reduction in the homeostatic drive to sleep as well as hyperarousal. Intrusion of alpha waves is common and may be due to a lower threshold for arousal to stimuli such as pain or noise. It is associated with awareness of thoughts during sleep, and with the perception that sleep is unrefreshing.

The peak melatonin secretion is reduced in primary insomnia in proportion to its duration rather than its severity. PET and SPECT scans have shown increased cerebral blood flow during sleep, with less reduction in the metabolic rate in the anterior cingulate and medial prefrontal cortex during wakefulness compared with NREM sleep.

The oxygen uptake is increased in stages 3 and 4 NREM sleep, even when arousals are allowed for, in those with primary insomnia compared to normal subjects. This suggests that the hyperarousal disorder underlying this condition affects both sleep and wakefulness. The heart rate is faster in all stages of sleep as well as in wakefulness in primary insomnia, and the pattern of heart rate variability indicates an increase in sympathetic and a reduction in parasympathetic activity. Hypertension is also commoner in those with insomnia than in normal subjects.

The serum level of noradrenaline is raised throughout the night in those with insomnia, particularly when their sleep efficiency is low, and it is likely that sympathetic activity is increased throughout the day as well. The ACTH level is raised throughout the day and night and there is a significant increase in plasma cortisol IL-6, and TNF alpha levels are increased, particularly in the daytime, but also during sleep.

These abnormalities may be detectable even before insomnia has become established. In subjects who undergo polysomnography and who subsequently develop insomnia, there is raised sympathetic activity with, for instance, an increased heart rate. This suggests that there is a trait to respond in this way to stressful situations.

Psychological disturbances

These are common during the episode of insomnia, but are completely reversible once it is relieved. They include:

1 Loss of concentration and deterioration of memory.

2 Irritability and mood disturbance including anxiety and depression. Anxiety and depression are present in more than 50% of those with chronic insomnia and may be either a cause or a result of the insomnia. A vicious cycle of insomnia and worsening anxiety and depression often develops. If insomnia persists despite treatment of depression or alcoholism or following cessation of antipsychotic drugs and schizophrenia, it is more likely that the underlying psychiatric disorder will relapse.

3 Loss of motivation.

4 Fear regarding long-term health effects of insomnia.

5 Intrusive ruminating thoughts at bedtime. These are often related to a fear of not sleeping or frustration or anger at the degree of insomnia and of not being able to function effectively, either at work or in family or social life.

Physical effects

These are also common and reversible once the insomnia is relieved. They include:

1 A sensation of physical weariness, fatigue or tiredness. This is distinct from excessive daytime sleepiness which mainly occurs in the minority of patients with insomnia in whom there is an organic cause.

2 Muscle aches. These are usually worse in the limbs, but may be diffuse and cause headaches and neckache. They are probably due to muscle tension associated with a lack of the normal inhibition of motor activity during sleep with the result that the muscles are contracting throughout sleep as well as during wakefulness.

3 Hypertension.

4 Short stature in children.

5 Increased risk of falls, particularly in the elderly.

Social effects

Insomnia has been shown to significantly impair the quality of life, particularly in the elderly. It is more common in lower socio-economic groups and is said to be associated with fewer episodes of promotion at work than in those without insomnia. This may be due to tiredness and poor work performance, but, equally, anxiety about the latter could be the cause of the insomnia. An excessive concern about responsibilities is thought to contribute to the insomnia of ambitious, high-achieving personalities.

Mortality

Individuals who sleep for less than 6 h per night have a shorter life expectancy than those who report sleeping

Table 7.3 Age and insomnia.

Childhood	Adolescence	Young and middle-aged adults	Old age
	Limit-setting disorders		
		Anxiety	
	Idiopathic insomnia		
		Drugs	
		Poor sleep hygiene	
	DSPS		
		RLS	
	Hyperarousal states		
	Depression		
			Menopause
		Dementia	
		Medical disorders	
		Neurological disorders	
	Narcolepsy		

DSPS, delayed sleep phase syndrome; RLS, restless legs syndrome.

for 7–8 h per night. This may be because diseases causing the sleep disturbance also shorten life expectancy, or because the high arousal state present in insomnia increases morbidity, and reduces the rate of recovery from other medical disorders.

Insomnia in children and adolescents

Insomnia or sleeplessness in children is a very common problem. Around 30% of 1 year olds wake at night and although the same number have a sleeping problem at the age of 5, this falls to around 10% in adolescence. Childhood sleepiness leads to parental sleep deprivation, mood changes, and frustration, which make it more difficult to cope with the child's disorder of sleep and can reinforce or help to perpetuate the problem.

It is almost invariably the parents' complaint about the child which leads to medical attention being sought rather than the child's complaint. It therefore reflects the attitudes of the parents, and other factors, such as parental depression. The threshold for seeking help varies considerably and it is important to assess not only parental attitudes to the child's sleep behaviour, but also the child's view of this, any fears about sleep or recall of adverse events during sleep.

The causes of insomnia vary according to the age of the child (Table 7.3).

Infancy

It is normal for infants to wake at night, but by around 6 months many children can sleep through the night. Sleepiness and crying in infants may also be due to 'colic', food or cow's milk allergy, gastro-oesophageal reflux, or chronic middle ear infections, which may not be readily apparent. Most children are able to sleep through the night after the age of 6 months without requiring feeding. Frequent waking at night requiring feeding to fall asleep again is usually due to a conditioned reflex rather than a physiological need. The frequency of night-time feeds should be gradually reduced.

1–4 years

Around 30% of children aged 1 year signal their awakenings at night to their parents by crying and this pattern may continue subsequently. It is usually the result of acquired behaviour patterns, which can be prevented or treated, particularly if they are tackled early. They are influenced both by the maternal behaviour and attitudes, and by the child's development.

The most effective strategy is behavioural management, whereby presleep routines lead to winding down of the child's activity become associated with the initiation of sleep. These routines include feeding, nappy changing, rocking or cuddling the child, and taking the child to bed with comforting toys and other objects. Going to bed should be associated with sleeping rather than playing. The parents should set limits on when the child goes to bed and how much subsequent attention the child has. If there is a problem in settling to sleep it may be necessary to gradually reduce the time spent with the child before sleep, to reduce the number of times that the parent checks the child during the night in response to crying, and to reward improvements in sleep behaviour. These measures require confidence from the parents in making adjustments.

4–12 years

Difficulty in initiating sleep may be due to behavioural factors similar to those at younger ages. The child may become irritable, with poor attention and poor school performance, which may lead to family tension. Idiopathic insomnia may develop at this age.

Night-time fears become increasingly common in middle childhood. These may take the form of fears of shadows, monsters or people apparently in the bedroom. These fears may be triggered by physical, psychological or family events and may be related to anxiety. They occasionally follow physical or emotional abuse. They often represent a type of separation anxiety and can be alleviated by sharing the bedroom with a pet, sibling or possibly a parent. Night-time fears should be distinguished from worries about family or school issues.

Frequent nightmares may lead to a fear of going to sleep. Nightmares develop around the age of 2–5 years and are commonest between the ages of 6 and 10 (page 189).

Waking during the night is unusual since the quality of sleep is greatest at around the age of 5 years, but may occur if there are physical disorders such as muscle cramps or 'growing pains', which are probably a manifestation of the restless legs syndrome during sleep.

Waking early in the morning may be a manifestation of an advanced sleep phase syndrome or depression. Early morning waking may also result from going to bed too early, or be due to a noisy or light sleep environment which prevents the child from sleeping later.

Adolescence

Insomnia due to failure of the parents to set limits in childhood usually improves in adolescence as control of the sleep patterns passes to the patient. He or she may choose to return to normal sleeping hours. Often, however, a pattern of a delayed sleep phase syndrome or of a short sleeper is adopted, and this may persist into adult life. These patterns are accentuated by behavioural factors, such as late night social activities, caffeinated drinks in the evening, alcohol, nicotine or recreational drugs, particularly amphetamines. Anxiety and depression frequently cause insomnia.

Drug treatment of insomnia in children should be limited to short-term courses. Antihistamines, chloral, benzodiazepines and related drugs have been used, although there is little evidence for their efficacy. Melatonin is also widely used in children, despite its potential effects on reproduction, but it only has a mild hypnotic effect and only improves circadian rhythms in certain specified conditions, such as the delayed sleep phase syndrome.

Insomnia in the elderly

Insomnia is common in the elderly. As many as 3–4% of subjects develop insomnia each year, and the complaint becomes progressively more frequent in females rather than in males with age, although paradoxically sleep is objectively better preserved in elderly women than in elderly men. This may be because men under-report insomnia to a greater degree. Other medical conditions, such as dementia, may reduce awareness of insomnia, but, conversely, the increased burden placed on the carers by the elderly insomniac is often the trigger that precipitates referral for medical care or transfer to a residential institution.

Insomnia in the elderly is usually multifactorial. Physiological arousals from sleep are more common and this increased fragility of sleep underlies the difficulty in maintaining sleep rather than initiating sleep which is particularly a problem in the elderly. Insomnia in the elderly is often associated with the following situations.

Chronic physical disabilities

These include rheumatoid arthritis, gastro-intestinal symptoms, pain and nocturia. In addition there are age-related sleep disorders which lead to insomnia, such as the restless legs syndrome and periodic limb movements in sleep and Parkinsonism.

Depression

Depression may be both the cause and the result of insomnia, and occurs in around 5% of the elderly population. It characteristically causes early morning awakening, but also leads to difficulty in maintaining sleep.

Maladaptive behaviour leading to poor sleep hygiene

A common sleep hygiene problem is lack of exposure to bright light. This is often reduced in the elderly because they remain indoors for longer and may have cataracts and macular degeneration which reduce the amount of light stimulating the retina. Exposure to bright light in the morning may also exacerbate the advanced sleep phase syndrome. Light exposure at night, even if it is brief, may reduce melatonin secretion and worsen insomnia. Lack of physical exercise, either due to a lack of opportunity, for instance in a residential home or because of physical restrictions, frequent daytime naps, particularly in the evenings, and excessive caffeine intake may all contribute to insomnia.

Treatment of insomnia in the elderly includes the following.

Sleep hygiene advice

Increased physical activity and exposure to bright light, ideally around 1000 lux for at least 1 h during the day, may help. Avoidance of naps in the evenings and caffeine at night is important. It is also important to avoid bright light during the night by, for instance, having a dimmer switch available.

Sedative drugs

Benzodiazepines may relieve the insomnia, but should only be used in the short term, and often cause sedation during the next day, with an increased risk of falls and accidents, including road traffic accidents. Shorter-acting drugs, such as zaleplon, zopiclone and zolpidem, are preferable in the elderly. Antihistamines and sedating antidepressants are frequently used, but may cause daytime sedation. Selective serotonin re-uptake inhibitors may improve depression if this is the cause of insomnia, but should be given in the morning to minimize the effect of their stimulating action on insomnia. Self-medication with alcohol is common, and while it may help to initiate sleep, it often causes insomnia later in the night.

Assessment

History

A careful history is essential to accurately assess insomnia (Chapter 3) (Table 7.4). The issues that should be considered are described below.

1 What is the nature of the insomnia? Is the complaint mainly about poor sleep, or feeling tired during the day? Is the insomnia at night due to a difficulty in initiating or maintaining sleep, or to early morning awakening, and is there a pattern of sleep reversal?

2 What are the subject's sleep–wake routines and sleep hygiene? The timing of sleep onset and waking up, and the regularity of these, is particularly important.

3 Why does the subject wake up? What is it that he or she is aware of on waking? Is there awareness of snoring, choking, vivid dreams, panicking, or symptoms such as headache, wheezing, a need to micturate, pain or discomfort? What does the subject do after waking? Are there any intrusive thoughts or does environmental noise prevent sleep from starting again? How long does the awakening last?

4 What is the time course of the insomnia? Is it acute or long-term, and if so at what age did it start? Is there any identifiable cause for the initiation of insomnia? Has it been cyclical since its onset and, if so, are these fluctuations associated with any identifiable factors? Are there features to suggest a circadian rhythm disorder?

5 Are there any factors that are perpetuating the insomnia? These include environmental noise or light, poor sleep hygiene, anxiety, depression, inappropriate drugs such as caffeine or excess alcohol before going to sleep, or medical disorders such as circadian rhythm disorders, dementia, or organic midbrain, hypothalamic or thalamic lesions.

6 What is the patient's attitude to the insomnia and what are the expectations of sleep? Are there any fears regarding its effects or psychological reactions to it such as a sense of loss of control?

Physical examination

Physical examination is usually normal in those with insomnia and contributes little to the assessment of its severity and causes, except in the minority with an underlying neurological disorder.

Investigations

A factor such as depression, anxiety, inappropriate drug treatment or poor sleep hygiene can often be identified and treated without further investigation.

Table 7.4 Diagnosis of the cause of insomnia from the history.

Diagnosis	History
Poor sleep hygiene	Erratic sleeping times, especially wake-up times Poor sleep environment, e.g. uncomfortable bed, noisy or light bedroom Shift worker High caffeine or other stimulant intake, especially in the evening
Hyperarousal state	Identifiable cause of onset of insomnia Excessive concern about sleep Rarely falls asleep in the day May show generalized anxiety features May have other disorder-specific symptoms, e.g. muscle pain and stiffness
Depression	EMW Early onset of sleep, often with daytime naps Other symptoms of depression
Neurological disorders	Insomnia may be profound Other neurological symptoms often present Sleep reversal in dementia Restless legs symptoms in evenings Daytime sleepiness and cataplexy suggest narcolepsy
Non-neurological medical disorders	Awakenings associated with recognizable symptom, e.g. angina, wheeze, nocturia Other symptoms of the underlying disorder Daytime sleepiness often accompanies insomnia
Circadian rhythm disorders	Regular pattern of DSPS or ASPS Irregular but recognizable pattern of non-24-h sleep–wake cycles Risk factor, e.g. shift work, transmeridian travel, blind, CNS lesion

ASPS, advanced sleep phase syndrome; CNS, central nervous system; DSPS, delayed sleep phase syndrome; EMW, early morning awakening.

Investigation in a specialist centre is required if insomnia persists despite treatment interventions or if there is doubt about its cause. Investigations may be needed to investigate either the degree or the causes of insomnia.

Demonstrate the degree of insomnia
A sleep diary and actigraphy in the home may be of value, but polysomnography may be needed, particularly to diagnose sleep state misperception.

Investigate the causes of the insomnia
This includes the following.
1 Questionnaires regarding anxiety and depression.
2 Polysomnography. This shows the extent and stages of sleep, and helps to elucidate the cause of insomnia (Table 7.5). It can be combined with temperature recording and melatonin and cortisol estimations to assess circadian rhythm disorders.
3 Imaging of brain. Computerized tomography (CT) and magnetic resonance imaging (MRI) scans are indicated if organic neurological disorders, including dementia, are being considered.

Principles of treatment

The causes of insomnia are often multifactorial, particularly in the elderly. They involve a combination of adverse environmental factors, maladaptive behaviour patterns and attitudes, and psychiatric problems which predispose towards insomnia or may be the result of it. Explanation, optimization of sleep hygiene and treatment of the causes of the insomnia are almost always required, but if these are insufficient, additional treatments should be considered (Fig. 7.2).

Explain, reassure and advise
Explanation, reassurance, and advice about modification of lifestyle and about accepting a degree of long-term insomnia if necessary may be helpful.

Table 7.5 Causes of insomnia requiring polysomnography.

Cause	Polysomnography findings
Organic causes: circadian rhythm disorder	Abnormal sleep-onset and wake-up times ± sleep architecture
PLMS	Limb movements and arousals
CSA and CSR	Abnormal respiratory patterns
Thalamic lesions	Abnormal sleep architecture
Sleep-state misperception	Normal sleep demonstrated
Multifactorial origin: e.g. combination of drug effects and a hyperarousal state, or poor sleep hygiene and chronic fatigue syndrome	Relative contributions of each factor

CSA, central sleep apnoea; CSR, Cheyne–Stokes respiration; PLMS, periodic limb movements in sleep.

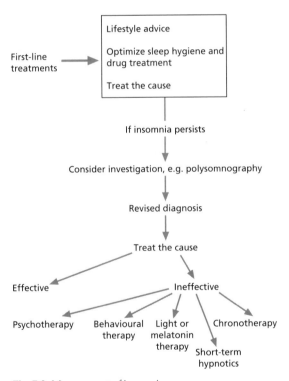

Fig. 7.2 Management of insomnia.

Optimize sleep hygiene

The quantity, quality and timing of sleep are affected by many everyday activities and attitudes (Table 1.4). Poor sleep hygiene is probably the most important cause of insomnia, but its significance is generally underestimated. In developed societies sleep is being increasingly squeezed into the time left over after family, social, work and recreational activities, with the result that insomnia, excessive daytime sleepiness and other sleep symptoms are becoming increasingly common.

The aim of sleep hygiene is to translate an understanding of the nature and control of sleep into practical advice about how to promote this through changes in lifestyle and the environment. It is especially important that the elderly counteract the loss of consolidation of the sleep pattern and their advanced sleep phase.

Sleep hygiene is useful in a wide range of sleep disorders [2] and combines advice about homeostatic, adaptive and circadian aspects of sleep control, how to avoid sleep deprivation and sleep fragmentation, and how to respond to awakenings from sleep if these occur. Some aspects of sleep hygiene fall into more than one of these categories, but in general it entails the following.

1 Altering the sleep environment so that the bed is comfortable and the bedroom warm, dark and quiet.

2 Improving sleep–wake patterns. This is required for most subjects with insomnia. Attention to increasing physical activity during the day, preparation for sleep (for instance by mentally winding down and taking a hot bath), and regular meals and sleep and wake times, may all be of help. Naps should be avoided, particularly in the evenings, and it is important to wake up at the same time each morning and also if possible to go to bed at the same time each evening.

3 Changing drug intake. Avoiding caffeinated drinks in the evenings and discontinuing other stimulants, such as glucocorticoids, and altering the timing of diuretics in order to minimize nocturia may all be of benefit.

Changes in sleep hygiene can be monitored by keeping a sleep diary and occasionally with actigraphy to assess the pattern of activity objectively. The ways in which poor sleep hygiene impairs sleep should be explained to the patient and a practical and personalized plan provided. Regular follow-up to monitor progress and to maintain motivation is important.

Treat the cause of insomnia

The commonest treatable causes of secondary insomnia are shown on Fig. 7.1.

Medical disorders

Medical disorders and symptoms due to, for instance, thyrotoxicosis, nocturnal asthma or angina should be treated.

Depression

It is important to treat depression and anxiety, which can both be either causes of insomnia or responses to it, before more complex aspects of management are considered. Antidepressants should only be used if features of depression are present and not as a routine treatment. Sedating tricyclic antidepressants, such as trimipramine, imipramine and doxepin, are particularly effective. Paroxetine is the most suitable of the SSRI antidepressants, several of which worsen insomnia even if it is due to depression (Table 7.6). The sedating action of mirtazapine is useful in treating insomnia.

Trazodone is widely used, especially in the USA, but it is probably less effective. Antidepressant drugs may successfully elevate the mood in depression, but insomnia may persist despite this. This combination increases the risk of a subsequent relapse of the depression.

Menopause

Insomnia associated with the menopause often responds to oestrogen replacement treatment. The duration of stages 3 and 4 NREM sleep is increased. Symptomatic improvement is most likely if hot flushes are relieved by the oestrogen.

Primary sleep disorders

Some sleep disorders causing insomnia, such as narcolepsy and periodic limb movements during sleep, require specialist assessment before initiating treatment (Chapters 6 and 9).

Drug-induced insomnia

Prescribed drugs causing insomnia should whenever possible be changed to an alternative which does not cause this problem. Caffeine and nicotine intake should be reduced if they are contributing to insomnia.

Table 7.6 Choice of benzodiazepine and related types of hypnotic.

Indication	Drug property	Drugs
DIS	Rapid onset	Triazolam
		Flunitrazepam
		Zaleplon
		Zolpidem
		Zopiclone
DMS	Intermediate duration	Temazepam
		Lormetazepam
		Oxazepam
		Zopiclone
		Zolpidem
EMW	Moderately long-acting	Temazepam
		Lormetazepam
		Flurazepam
		Nitrazepam
EMW with anxiety	Long-acting	Nitrazepam
		Diazepam
		Clorazepate
		Clonazepam
		Oxazepam

DIS, difficulty in initiating sleep; DMS, difficulty in maintaining sleep; EMW, early morning awakening.

Shift work

Counter-measures should be employed to minimize the insomnia and excessive sleepiness associated with shift work (page 123).

Hypnotic treatment

The aim of hypnotic treatment is not only to improve the quality and duration of sleep, but also to increase the degree of alertness during the day, and to relieve any hyperarousal state. Unfortunately, with many hypnotics the dose needed to improve sleep at night also causes sedation during the day. Short-acting benzodiazepines, zaleplon, zolpidem and zopiclone avoid this complication. They are of particular value in the elderly, in whom the metabolism of benzodiazepines is slowed and sedation during wakefulness may lead to confusion, amnesia and ataxia, leading to falls. Long-acting hypnotics may also impair psychomotor performance during the day in younger subjects and lead to accidents related to driving and handling moving machinery.

Tolerance develops to most hypnotics with prolonged use and because of this it is usually recommended that treatment should not exceed 1 month in duration. This is often sufficient to break the pattern of insomnia, especially when hypnotic treatment is used in conjunction with other measures. This is also sufficiently long to cope with temporary exacerbations of chronic insomnia and with transient and cyclical insomnia. Occasionally, however, longer-term treatment is required, in which case the benefits of treatment have to be weighed against the risks of tolerance, dependence and withdrawal symptoms. These may be reduced by giving the hypnotic intermittently, for instance for only 3–5 days each week.

Hypnotics should be avoided wherever possible in children, during pregnancy and also while breastfeeding, since many drugs – for instance, benzodiazepines – cross the placenta and enter breast milk. Most hypnotics interact with other similar drugs and alcohol to accentuate their hypnotic effect and daytime sedation. There is a risk of respiratory depression and induction of obstructive sleep apnoeas, and wherever possible hypnotics should be avoided in the presence of risk factors for these conditions.

The most effective drugs for transient insomnia are quick-acting hypnotics, such as diazepam, zopiclone, eszopiclone and zolpidem.

The most suitable drugs for treating chronic insomnia, with and without anxiety [3, 4], are discussed in detail in Chapter 4.

1 *Benzodiazepines and similar drugs* (Tables 4.6 and 7.6). These are the most commonly used hypnotics.
2 *Barbiturates*. These are now very rarely used.
3 *Antihistamines*. Sedating antihistamines such as chlorpheniramine, promethazine and diphenhydramine lead to daytime sleepiness as well as anticholinergic side-effects.
4 *Chloral*. This is a mild hypnotic which may be useful in children and the elderly.
5 *Melatonin*. Exogenous melatonin is a mild hypnotic but this effect is only apparent if it is taken during the day. It also advances the sleep phase if it is given in the evening, and long-term treatment entrains the circadian sleep rhythm. It has limited effectiveness in insomnia [5], but should be considered in circadian rhythm disorders (Chapter 5).
6 *Alcohol*. This is frequently used to facilitate sleep, but causes problems including REM sleep rebound late in the night.
7 *Herbal remedies*. These are commonly used but neither their efficacy nor their long-term safety has been established.

Cognitive behavioural therapies

Insomnia responds much better to specific psychotherapy and behavioural therapies directed towards the aims, beliefs and behaviour about insomnia than it does to conventional psychotherapy. The aim is to reverse the maladaptive thoughts and behaviour patterns that perpetuate insomnia [6]. Treatment is often combined with sleep hygiene advice [7].

The techniques of cognitive behavioural therapy are, however, time consuming, expensive and require a skilled therapist. The treatments should be individualized for each patient, but can be delivered in group therapy. The optimum duration and frequency of treatment have yet to be established [8]. Follow-up is required to deal with problems that may arise and to motivate the patient to continue with treatment.

It is uncertain which modes of behavioural therapy are most effective for the different types of insomnia. Cognitive therapy requires a good relationship between the patient and the therapist and is most effective if the patient has an active and coping style.

It may be best to combine cognitive behavioural therapy with a course of up to 1 month of hypnotic treatment in order to break the established patterns of thoughts and behaviour, as well as to give rapid relief of insomnia which can then be maintained by the cognitive behavioural therapy. A similar approach using a beta blocker such as propranolol, to reduce the level of arousal, may help. The addition of modafinil to improve the ability to cope with initial sleepiness during the day during cognitive behavioural therapy and to increase daytime activity, and thereby promote sleep at night, may be effective.

The most important individual techniques are described below.

Cognitive therapy

Chronic insomnia is characterized by intrusive thoughts and worries and often a racing mind. In contrast good sleepers often think of nothing in particular before falling asleep. Concerns about not sleeping, or the urgency for sleep, the extent of the consequences of poor sleep and the need to control sleep all lead to frustration, performance anxiety, arousal and difficulty in initiating sleep.

Cognitive therapy aims to change these maladaptive thoughts, which need to be accurately identified, discussed with the patient, and then realistic expectations set. The patient should become able to accept and tolerate times of sleepiness without becoming emotionally distressed or frustrated.

Cognitive therapy includes techniques which enhance the ability to cope with stresses which may be contributing to insomnia, and it aims to change the assumptions and perceptions about insomnia [9].

Mental relaxation

Many insomniacs are excessively concerned with activities of the previous day or the next day, and it is important that these concerns are minimized by allowing time before going to bed to sort out problems that have arisen or may arise. Encouragement to relax, to ignore irrelevant thoughts and to visualize a reassuring or pleasant scene is important. Mental relaxation techniques including meditation and yoga may be of help.

Physical relaxation

Physical tension, particularly shortly before bedtime, is common in insomnia. A programme of relaxation exercises shortly before attempting to fall asleep may be effective, especially in DIS. Meditation, deep breathing and biofeedback techniques may be useful.

Stimulus control therapy

The principle of this treatment is to condition the patient to associate being in bed with successful attempts at falling asleep and maintaining sleep. It aims to interrupt the negative link between the patient's thoughts about sleep by encouraging sleep-promoting behaviour.

Mental conditioning to associate the bedroom with sleep and not with other activities, apart from sexual activity, should be reinforced by not allowing, for instance, video or television watching, working, eating or computer activities in the bedroom.

The subject should only go to bed when he or she feels sleepy and not according to the time. He or she should get out of bed if wakefulness persists for more than 15–30 min, or if wakefulness during the night occurs for this long. It is best to leave the bedroom and carry out a non-stimulating activity such as reading or listening to music before returning when feeling sleepy again.

These techniques enable control to be exerted over the problem which then becomes more manageable, although a degree of sleep restriction may be induced.

Sleep restriction

Many subjects with insomnia try to compensate for this by spending more time in bed to provide enough opportunity for sleep, and particularly by staying in bed trying to sleep while this is difficult. This not only induces abnormal circadian rhythms, but also causes frustration.

Sleep restriction assumes that sleep deprivation will lead to deeper and more continuous sleep which, in turn, will reverse the negative conditioning which perpetuates insomnia. Sleep restriction techniques reduce the time in bed in order to increase sleep efficiency.

A sleep–wake diary is kept and the initial time spent in bed should represent the average time asleep or felt to be asleep, but not less than 4.5 h. This is gradually increased as long as the subjective sleep efficiency remains above 80–85% for five nights in every seven. A constant awakening time is adhered to irrespective of the time of going to bed. Fifteen to thirty-minute increments of sleep time are usual and no daytime naps are allowed.

There may be an initial worsening of daytime sleepiness but this gradually improves over a period of months.

Chronotherapy

Chronotherapy is the manipulation of sleep and waking times by resetting the sleep cycle and then maintaining the change. It is in effect similar to a time zone transition but changes in the sleep cycle are made gradually in order to avoid symptoms similar to jet lag.

Many insomniacs regularly go to bed too early and this contributes to DIS. A regular waking time helps to establish a regular circadian pattern and this should be continued even at weekends. Compliance with chronotherapy regimes is arduous and often limits the benefits that are obtained.

The indications for chronotherapy are as follows.
1 To prevent and minimize the effects of jet lag. Chronotherapy induces a progressive adjustment to the new environmental time before and after arrival at the destination.
2 Delayed sleep phase syndrome. Putting the bedtime back 3 h each night, and waking up 3 h later, until the desired sleep and waking times are reached is often effective. This requires a motivated patient and determination to maintain the rhythm.
3 Advanced sleep phase syndrome.

Light therapy (phototherapy, luminotherapy)

Light therapy is useful in insomnia due to circadian rhythm disorders such as jet lag, shift work and delayed and advanced sleep phase syndromes (see Chapter 5). It has also been used in the evening to delay the sleep phase and improve early morning waking, for instance in depression. Its effectiveness in this situation is uncertain and is probably only transient.

Primary insomnia (hyperarousal states)

Overview

Primary insomnia is the second commonest cause, after poor sleep hygiene, of chronic insomnia [10].

Table 7.7 Causes of primary insomnia.

Sleep-state misperception
Psychophysiological insomnia
Anxiety states
Attention deficit hyperactivity disorder
Chronic fatigue syndrome
Fibromyalgia
?Idiopathic insomnia

The hyperarousal state associated with primary insomnia is usually present throughout wakefulness as well as during sleep, and may be due to an increase of the activity of the ascending reticular activating system or possibly to a reduction in the adaptive drive to sleep.

Causes

Several clinical patterns of insomnia have been identified and given distinct names (Tables 7.7, 7.8). There is, however, considerable overlap and their classification is unsatisfactory. They all have similar causes which can be broken down into the following.

Predisposing factors

1 Constitutional factors. These probably have a genetic basis.

Table 7.8 Comparison of hyperarousal states.

Characteristic	Psychophysiological insomnia	Anxiety states	Chronic fatigue syndrome	Fibromyalgia
Age of onset (years)	20–40	Any age	Young adults	Young adults
Gender	M < F	M < F	M < F	M < F
Trigger	Stressful event	Nil or stress	Often infection	Nil
Psychological effects	Anxiety about sleep	Generalized anxiety	Poor concentration and memory	Generalized anxiety
Somatization of symptoms	++	±	Fatigue	Muscle aches, point tenderness
Polysomnography				
–TST	↓	↓	↓	↓
–SL	↑	↑	↑	↑
–1 and 2 NREM sleep	↑	NAD	?	↑
–REM sleep		NAD	↑	
–Alpha intrusion	+	–	+	+
–Awakenings	↓	↑	?	↑

F, Female; M, Male; NAD, normal; NREM, non-rapid eye movement; REM, rapid eye movement; SL, sleep latency; TST, total sleep time.

2 Abnormal circadian rhythms, e.g. shift work or a delayed sleep phase syndrome which predisposes to difficulty in initiating sleep.

3 Personality differences. A personality pattern with intrusive and ruminating thoughts and internalization or somatization of stress and a tendency to depression is present in around 75% of those with chronic insomnia.

4 Age. Elderly subjects are more vulnerable to develop disturbed sleep and may have an advanced sleep phase pattern and an earlier circadian phase.

5 Susceptibility to specific diseases. Disorders whose symptoms are exacerbated by sleep such as peptic ulcer, rheumatoid arthritis or asthma predispose to insomnia.

Precipitating factors

Seventy-five per cent of those with chronic insomnia link the onset of their sleep disorder to a stressful event. This may be a difficulty in a close relationship, bereavement, a change in school or employment, or the onset of a medical disorder. The stress leads to both physiological and psychological arousal, which is more likely to precipitate insomnia if the predisposing factors listed above are present. If they are absent, or if the patient adapts to the stress, insomnia may only be transient.

Perpetuating factors

These become more important than the predisposing and precipitating factors once chronic insomnia has become established. Many subjects with insomnia have a coping pattern which involves avoidance and denial. This does not deal with stresses, but tends to perpetuate what in other subjects might be only a transient sleep disturbance An excessive concern about a lack of sleep may lead to anxiety with intrusive thoughts which initiate a vicious cycle of insomnia, hyperarousal and an inability to relax. This may develop into an introspective obsession with the difficulty in sleeping (psychophysiological insomnia).

Secondary behavioural changes which lead to poor sleep hygiene may be adopted. Fear of not being able to sleep may lead to an earlier bedtime or an attempt to reduce 'overstimulation' by avoiding social contact. An excess of caffeine or alcohol in the evenings may contribute to insomnia. Irregular sleep–wake habits and naps during the day may worsen the night-time sleep pattern. The inability to sleep at night may lead to a conditioned reflex whereby going to bed is associated with the anticipation of staying awake rather than falling asleep.

The disability resulting from insomnia may provide a secondary gain by helping to avoid work, family responsibilities, or interactions with other people. It may also attract an increased level of care from others which may tend to perpetuate the insomnia.

Sleep-state misperception (pseudo-insomnia, subjective insomnia)

Sleep-state misperception is due to an inaccurate perception of the time spent asleep. There is a wide range of accuracy of perception of sleep in those with insomnia, but it is common for the sleep latency to be exaggerated and sleep efficiency to be underestimated. Sleep-state misperception probably represents the extreme end of the range of misperception and interestingly it may be associated with similar physiological changes to those seen in primary insomnia, despite apparently normal sleep.

Sleep-state misperception usually occurs in young adults, especially females. Their complaint is of a difficulty in sleeping at night, especially difficulty in initiating sleep and difficulty in maintaining sleep, or occasionally even of not sleeping at all. This may be associated with daytime fatigue and mood changes. Investigations do not reveal any sleep abnormality.

Polysomnography shows a normal sleep duration, sleep latency and architecture, with few arousals. A similar degree of poor sleep is usually reported during the study as during sleep at home. MSLTs are normal.

The diagnosis is made by a combination of the history of insomnia with normal polysomnography and the absence of any other sleep disorder. The condition should be distinguished from short sleepers, DSPS, psychophysiological insomnia and malingering, in which the subject is aware that there is no true insomnia. The demonstration of a normal sleep pattern, treatment of any associated anxiety or depression, and help in improving the accuracy of perception of sleep may be of benefit.

Psychophysiological insomnia (conditioned insomnia)

Overview

An apprehensive over-concern about sleep perpetuates insomnia.

Occurrence

This is common, and probably accounts for around 15% of chronic insomnias. It is more common in women than in men, and the usual age of onset is 20–40 years.

Pathogenesis

The cardinal feature is an emotional trigger or precipitating event which may be stressful and which initiates the insomnia. Even after the stress abates the insomnia persists and a specific anxiety develops regarding sleep. Confidence about the ability to fall asleep deteriorates and in effect a specific sleep neurosis or somatized performance anxiety develops. Negative conditioning increases the anxiety and the level of arousal, making sleep more difficult.

Presleep rituals such as brushing the teeth become associated mentally with the failure to fall asleep. This becomes extended to anything associated with sleep, particularly the bedroom. Sleep is better elsewhere, for instance in a hotel room, during holidays, or even in a sleep laboratory or while watching television in the living room, where the expectations regarding sleep are lower. The continual application of excessive efforts to try to fall asleep raises the state of arousal, reinforces the apprehension about sleep, and the sense of difficulty about sleeping. Secondary sleep hygiene maladaptations may also develop.

Clinical features

These patients have often been poor sleepers before the initiating event, which is usually recalled as focusing their attention on their sleep problem. They often minimize any emotional response to their sleep difficulty. They do not become excessively sleepy during the day, but complain of daytime fatigue, lack of energy, poor memory, poor concentration and physical symptoms such as tension headaches and dizziness. During the night they lie awake with intrusive thoughts and a sensation of restlessness. Psychophysiological insomnia usually remains stable for long periods but improves on holiday. It may lead to depression, loss of motivation and concentration.

Investigations

Polysomnography shows a prolonged sleep latency with a short total sleep time, increased stages 1 and 2 NREM sleep with alpha intrusion, frequent awakenings and positional shifts during the night. There is a reversed first night effect in that sleep is better in the sleep laboratory than at home, but unlike sleep-state misperception this satisfactory sleep is acknowledged. Multiple sleep latency tests are normal.

Differential diagnosis

Psychiatric disorders, circadian rhythm disorders, poor sleep hygiene and insomnia due to other causes should be excluded. Psychophysiological insomnia differs from generalized anxiety states, in which anxiety pervades all aspects of life, since in psychophysiological insomnia it is focused only on the sleep problem.

Treatment

Excessive alcohol is often taken regularly, but is of little value. Hypnotics may have a place in short courses to try to break the pattern of the insomnia. Long-acting benzodiazepines and antidepressants are both often effective. Sleep hygiene advice may help and cognitive behavioural therapy, including relaxation, stimulus control and sleep restriction treatments, may be of value.

Anxiety states

Clinical features

Anxiety states are characterized by excessive worrying, fear or guilt and an unrealistic apprehension about common life situations. Generalized anxiety may be somatized causing muscle tension, palpitations, breathlessness, fatigue, sweating and loss of concentration. There is no change in circadian rhythms but DIS with intrusive thoughts is common. Anxiety associated with panic attacks may cause frequent awakenings from sleep and a complaint of insomnia.

Investigations

Polysomnography is rarely required, but reveals a short total sleep time, increased sleep latency, reduced sleep efficiency, an increased number of arousals from sleep, and normal NREM and REM sleep proportions.

Treatment

Long-acting benzodiazepines are often effective in improving insomnia and relieving daytime anxiety.

Attention deficit hyperactivity disorder (ADHD)

This is characterized by poorly sustained attention, impulsivity, hyperactivity, irritability and a hyperarousal state. It is commonest in children, but may persist into adult life and is three to six times commoner in males than in females. Difficulty initiating sleep, frequent awakenings and being physically restless during sleep are common complaints but sleepiness during the day is rare.

The clinical features of ADHD can be mimicked by sleep fragmentation due to the restless legs syndrome, obstructive sleep apnoeas, and occasionally narcolepsy which leads to frequent awakenings during sleep. Polysomnography may be required to confirm these diagnoses. In ADHD it may be normal or show a low sleep efficiency, reduced total sleep time, an increased number of sleep cycles during the night and an increase in the duration of REM sleep. Limb movements are frequent in stages 1 and 2 NREM sleep.

Chronic fatigue syndrome (CFS, post-viral fatigue syndrome, myalgic encephalomyelitis, ME)

Clinical features

This condition is commonest in young adults and is characterized by unexplained fatigue which lasts for more than 6 months. This is often associated with insomnia, unrefreshing sleep, daytime fatigue and lack of energy which is not relieved by sleep or rest and which is worsened by exercise. Memory, concentration and attention span deteriorate.

There may be a genetic factor or personality type which predisposes to CFS in the presence of an initiating event, which may be a viral infection such as the Epstein–Barr virus, or emotional stress. The characteristic response in CFS is a hyperarousal state with abnormalities of pituitary and other aspects of endocrine function. It may be complicated by depression and anxiety.

Investigations

Polysomnography may be required to establish the cause of the sleep symptoms. It shows a prolonged sleep latency with reduced sleep efficiency and often alpha intrusion into NREM sleep. Rapid eye movement sleep latency is normal, but the duration of REM sleep is reduced, and there is an increased frequency of arousals and awakenings from sleep. Multiple sleep latency tests are normal.

These changes occur even in the absence of depression and anxiety, but these can cause sleep disturbances which are superimposed on those of CFS. The sleep abnormalities of CFS may be related to changes in immune function, such as increases in IL-1, which frequently occur.

Treatment

There is no specific treatment to reverse the sleep abnormalities of CFS, but it is important to treat any depression and anxiety, and to recognize and treat problems with sleep hygiene which are common and which may contribute to the sleep disturbance. Frequent naps are often taken during the day, together with a lack of exercise and little exposure to light. These maladaptations may be the most important factors in the sleep disturbance.

Cognitive therapy may help in gradually increasing the level of activity and in achieving carefully structured goals. Tricyclic antidepressants may be of benefit and the condition usually improves gradually over months or years.

Fibromyalgia

Clinical features

This is a poorly defined syndrome which is commoner in females than in males and usually develops in young adults. Its characteristic features are fatigue with tenderness over various points, particularly in the chest and abdomen, and diffuse musculoskeletal pain and stiffness. This is usually worst around the neck and shoulders on waking, whereas in normal subjects the pain threshold is highest on waking.

Sleep is usually felt to be light and unrefreshing and this correlates with the number of tender points. Tiredness is common during the day, but it is unusual for sleep to be entered. Fibromyalgia may have a similar pathogenesis to the chronic fatigue syndrome, with hyperarousal, changes in endocrine function and in autonomic responses, abnormal reactions to stress, and a particularly increased sensitivity to pain.

Investigations

Polysomnography may be required to elucidate the cause of the sleep symptoms. It shows a prolonged sleep latency, an increased number of arousals from sleep, prolonged stage 1 NREM sleep, few sleep spindles, reduced stages 3 and 4 NREM sleep, and alpha intrusion, particularly into stages 3 and 4 NREM sleep. The duration of REM sleep is reduced. The extent of alpha activity is related to the severity of the musculoskeletal pains and to the awareness of sleeping lightly. Multiple sleep latency tests are normal.

Treatment

Pain relief and improvement in sleep hygiene often help to relieve symptoms, but low-dose tricyclic antidepressants and cognitive therapy may be of benefit.

Table 7.9 Comparison of idiopathic insomnia, limit setting difficulty and DSPS.

Characteristic	Idiopathic insomnia	Limit setting difficulty	Delayed sleep phase syndrome
Age of onset	Childhood	Childhood	Adolescence
Trigger	Nil	Poor sleep hygiene enforcement	Nil or poor sleep hygiene enforcement
Sleep onset time	Variable	Variable	Constant and late
Poor sleep hygiene	Follows insomnia	Alters in adolescence	May improve in adult life
Natural history	Constant and lifelong	Alters in adolescence	May improve in adult life
Psychological changes	Secondary anxiety and depression	Attention seeking	Nil

Idiopathic insomnia

Overview

This condition is characterized by the early onset of insomnia without any underlying psychological or psychiatric abnormalities or other detectable cause (Table 7.9).

Occurrence

It is uncommon but may be familial. The onset is usually in early childhood and it persists throughout adult life without remission.

Pathogenesis

No physical or psychological cause has been detected, but idiopathic insomnia may represent the wakeful end of the normal range. It is probably heterogeneous and in some patients minor organic neurological abnormalities such as dyslexia or hyperkinesis have been detected. A reduction in 5HT turnover has been found in some patients.

Clinical features

Insomnia may be severe with as little as 3–4 h sleep being obtained each night and with frequent awakenings. The subject wakes feeling unrefreshed and feels tired and irritable during the day, but excessive daytime sleepiness is not a feature. Poor attention, mood disorders, lack of motivation and secondary anxiety occur, often with somatic symptoms and depression. Secondary maladaptive sleep hygiene patterns are common, but follow, rather than predate, the insomnia.

Investigations

The waking EEG may show a diffuse abnormality such as ragged rather than sinusoidal alpha waves at night. The sleep latency may be markedly prolonged with a reduction in total sleep time and sleep efficiency, often with poor definition of individual sleep stages. The duration of stages 3 and 4 NREM sleep is often markedly reduced and there is alpha intrusion.

Sleep spindles are poorly formed and there are few eye movements in REM sleep, which is often prolonged.

Differential diagnosis

Diagnosis requires the establishment of a childhood onset of insomnia prior to any detectable cause or psychological changes. Insomnia is chronic and stable and independent of any sleep hygiene abnormalities. It should be distinguished from short sleepers, who do not complain of any sleep problem or daytime fatigue, anxiety states, and psychophysiological insomnia.

Treatment

Alcohol and other hypnotics are often taken to assist sleep, and caffeine to help keep awake during the day, but none of these treatments are very effective. Behavioural therapy may be of some help.

Psychiatric disorders

Anorexia nervosa

Anorexic patients rarely complain of insomnia but often wake early in the morning. Psychiatric problems may contribute to the changes in sleep pattern, but weight loss is associated with polysomnographic findings of a short total sleep time, reduced sleep efficiency, frequent awakenings and to a variable extent with lengthening of stages 1 and 2 and shortening of stages 3 and 4 NREM sleep [11]. These abnormalities improve as weight is regained.

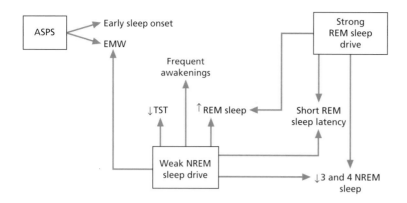

Fig. 7.3 Changes in sleep control in depression. ASPS, advanced sleep phase syndrome; EMW, early morning awakening; NREM, non-rapid eye movement; REM, rapid eye movement; TST, total sleep time.

Depression

Clinical features

Insomnia is a common and occasionally the initial symptom of depression. It is not related to the number of depressive episodes or to the duration of the depression, but is more common in older subjects. There is usually little difficulty in initiating sleep, but there are frequent awakenings during the night and early morning awakening, often after an unpleasant dream, especially in endogenous depression. Sleep is often unrefreshing and frequent naps may be taken during the day, especially in younger subjects.

There is a tendency towards an advanced sleep phase syndrome in depression (Fig. 7.3) which may contribute to early morning awakening [12]. In contrast, depression in the seasonal affective disorder causes excessive daytime sleepiness and a delayed sleep phase syndrome. Changes in circadian rhythms such as cortisol secretion are common in depression. Melatonin secretion is reduced in depression, possibly because of reduced 5HT and noradrenaline stimulation of the pineal gland. The amplitude of the diurnal temperature rhythm is lessened and core body temperature at night is higher than in normal subjects. The reduction in REM sleep latency correlates with both of these abnormalities.

Investigations

Polysomnography is occasionally required to establish the relative contributions of depression and other conditions that may contribute to the sleep symptoms. Polysomnography is usually normal in depression occurring before puberty and may only be slightly abnormal in adolescence. In adults, especially the elderly, it characteristically reveals a short total sleep time, increased sleep latency with a short REM sleep latency (usually 20–40 min), an increase in the duration of REM sleep, particularly in the first half of the night, and a reduction in stages 3 and 4 NREM sleep with an increase in stages 1 and 2, and frequent awakenings [10].

These abnormalities are most obvious during an episode of depression, but they rarely disappear completely even between episodes, and the REM sleep latency in particular usually remains short. Similar findings are often seen in close relatives who have not been and are not depressed. They may represent a 'trait' for depression rather than the state of depression.

The increase in REM sleep is due to both an increase in the drive to REM sleep and a weak NREM sleep drive. The REM sleep drive appears to be proportional to the severity of the depression. The NREM sleep drive becomes weaker with age and this may underlie the increased frequency of sleep abnormalities in older subjects with depression. It also leads to a shorter sleep time and briefer NREM sleep episodes with an increase in the number of awakenings from sleep, although some of these may be related to anxiety.

Treatment

Sleep deprivation leads to mood elevation in depression and even to mania in bipolar disorders [13]. This effect is particularly felt if sleep is lost during the second half of the night when REM sleep is most prolonged, and the improvement in mood is a predictor of response to antidepressant drug treatment. Sleep deprivation increases the homeostatic drive to NREM sleep. Loss of REM sleep and a longer REM sleep latency are also features of most antidepressant drugs, and of electroconvulsive treatment, suggesting that REM sleep generation is closely linked to the development of depression.

The neurotransmitter basis of depression is uncertain, but probably relates to the balance between the REM sleep promoting influence of the cholinergic mechanisms in the pons, particularly those related to the pedunculopontine and laterodorsal tegmental (LDT/PPT) nuclei, and the REM sleep inhibiting influence of other centres, particularly the noradrenergic locus coeruleus and the dorsal raphe nuclei which produce 5HT at their synapses. The theory that depression is due to a deficiency of these two latter chemicals (the monoaminergic theory of depression) may explain why tricyclic and SSRI antidepressants improve the sleep pattern in depression during the first night, but changes in mood may take around 2 weeks and be due to alterations in the function of the receptors for these neurotransmitters.

Antidepressants with a sedative action, such as clomipramine, trimipramine, dothiepin and mirtazapine, are indicated particularly when insomnia is a major problem in depression, but mood and other changes may improve, while insomnia persists. In this situation combining an antidepressant with either hypnotic or cognitive behavioural therapy may be effective [14].

Early morning awakening may respond to light therapy in the evening and possibly to melatonin.

Mania and manic depression (bipolar disorder)

Mania often leads to a feeling of being refreshed after only 3–4 h of sleep at night. It may even prevent sleep for several days, but the subject then becomes exhausted. The total sleep time is shortened, sleep latency is prolonged, there is a short REM sleep latency, the duration of stages 3 and 4 NREM sleep is often normal, but there can be a gross alteration in the sleep architecture. Abnormalities of circadian rhythms include changes in the diurnal cortisol secretion pattern.

Sleep deprivation tends to elevate the mood, as in depression, and this may worsen the mania and lead to further sleep restriction. Treatment with benzodiazepines or sedating antipsychotics improves the insomnia in bipolar disorder. This also improves with lithium, but more slowly.

Excessive daytime sleepiness only occurs in the depressive phase of bipolar illnesses.

Obsessive–compulsive disorders

Patients often complain of insomnia and frequent awakenings at night, and the rituals that they need to carry out before sleep may disturb the quality of sleep. The total sleep time is reduced, the duration of stage 4 NREM sleep is shortened, REM sleep latency is reduced and awakenings are frequent.

Post-traumatic stress disorder

Clinical features

This condition follows either a military or a civilian traumatic event and is characterized by repetitive re-experiencing of this through intrusive thoughts, flashbacks and 'nightmares'. These occur especially between 12.00 midnight and 3.00 AM, in contrast to typical nightmares which occur later in the night. They may arise either from REM sleep or usually stages 1 or 2 NREM sleep. The content is related to the traumatic event, although it may be disguised or generalized. These 'nightmares' may be repetitive and other dreams are rarely recalled.

A hyperarousal state develops with insomnia and difficulty in both initiating and maintaining sleep. The perception of the severity of insomnia is often accentuated, and panic attacks and depression, which may worsen insomnia, are frequent.

These subjects are often restless sleepers and, in association with sudden awakenings from the 'nightmares', make violent movements, for instance diving out of bed.

Investigations

The diagnosis is usually made clinically. Polysomnography shows variable findings, but if the disorder is severe there is usually a prolonged sleep latency, low sleep efficiency due to long awakenings during the night as well as to microarousals, an increase in stage 1 NREM sleep and reduced stages 3 and 4 NREM sleep with a normal or prolonged REM sleep latency and a short duration of REM sleep. There may be an increase in the ratio of phasic to tonic REM sleep. Muscle twitches during REM sleep are common and limb movements, which may be periodic, are more frequent in NREM sleep than in normal subjects. Gross body movements are particularly frequent in stage 2 NREM sleep.

Treatment

Behavioural therapy and psychotherapy may be of help, especially when combined with antidepressants, particularly the SSRIs, or venlafaxine. Prazosin is effective in relieving 'nightmares' and associated motor abnormalities.

Schizophrenia

Clinical features

Schizophrenia may cause difficulty in initiating sleep and difficulty in maintaining sleep, especially before and during acute exacerbations. This may be associated with sleep reversal, but there are no changes in circadian rhythms [15].

Bizarre thoughts and distortions of reality during wakefulness may resemble dreams. This led to the theory that schizophrenia was due to REM sleep intrusion into wakefulness and that it was similar to narcolepsy, but this is unlikely. The dreams of schizophrenics during sleep often feature strangers.

Daytime sleepiness is usually related to psychotropic drugs used for symptom control rather than to the schizophrenia itself.

Investigations

Polysomnography has shown variable results, but in general the total sleep time is reduced, sleep latency is increased, sleep efficiency is low and the number of arousals is increased. Rapid eye movement sleep latency is occasionally shortened and the duration of stages 3 and 4 NREM sleep is reduced, especially during psychotic episodes.

Neurological disorders

The site of a neurological lesion is important in determining the clinical features associated with the insomnia, although in many disorders the neurological abnormalities are diffuse. The most important types of damage are as follows.

Hypothalamic lesions

Lesions such as tumours in the anterior hypothalamus may cause insomnia. They may derange the function of the suprachiasmatic nuclei as well as reducing the homeostatic drive to sleep. Head CT and MRI scans may be required.

Thalamic lesions

Thalamic lesions may prevent NREM sleep from being initiated and maintained, but the clinical pattern varies according to which nuclei within the thalamus are affected. Lesions of the mediodorsal and anterior thalamic nuclei lead to a combination of features known as agrypnia excitata [16]. This comprises insomnia with vivid dreams and hallucinations which are physically enacted. There is also generalized motor agitation with irregular movements and tremors, confusion and sympathetic over-activity with tachycardia, hypertension, fevers and sweating. Agrypnia excitata is a feature particularly of fatal familial insomnia, Morvan's fibrillary chorea and delirium tremens. Agrypnia excitata has similarities to status dissociatus, in that the boundaries between sleep states and wakefulness become obscured.

Fatal familial insomnia

Pathogenesis

This autosomal dominant disorder is due to a mutation at codon 178 of the prion protein gene, in which asparagine is substituted for aspartate coupled with the presence of methionine rather than valine at position 129 [17]. This leads to production of an abnormal form of a glycoprotein (prion protein) which is resistant to proteases and leads to neuronal death, particularly in the mediodorsal and anterior thalamic nuclei. Progression of the disease is more rapid in methionine homozygotes than methionine-valine heterozygotes.

Clinical features

This condition is equally common in males and females. It is usually familial but occasionally sporadic, and usually appears between the ages of 40 and 70 years. Progressively worsening insomnia is associated with vivid dreams and motor activity similar to that of the REM sleep behaviour disorder. The fall in total sleep time is associated with disintegration of the sleep structure with no discernible NREM or REM sleep. The normal 24-h rest–activity cycle is lost and the circadian cortisol rhythm disappears. Autonomic and motor abnormalities appear, but cognitive function is retained until stupor and eventually coma develop shortly before death. This usually occurs 6–24 months after the onset of the condition.

Differential diagnosis

The differential diagnosis includes the REM sleep behaviour disorder, although this does not have any autonomic abnormalities, dementia, particularly due to Alzheimer's disease, Creutzfeldt–Jakob disease and occasionally schizophrenia.

Treatment

There is no effective treatment.

Creutzfeldt–Jakob disease

This is usually sporadic, but is occasionally familial. It is due to the same codon 178 mutation as in fatal familial insomnia, but polymorphism at other codons, such as 129, leads to a different phenotypic expression of the genetic abnormality. The cerebral cortex is usually predominantly affected, but in a subtype of the disease there is extensive thalamic atrophy. In these subjects insomnia is a prominent feature, in addition to the dementia and motor abnormalities. There is a progressive loss of both NREM and REM sleep with absence of spindles and K-complexes, and eventually there is no recognizable NREM or REM sleep.

Morvan's fibrillary chorea

This rare condition is the result of abnormalities of the voltage gated potassium channels usually due to the production of auto-antibodies due to malignancy. It represents a form of limbic encephalitis. There is a reduction in sleep spindles and stages 3 and 4 NREM sleep, but muscle tone during REM sleep is retained and dream enactment similar to the REM sleep behaviour disorder is common. Insomnia, hallucinations, intense anxiety and delirium are characteristic. Hypertension, tachycardia, sweating and fever are common. The disorder may remit or progress and may respond to plasma exchange.

Delirium tremens

This is usually the result of acute withdrawal from alcohol, leading to abnormalities in the anterior thalamus and cingulate cortex. Vivid hallucinations, motor hyperactivity, autonomic activation and confusion are characteristic. Insomnia may be profound. Hallucinations are due to intrusion of REM sleep into wakefulness with enactment similar to that seen in the REM sleep behaviour disorder.

Thalamic infarction

This is the commonest thalamic lesion and, like tumours and trauma, more commonly causes insomnia than excessive daytime sleepiness. This is probably due to a loss of the ability of the thalamus to synchronize the cortical activity which is required to enter and maintain NREM sleep. Anencephalic infants without a thalamus appear to sleep, probably because they have little cerebral cortex, and so do not require organized thalamic activity to regulate its activity.

Basal forebrain lesions

Lesions in the basal forebrain may cause insomnia.

Cerebral cortex disorders

Dementia

Clinical features

Insomnia is common in the elderly, probably due to degeneration of the sleep-regulating mechanisms, but these effects are exaggerated in dementia due to degenerative disorders, particularly Alzheimer's disease [18], and in multi-infarct dementia. The clinical features vary according to the distribution of the degeneration, and in particular whether the homeostatic sleep control mechanisms or other regions of the brain are mainly involved. The suprachiasmatic nuclei appear to be normal and the diurnal pattern of cortisol secretion is normal.

There is a loss of the sleep–wake cycle and of the normal sleep architecture (see Table 7.10). Daytime naps are frequent and occasionally there is sleep reversal if the dementia is severe. 'Sundowning' is a characteristic particularly of Alzheimer's disease, in which there is agitation, particularly in the afternoon or early evening, associated with wandering and an exacerbation of any behavioural abnormalities. It may be more frequent in the winter when there is less exposure to light, and improves with light therapy of 5000–10 000 lux in the evenings, which causes a sleep phase delay.

An advanced sleep phase is common in dementia and the time spent awake at night is increased. Confusion and wandering at night are common and may be exacerbated by adverse environmental conditions and poor sleep hygiene.

Investigations

Polysomnography is rarely required, but shows that the sleep efficiency may be reduced to around 60% by the frequent awakenings, which are often prolonged. The duration of stage 1 NREM sleep is lengthened and stages 3 and 4 are shortened. Sleep spindles are few in number, and slow in frequency, and there are few K-complexes. There is an increase in REM sleep latency and the duration of REM sleep is reduced. Periodic limb movements are common, possibly due to a reduction in dopamine and acetylcholine as neurotransmitters, and obstructive and central sleep apnoeas and Cheyne–Stokes respiration are frequently seen.

Characteristic	Dementia	Depression
TST	↓	↓
Awakenings	↑↑	↑
EMW	+	+
Sleep latency	–	↑
1 and 2 NREM sleep	↑	↑
3 and 4 NREM sleep	↓	↓
REM sleep latency	↑	↓
REM sleep	↓	↑
Daytime naps	++	±

Table 7.10 Effects of dementia and depression on sleep.

EMW, early morning awakening; NREM, non-rapid eye movement; REM, rapid eye movement; TST, total sleep time.

Treatment

Improvement in sleep hygiene is the most important aspect of management. Regular sleep–wake patterns, exposure to light during the day, encouragement to take exercise and avoidance of stimulants such as caffeine may be of help. Short-acting hypnotics such as chloral or zopiclone in low dose may be indicated, but drugs which induce daytime sedation should be avoided. Treatment of any depression and any other primary sleep disorder may be helpful [19].

Brain injury

Insomnia may follow brain injuries and be due to pain and other symptoms directly related to the trauma, anxiety, depression, post-traumatic stress disorder, a delayed sleep phase syndrome or a non-24-h sleep–wake rhythm associated with deterioration in vision. The post-concussion syndrome is associated with insomnia and occasionally there appears to be physical damage to the wake-promoting regions in the brain, leading to a marked reduction in stages 3 and 4 NREM sleep and REM sleep.

Frontal lobotomy (leucotomy)

In this procedure the frontal lobes are severed from the rest of the cerebral cortex. It has been used in the past for severe depression with anxiety. It causes temporary insomnia, but after around 10 years there is an increase in the duration of stages 3 and 4 NREM sleep.

Encephalitis

Encephalitis usually leads to excessive daytime sleepiness, but may cause insomnia if it damages the mechanisms that are involved in sleep initiation or maintenance.

Encephalitis lethargica can cause insomnia and encephalitis due to cerebral involvement in Whipple's disease can cause severe insomnia without any recognizable stages 3 and 4 NREM or REM sleep.

Movement disorders

Many of the movement disorders of wakefulness cause insomnia. The most important are idiopathic Parkinsonism, multiple system atrophy, progressive supranuclear palsy, Huntington's disease, torsion dystonia and Tourette's syndrome (Chapter 9).

Idiopathic Parkinsonism is associated particularly with difficulty in maintaining sleep and early morning wakening insomnia and may cause an advanced sleep phase syndrome and even sleep reversal. Several factors contribute to these problems.

1 Poor sleep hygiene due to disabilities related to the physical effects of Parkinsonism.

2 Sleep fragmentation. This may be due to stiffness, discomfort and pain during sleep. There are fewer position shifts during sleep than in normal subjects because of difficulty in initiating movements. There may be complaints of being unable to turn over during sleep and of difficulty in getting out of bed, for instance to urinate. There is also difficulty in swallowing saliva and drooling. Leg cramps are frequent and back pain and excessive sweating may disturb sleep.

3 Depression. This is a common complication particularly in the later stages of Parkinsonism. It responds best to selective serotonin re-uptake inhibitor antidepressants.

4 Drugs. L-dopa and dopamine agonists may cause insomnia if they lead to frequent vivid dreams and nightmares.

5 Persistence of motor disorder. The Parkinsonian tremor is most prominent at the moment of arousal from sleep or at transitions from deeper to lighter stages of sleep and in stages 1 and 2 NREM sleep.

Narcolepsy

Insomnia is a common but under-recognized symptom of narcolepsy (Chapter 6).

Restless legs syndrome and periodic limb movements in sleep

These may cause insomnia and excessive daytime sleepiness (Chapter 9). Insomnia is unusual in most other motor abnormalities during sleep unless they are very frequent.

Non-neurological medical conditions

This is an important, but heterogeneous, group of conditions which frequently cause secondary insomnia. Many of them are further discussed in Chapter 12. Sleep can be prevented, fragmented or terminated by symptoms such as: pain, for instance from rheumatoid arthritis; discomfort, which is common, for example, in Parkinsonism and multiple sclerosis at night; and nocturia. Symptoms due to autonomic changes during sleep, such as those related to nocturnal angina, asthma and peptic ulceration, may cause insomnia, although the complaint may be primarily of the specific symptom rather than of insomnia. Sleep can also be disrupted by disorders that occur only during sleep, such as central and obstructive sleep apnoeas.

Of these organic causes, the most important are the following.

Respiratory disorders

Examples of respiratory disorders that may lead to insomnia are obstructive and central sleep apnoeas, Cheyne–Stokes respiration, asthma, chronic bronchitis and emphysema. These more commonly cause excessive daytime sleepiness than insomnia.

Cardiovascular disorders

Nocturnal angina and occasionally dysrhythmias may disturb sleep.

Gastro-intestinal disorders

Symptoms from peptic ulcers may cause awakenings from sleep. Poor quality of sleep is associated with the irritable bowel syndrome.

Musculoskeletal disorders

Any musculoskeletal disorder that causes pain, stiffness, or limited mobility during sleep may lead to insomnia. This may be difficulty in initiating sleep but is more commonly difficulty in maintaining sleep. Insomnia in fibromyalgia is accentuated by a hyperarousal state, and rheumatoid arthritis may be complicated by the restless legs syndrome and periodic limb movements in sleep, possibly because of its associated iron-deficiency anaemia.

Excessive daytime sleepiness may also develop in rheumatoid arthritis as a result of obstructive sleep apnoeas due to crico-arytenoid arthritis or obesity caused by glucocorticoid treatment, opiate analgesics or poor sleep hygiene induced by the lifestyle limitations imposed by the arthritis. Excessive daytime sleepiness in musculoskeletal disorders should be distinguished from depression and physical tiredness due to the underlying disorder.

Metabolic disorders

An example of a metabolic disorder that may lead to insomnia is chronic renal failure (page 288). Insomnia is a frequent problem, with a short total sleep time with disorganized sleep architecture and frequent arousals. The sleep architecture improves following dialysis and renal transplantation, suggesting that most of the abnormalities are due to a metabolic disturbance. This may underlie the association between chronic renal failure and the restless legs and periodic limb movements in sleep, but nocturia also causes arousal from sleep.

Endocrine disorders

Premenstrual insomnia

This commonly occurs in the week before each menstrual period, and is often partly due to physical symptoms such as abdominal pain, but a fall in progesterone secretion may also contribute. Polysomnography premenstrually shows frequent sleep-stage transitions and arousals and a reduced sleep efficiency.

Pregnancy insomnia

This usually worsens as the pregnancy progresses. Pregnancy insomnia may be due to nausea, backache, urinary frequency, heartburn, cramps, discomfort and fetal movements. Vivid dreams and nightmares are common. The postnatal need to respond to and care for the child at night, and occasionally postnatal depression, may perpetuate the insomnia so that it becomes established as a long-term difficulty.

Menopausal insomnia

Spontaneous awakenings from sleep are often associated with night sweats or hot flushes which respond to oestrogen replacement treatment. The condition usually resolves after several months but occasionally only after several years. Depression may contribute to the insomnia.

Thyrotoxicosis

This causes difficulty in initiating sleep and early morning awakening with a reduction in total sleep time and an increase in the duration of stages 3 and 4 NREM sleep. Hyperactivity with a high level of arousal is usual, and excessive daytime sleepiness is not a feature.

Diabetes mellitus

Polyuria, paraesthesiae from a peripheral neuropathy, and nocturnal cramps all cause awakenings from sleep.

Cushing's syndrome

This is manifested by difficulty in maintaining sleep and early morning awakening which are similar to the effects of administered glucocorticoids. The insomnia may be mediated by interactions with cytokines.

References

1 Jensen E, Dehlin O, Hagberg B, Samuelsson G, Svensson T. Insomnia in an 80-year-old population: relationship to medical, psychological and social factors. *J Sleep Res* 1998; 7: 183–9.

2 Stepanski EJ, Wyatt JK. Use of sleep hygiene in the treatment of insomnia. *Sleep Med Rev* 2003; 7(3): 215–25.

3 Wagner J, Wagner ML. Non-benzodiazepines for the treatment of insomnia. *Sleep Med Rev* 2000; 4(6): 551–81.

4 Mendelson WB, Roth T, Cassella J, Roehrs T, Walsh JK, Woods JH, Buysse DJ, Meyer RE. The treatment of chronic insomnia: drug indications, chronic use and abuse liability. Summary of a 2001 New Clinical Drug Evaluation Unit Meeting Symposium. *Sleep Med Rev* 2004; 8: 7–17.

5 Rogers NL, Dinges DF, Kennaway DJ, Dawson D. Potential action of melatonin in insomnia. *Sleep* 2003; 26(8): 1058–9.

6 Edinger JD, Wohlgemuth WK, Radtke RA, Marsh GR, Quillian RE. Does cognitive-behavioral insomnia therapy alter dysfunctional beliefs about sleep? *Sleep* 2001; 24(5): 591–8.

7 Montgomery P, Dennis J. A systematic review of non-pharmacological therapies for sleep problems in later life. *Sleep Med Rev* 2004; 8: 47–62.

8 Harvey AG, Tang NKY. Cognitive behaviour therapy for primary insomnia: can we rest yet? *Sleep Med Rev* 2003; 7(3): 237–62.

9 Cervena K, Dauvilliers Y, Espa F, Touchon J, Matousek M, Billiard M, Besset A. Effect of cognitive behavioural therapy for insomnia on sleep architecture and sleep EEG power spectra in psychophysiological insomnia. *J Sleep Res* 2004; 13: 385–93.

10 Bonnet MH, Arand DL. Hyperarousal and insomnia. *Sleep Med Rev* 1997; 1: 97–108.

11 Nobili L, Baglietto MG, Beelke M, Carli F De, Comite R Di, Fiocchi I, Rizzo P, Veneselli E, Savoini M, Zanotto E, Ferrillo F. Impairment of the production of delta sleep in anorectic adolescents. *Sleep* 2004; 27(8): 1553–9.

12 Adrien J. Neurobiological bases for the relation between sleep and depression. *Sleep Med Rev* 2002; 6(5): 341–51.

13 Giedke H, Schwarzler F. Therapeutic use of sleep deprivation in depression. *Sleep Med Rev* 2002; 6(5): 361–77.

14 Jindal RD, Thase ME. Treatment of insomnia associated with clinical depression. *Sleep Med Rev* 2004; 8: 19–30.

15 Monti JM, Monti D. Sleep in schizophrenia patients and the effects of antipsychotic drugs. *Sleep Med Rev* 2004; 8: 133–48.

16 Lugaresi E, Provini F. Agrypnia excitata: clinical features and pathophysiological implications. *Sleep Med Rev* 2001; 5(4): 313–22.

17 Gambetti P. Fatal familial insomnia and familial Creutzfeldt–Jakob disease: a tale of two diseases with the same genetic mutation. *Curr Top Microbiol Immunol* 1996; 207: 19–25.

18 Reynolds CF, Hoch CC, Stack J, Campbell D. The nature and management of sleep/wake disturbance in Alzheimer's dementia. *Psychopharmacol Bull* 1988; 24: 43–8.

19 McCurry SM, Reynolds CF III, Ancoli-Israel S, Teri L, Vitiello MV. Treatment of sleep disturbance in Alzheimer's disease. *Sleep Med Rev* 2000; 4(6): 603–28.

8 Dreams and Nightmares

Introduction

Experiences during sleep include abnormalities of awareness, sensations, thoughts and emotions. Dreams and nightmares can be distinguished from other conditions by their narrative or sequence of events, and are recalled immediately on waking. Once arousal has taken place the awareness of a dream or nightmare is strictly speaking no longer occurring in sleep. The same applies to other experiences from sleep, such as recall of pain, the sensation of breathlessness with obstructive sleep apnoeas, or the feeling of a need to move the legs with the restless legs syndrome.

Neurophysiology

Dreams appear to be initiated in REM sleep by pontine centres, particularly the LDT/PPT. These are responsible for muscle atonia and project to the cerebral cortex, which in REM sleep, unlike NREM sleep, is receptive to input from the brainstem. The exception to this is that there is little activity in the ascending pain pathways during REM sleep. This is probably responsible for the rarity of the sensation of pain in dreams.

The cerebral activity during REM sleep is largely independent of environmental stimuli and reflects the internal processing of information reaching the cortex from the brainstem, including the limbic system. The cerebral cortex is selectively active during REM sleep [1]. There is no primary sensory cortical activation and the dorsolateral prefrontal cortex is also inactive. In contrast the limbic system and orbitomedial prefrontal cortex are active. Retention of social awareness during dreams is due to persisting functioning of the orbito-medial frontal cortex.

The non-functioning of the dorsolateral prefrontal cortex, which is involved in executive and planning functions, is probably responsible for loss of logical connections and the time distortion of dreams. The strong visual component relates mainly to occipital lobe activity. The fusiform gyrus, which is responsible for face recognition, interacts with the medial occipital and temporal cortex, which is involved with visual imaging and auditory sensations. The inferior parietal lobe adds spatial awareness to dreams. Activation of the amygdala is probably responsible for much of the emotional content of dreams.

In general, simple forms of unfamiliar faces and brief visual images arise in the occipital cortex, whereas images of animals and familiar figures, with other modalities such as the sensation of being watched and of voices, arise in the pons. The bizarre nature of images in dreams is probably due to partial loss of frontal supervision of mentation and also to the loose mental associations which are characteristic of REM sleep.

Dreams during NREM and REM sleep

There has been considerable debate as to whether dreams occur only or predominantly in REM rather than NREM sleep [2]. This is made more complex by the existence of mixed NREM/REM sleep states, particularly later in the night when fragments of REM sleep appear to intrude into NREM sleep [3]. These episodes occur most frequently either just before or after episodes of REM sleep, or at times when, from the 90-min ultradian REM sleep cycle, it would be anticipated that an episode of REM sleep would have taken place. NREM sleep closest to a previous episode of REM sleep has the greatest dream content, especially late in the night. This suggests that REM sleep processes extend into what is classified conventionally as NREM sleep and that there is not an instantaneous change from REM to NREM sleep and vice versa during the night.

In pure NREM sleep there is awareness of 'dreams' which often involve verbal problem solving and have a simple content, whereas REM sleep dreams have more narrative, motion and emotional content. The thought content in REM sleep dreams declines during the night as the internal visual imagery increases, probably exponentially.

Dreams during wakefulness

Dream-like hallucinations

The processes responsible for dreams can be activated outside sleep by, for instance, drugs and by sensory, food or sleep deprivation, as well as in psychiatric and neurological disorders. In these situations sensory processing is disordered, and leads to unusual perceptions. These may be primarily visual, as in peduncular hallucinosis due to midline lesions of the midbrain, or in the Charles Bonnet syndrome in which visual hallucinations occur despite blindness. Degenerative disorders such as fatal familial insomnia, Parkinson's disease and Lewy body disease are also associated with hallucinations during wakefulness which are analogous to dreaming in sleep.

Hypnagogic and hypnopompic hallucinations (pre- and post-sleep dreams)

Dreams normally occur during sleep but they may arise before any other features of sleep have developed. This occurs in normal subjects who are extremely sleep deprived, particularly of REM sleep, and may occur with jet lag due to east–west travel, since this induces an acute advanced sleep phase and sleep-onset REM sleep. It is, however, commonest during drowsiness in narcolepsy, in which the hallucinations are particularly vivid. The images and forms that these presleep dreams, or hypnagogic hallucinations, take may be so realistic that it may subsequently be impossible to be sure whether the events were true or were simply dreamt.

Similar dreams can occur at the transition from sleep to wakefulness, particularly at the end of the night (hypnopompic hallucinations). These are commoner in normal subjects than hypnagogic hallucinations, but are also a feature of narcolepsy.

The content of these experiences is often auditory, with repetitive sounds or voices, visual, including shadowy outlines or shapes of people, a sense of pressure or of floating or flying, or the awareness of the presence of a person or spirit, such as a demon. The latter is often associated with fear which may be intense. 'Out of body' experiences are probably due to changes in the processing of proprioceptive sensory input and are often associated with lucid dreams and sleep paralysis.

Dream analysis techniques

Most studies of dreams have had significant methodological problems but the following techniques have been commonly used.

1 *Recall of most recent dreams.* The date and content of the dream are recorded. This can be used to assess how a group differs from normal and to assess the effects of treatment.

2 *Dream diaries.* These are uninfluenced by the aims of the researcher.

3 *Waking tests.* The subject is woken, usually in a sleep laboratory, and questioned about the dream content. Recall rapidly falls if wakening is gradual so it is important to wake the subject rapidly.

4 *Recall training.* The subjects are trained to recall their dreams after waking naturally and not, for instance, with an alarm. They should lie still with their eyes closed, rehearse the last dream image and give it a title to increase recall and then write down the content of the whole dream immediately afterwards.

5 *Dream summarizing scales.* These compare dreams using predetermined lists of items. They can be analysed blind by a reader who knows nothing about the subject. If the analyst is known to the subject this may introduce bias according, for instance, to the genders of the dreamer and analyst. Over a hundred dreams are usually required to provide statistically valid content analysis.

6 *Text analyses.* These analyse not just assess dream content, but also action and emotion.

Dream recall

It is usual to have around 40 REM sleep episodes each week, but only to recall two to three dreams each week. Dream recall usually fades rapidly after the onset of wakefulness, suggesting that dreams are not incorporated into either short- or long-term memory.

Dream recall is increased in the following situations.

1 Narcolepsy in which REM sleep intrudes into partial wakefulness.

2 Insomnia. Dream recall increases in proportion to the number of awakenings during the night [4].

3 Abrupt wakenings from REM sleep. This is usually due to environmental stimuli such as noises. Sleep fragmentation caused by obstructive sleep apnoeas only occasionally leads to dream recall, probably because of the extent of the fragmentation of REM sleep which prevents dreams from becoming fully formed.

4 Pregnancy.

5 Fever.

6 REM sleep rebound due to either REM sleep deprivation or withdrawal of drugs, such as tricyclic antidepressants, benzodiazepines, barbiturates or alcohol.

Recall of dreams is less frequent in the following situations.

1 Old age, despite the duration of REM sleep remaining constant in old age.

2 Sleep inertia. Drowsiness or confusion on arousal may inhibit recall of dreams.

3 Depression.

4 Pontine degeneration. Dream recall may be absent in conditions such as progressive supranuclear palsy and multiple system atrophy, particularly of the olivopontocerebellar atrophy type. Loss of dream recall is usually associated with loss of saccadic eye movements, although pursuit movements are retained.

5 Lesions affecting particularly the inferior parietal lobe, the frontal lobes bilaterally or the posterior dominant hemisphere.

6 Hydrocephalus.

7 Drugs, e.g. benzodiazepines, barbiturates, alcohol.

Narrative content

The types of dreams typically associated with REM sleep are more than just the usual type of experience characteristic of wakefulness and they differ from the mundane, logical 'dreams' of NREM sleep [5].

Dreams are a self-report of mental activity and thinking which is based on life experiences, but they have several unusual features. First, dreams, unlike waking thoughts, are involuntary. Second, they involve considerable imagination and are unpredictable and in some ways show the chaotic organization that is characteristic of many physiological aspects of REM sleep (page 28). They often expand or unfold in an illogical way, and are not constrained by normality. Events are not accurately perceived or represented [6], but are orderly and not random. Illogicality is accepted passively by the dreamer, suggesting that there is a different pattern of information processing than in wakefulness. The associations between ideas and events are much weaker or looser than in the more logical thought processes of wakefulness and probably of NREM sleep. Despite the illogicality there is a sense of social awareness during dreams in that the thoughts and actions of other people in response to the dream content are realistically assessed.

The content of dreams reflects the current concerns of the subject and previous experiences [7]. Emotional events of the previous week are strongly represented. Dreams are reactive and are more closely linked to pre- than post-sleep thoughts and emotions. Previous experiences are often recreated. Some external stimuli occurring during sleep are ignored and others are incorporated into the dream narrative in a modified form. These are almost always self-centred or personal, and death of the dreamer never occurs in the dream.

There is a limited number of main themes of dreams. These are connected to basic biological needs that are common to all individuals. Aggressive or hostile behaviour towards others or towards the dreamer, resulting in dominance or submission, may manifest in dreams by various actions and emotions. Dreams that have a content of bonding to other people, or a sexual content, or that are related to feeding are common.

Many people have repetitive dreams or dream themes and the frequency of repetitive dreams is related to the intensity of the individual's concern about the topic. The content of the dreams also varies according to the following factors.

Age

Young children frequently dream of animals, but this becomes less common in teenage years, especially in industrialized societies rather than in hunter–gatherer communities. There is little change in dream content with age after around 16–18 years, although recall declines in the elderly. Dreams involving guilt or sexual activity are more common in young adults, and in the elderly death-related dreams are frequent. The frequency of dreams of individual members of the family remains constant throughout life.

Culture

There are many cross-cultural similarities in dream content, although the interpretation of dreams varies widely, and in some cultures is more religious than in others.

Race

This has little effect on dream content.

Gender

Males have more aggressive content to their dreams than females whose dreams tend to be friendlier and involve both males and females equally. Dreams during the first half of the menstrual cycle before ovulation tend to have a more positive emotional content than post-ovulation dreams when the progesterone level is rising. During menstrual periods the emotional content of dreams tends to be intensified and the dreams may be more hostile [8].

Dreams occurring early in the night tend to be shorter, less complex and have less emotional content than those later in the night when the drive to enter REM sleep is stronger. The exception to this is narcolepsy in which the initial dream at night has the most emotional content. It is common for the same event to figure in a series of dreams during the night and for it to become gradually more distorted as the associations between dream and reality become looser during the night. This is probably because of the predisposition in REM sleep to form weak mental associations between events, so that the reality underlying the dream becomes progressively harder to distinguish in dreams later in the night. The presence of objects or problems during successive dreams in a single night may represent the problem being worked on and resolved during sleep.

Sensory content

Dreams are usually multimodal with a combination of several sensations. Around 75% of subjects dream in colour and visual dreams are retained following the onset of blindness for at least 10 years. Non-visual dreams only occur in those who become totally blind before the age of 5. There is an auditory component to dreaming in around 75% of subjects. Sensations of falling, levitation or occasionally flying are common and are probably due to inhibition of muscle spindle activity or occasionally to changes in vestibular function. This type of dreaming is most common in narcolepsy.

Sensations of touch and taste only occur in around 1% of dreams and smell is even less frequent. There may be a sensation of suffocation or panic in obstructive sleep apnoeas related to the difficulty in breathing, and perhaps in 'vulnerable' personalities when they are in the supine position. Pain is rare in dreams unless the subject is in pain, for instance, from extensive burns [9], and the sensation of pain during dreams is also associated with persistence of pain during the day.

These sensory differences reflect the ability of the brainstem and thalamus to differentially gate the sensory pathways to the cerebral cortex. The varying tempo of dreams, which often start slowly, speed up and then slow down, and their occasional discontinuities may reflect variations in the patterns of activity in the cortical association areas.

Emotional content

A characteristic feature of dreams is their emotional content, presumably due to activation of the limbic system. The types of emotion are similar to those experienced during wakefulness, but vary considerably in intensity. In some people there is no emotional content at all, whereas in others it is so intense that dreams are felt to be exhausting.

The mood of the subject influences the degree of pleasantness of dreams. They frequently have a negative tone in depression and a hostile component in schizophrenia. An aggressive reaction to a perceived threat is characteristic of the REM sleep behaviour disorder. Intense fear and anxiety in response to a potentially harmful situation is characteristic of nightmares.

Dream vividness

Dreams vary in their vividness, and in their extreme form can be so realistic that the subject is unaware whether the events in the dream have actually taken place or not. This is a feature particularly of narcolepsy, REM sleep behaviour disorder and the post-traumatic stress disorder, as well as with drugs such as L-dopa and lipophilic beta blockers such as propranolol, metoprolol, labetalol and pindolol.

Lucid dreams

Lucid dreams are characterized by both awareness of being awake and an ability to direct the course of the dream. This is commonest in narcolepsy, but occurs occasionally in over 50% of the normal population, and more than once a month in around 15%.

Lucid dreaming is due to a mixed REM sleep/wake state in which the conscious control of wakefulness is present but does not terminate dream mentation. Lucidity training has been used effectively to control nightmares.

Dream timing

It is unusual for dreams to occur soon after falling asleep since the normal REM sleep latency is around 90 min. They are most frequent, prolonged and complex later in the night when REM sleep duration is greatest. In narcolepsy, however, dreams may occur even in the waking state while drowsy before sleep (hypnagogic hallucinations) and in a similar condition after waking (hypnopompic hallucinations).

Physical enactment of dreams

In REM sleep most of the skeletal muscles, except for instance the diaphragm, are intensely inhibited and the only movements that are seen are occasional twitches or jerks when the inhibition of muscle tone is temporarily lost. Motor inhibition prevents the dream experiences from being physically enacted. The exceptions are REM sleep behaviour disorder and status dissociatus when motor inhibition is lost and the aggressive content of the dreams is physically enacted. Dreams are also enacted in agrypnia excitata where the dreams represent REM sleep intrusion into wakefulness, and post-traumatic stress disorder when the 'nightmares' arise from NREM rather than REM sleep.

Consequences of dreams

Dreams are thought to represent the amalgamation of new experiences and ideas into existing neural networks. Dreams may alter the mood of the dreamer and facilitate solution of problems from the previous day. The loose association of ideas in REM sleep opens the opportunity for creative associations to be made and this type of information processing may be particularly important in children. It may lead to finding creative new solutions to current problems.

Dreams affect the emotional state of the dreamer on waking and may as a result affect behaviour. The nature of the dream mentation does appear to reflect the state of the subconscious mind as well as specific experiences and ideas that feature in the dreams. Most theories about the interpretation of dreams mainly reflect the mental constructs of the interpreter.

Nightmares

Overview

Nightmares are dreams which are terrifying and lead to intense anxiety or fear on arousal from sleep. They occur in REM sleep but because of the intense motor inhibition they rarely lead to any detectable movement until arousal has occurred.

Occurrence

Nightmares are equally common in males and females in childhood, but are more common in females in adult life. They usually arise between the ages of 2 and 5 years, occur in 10–50% of 3–6 years olds and are most frequent between the ages of 6 and 10. They

Table 8.1 Causes of nightmares.

Sleep deprivation causing REM sleep rebound
Narcolepsy
REM sleep behaviour disorder
Schizophrenia and schizoid personalities
Anxiety states
Drugs, e.g. L-dopa, beta blockers
Drug withdrawal, e.g. antidepressants, alcohol

occur occasionally in 40–50% of adults and less frequently in the elderly. The most common causes are shown in Table 8.1.

Clinical features

Nightmares are often long and complex but are only recognizable and recalled if the subject awakens from sleep. There is little autonomic over-activity, although around 40% of subjects have an increased heart rate on wakening, which is not related to the activity, such as running or fighting, of the nightmare. There is no motor enactment during the nightmare, except in the REM sleep behaviour disorder, in which muscle tone is retained. There are, however, gross body movements after arousal from sleep.

The subject is not confused on awakening, has vivid recall of the nightmare and often has difficulty in returning to sleep. Nightmares occur most frequently and intensely during the last third of the night when REM sleep is more prolonged. The degree of distress caused by nightmares is greater in those with anxiety states, but the frequency of nightmares is not related to anxiety or any other psychological disorder.

Investigations

Polysomnography is rarely required but may show increased REM density for around 10 min before an abrupt awakening from the nightmare, together with some respiratory and heart rate variability. Nightmares almost invariably arise from REM sleep, except in the post-traumatic stress disorder, where they may occur in stages 1 or 2 NREM sleep as well.

Differential diagnosis

1 REM sleep behaviour disorder.
2 Nocturnal panic attacks.
3 Epilepsy. The aura may be mistaken for a nightmare.
4 Sleep terrors. These have little dream imagery and occur early in the night (Table 8.2).

Characteristic	Nightmare	Sleep terror
Age of onset	Usually 3–6 years	Usually 2–6 years
Gender	M = F	M > F
Time in night	Last third	First third
Dream content	Long and complex, terrifying	Nil
Recall	Good	Very little
Behaviour	No movement	Very active
Autonomic response	Little	Intense
Post event	Orientated	Confused

Table 8.2 Nightmares and sleep terrors.

Problems

Nightmares are frightening for the patient [10], and can induce a fear of going to sleep. They cause nocturnal awakenings from which it may be difficult to re-enter sleep.

Treatment

Treatment is not usually required, but any drugs that predispose to nightmares, such as L-dopa or beta blockers, may need to be discontinued and those with a REM sleep suppressant action should be tailed off slowly. Reduction of stresses that have precipitated the nightmares and improvement in sleep hygiene may be of help.

Cognitive behavioural therapy may be of benefit. This is based on the assumption that nightmares are a learned behaviour or a conditioned process. The initiating factor such as a traumatic or childhood event is de-emphasized and shown to be irrelevant to any actions needed by the patient to change the dream content. Relaxation techniques, desensitization through the subject experiencing fearful situations, and imagery rehearsal therapy may be effective. In imagery rehearsal therapy the dreamer is taught to change the content of the nightmares into any form that is preferred. It is a form of lucid dream training and requires frequent repetition to be effective. The efficacy is not related either to the chronicity of the nightmares or to their content. It reduces both the distress and the frequency of the nightmares and can shorten the sleep latency and increase sleep efficiency.

If nightmares persist despite these techniques, REM sleep suppressant drugs such as tricyclic antidepressants may be required.

Differential diagnosis of dreams

Dreams have characteristic features, but can be confused with other sensory experiences during sleep (Table 8.3).

Sensory hypnic jerks

Hypnic jerks are common (page 198), but their sensory equivalents are under-recognized. A sensation of falling or occasionally floating is common. Flashes of light, or even fragments of visual hallucinations, may occur, and usually accompany the motor jerk. Auditory sensations such as snapping noises or loud bangs may be heard and may be associated with a sensation of bursting in the head. These are often

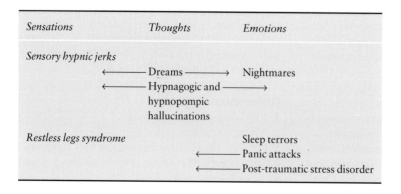

Table 8.3 Sensations, thoughts and emotions in sleep and on arousal.

frightening and are probably responsible for what has been termed the 'exploding head syndrome'.

These sensations occur at the transition from wakefulness to stage 1 or 2 NREM sleep, and are followed by an arousal to wakefulness, often with a tachycardia. They may generate a fear of initiating sleep if they recur frequently.

Investigations are not usually required and reassurance is usually sufficient.

Arousal disorders

Vivid, often frightening, but poorly defined sensations may be perceived, particularly in adults. Occasionally complex imagery may be recalled.

Nocturnal epilepsy

An ill-defined frightening sensation, often of a near-death experience, is characteristic of nocturnal frontal lobe epilepsy. Temporal lobe epilepsy may be manifested by recurrent dreams.

Nocturnal visual hallucinations

Nocturnal visual hallucinations may arise from stages 2 and 3 NREM sleep, and on waking vivid complex visual figures, usually of people or animals, are seen. There is little movement, no dream recall and the figures vanish if the light is switched on. The hallucinations may be frightening, and may be associated with anxiety states, betablockers and Lewy body disease. They are similar to the hallucinations during wakefulness in the Charles Bonnett syndrome and peduncular hallucinosis.

Post-traumatic stress disorder

'Nightmares' occur in around 75% of patients, particularly in stages 1 and 2 NREM sleep rather than REM sleep. They have a recurrent content, related to the previous traumatic event. They are experienced intensely and the frequency of the dreams is proportional to the intensity of the concern about the event. They occur particularly early in the night and are associated with gross body movements [11].

Alpha blockers such as prazosin are effective, but beta blockers worsen the nightmares.

Dreams in neurological disorders

Disorders of REM sleep

1 Narcolepsy.
2 REM sleep behaviour disorder.
3 Status dissociatus.
4 Agrypnia excitata.

Disorders of pons

Idiopathic Parkinsonism

Vivid dreams are a feature of Parkinsonism. They usually have a strong visual content and are particularly marked during treatment with L-dopa or dopaminergic agents.

Visual hallucinations also occur during wakefulness in around 25% of those with idiopathic Parkinsonism but especially in Lewy body disease. They often involve strangers, but are not frightening. They are probably due to brief episodes of REM sleep intruding into wakefulness and occur particularly in those who have sleep-onset REM during polysomnography [12] and REM sleep demonstrated during naps in the day. Cataplexy does not occur.

Progressive supranuclear palsy

Dreams are few or absent.

Disorders of cerebral cortex

Dreams are infrequent with lesions of the inferior parietal lobe, bilateral frontal lobe disorders and those involving the posterior dominant hemisphere.

Dreams in psychiatric disorders

Anxiety

Waking with anxiety and autonomic hyperactivity which is out of proportion to the content of the dream is typical. The subject immediately regains full alertness and has good recall of the dream or nightmare. There may also be nocturnal panic attacks arising from stages 2 and 3 NREM sleep which do not have any dream content.

Depression

Dreams usually have a negative emotional content throughout the night, but if the tone of the dreams improves during the night the depression is more likely to persist. Dreams are shorter than normal and recall is reduced. They tend to become less complex later in the night and intense dreams and nightmares are unusual. Patients who feel suicidal are slightly more likely to have dreams of death.

Obsessive–compulsive disorder

The dreams do not contain rituals similar to those that are performed during the day.

Eating disorders

In anorexia nervosa, dreams of the feminine role and

food rejection are common. In bulimia dreams of food and eating are frequent, but have a negative tone.

Schizophrenia

Dreams during sleep should be distinguished from hallucinations during wakefulness. Dreams rarely include friends, but commonly feature strangers. Dreams may picture living in an alienated world which is often hostile to the schizophrenic.

Autism and Asperger's syndrome

There is little dream content in these conditions.

Drug-induced dreams

Most drugs that influence dreams and nightmares act on the cholinergic, aminergic or related neurotransmitters. An increase in cholinergic activity in the pons tends to promote REM sleep and is associated with intense multimodality dreams or hallucinations during wakefulness. In contrast an increase in noradrenergic activity, as in the post-traumatic stress disorder, leads to simpler repetitive intense dream- or nightmare-like events.

The main groups of drugs that increase the frequency and intensity of dreams are as follows.
1 Cholinergic drugs. Cholinesterase inhibitors, such as rivastigmine, anticholinesterases and other cholinergic drugs, all tend to promote dreams.
2 Adrenergic agonists and blockers. Alpha agonists such as captopril increase dreams whereas alpha blockers, such as prazosin, which is a short-acting lipid soluble drug, suppress the 'nightmares' of the post-traumatic stress disorder.

Lipophilic beta blockers, such as propranolol, metoprolol, labetalol and pindolol, increase dreams and nightmares more than lipophobic drugs such as sotalol and atenolol.
3 Dopaminergic drugs and antagonists. L-dopa, dopamine receptor agonists such as cabergoline, and other dopaminergic agents such as amantadine all increase dream frequency and may lead to nightmares. Amphetamines and related drugs cause an increase in intensity of dreams. Cocaine increases dream intensity and emotional content, and this is linked to the feeling of euphoria during wakefulness.

Antipsychotic drugs such as chlorpromazine are dopamine antagonists, but also increase dream frequency and intensity.
4 Antidepressants. Monoamineoxidase and tricyclic antidepressants increase the frequency of dreams.

Selective serotonin re-uptake inhibitors also lead to intense, vivid and realistic dreams, although they are REM suppressant [13]. Withdrawal of these drugs leads to REM sleep rebound with bizarre dreams and may induce the REM sleep behaviour disorder. SSRI antidepressants also cause frequent eye movements, particularly in stage 2 NREM sleep, which may be a permanent effect of only temporary treatment.
5 Opioids, e.g. tramadol, buprenorphine.
6 Antihistamines, e.g. chlorpheniramine.
7 Anti-epileptics, e.g. lamotrigine, sodium valproate.
8 Anaesthetics, e.g. ketamine.
9 Antibiotics, e.g. ciprofloxacin, erythromycin, ganciclovir.
10 Nonsteroidal anti-inflammatory drugs, e.g. naproxen.
11 Withdrawal of REM suppressant drugs, e.g. benzodiazepines and related drugs, barbiturates and alcohol.

References

1 Hobson JA, Pace-Schott EF. The cognitive neuroscience of sleep: neuronal systems, consciousness and learning. *Neuroscience* 2002; 3: 679–93.
2 Takeuchi T, Miyasita A, Inugami M, Yamamoto Y. Intrinsic dreams are not produced without REM sleep mechanisms: evidence through elicitation of sleep onset REM periods. *J Sleep Res* 2001; 10: 43–52.
3 Suzuki H, Uchiyama M, Tagaya H, Ozaki A, Kuriyama K, Aritake S, Shibui K, Tan X, Kamei Y, Kuga R. Dreaming during non-rapid eye movement sleep in the absence of prior rapid eye movement sleep. *Sleep* 2004; 27(8): 1486–90.
4 Schredl M, Schafer G, Weber B, Heuser I. Dreaming and insomnia: dream recall and dream content of patients with insomnia. *J Sleep Res* 1998; 7: 191–8.
5 Fagioli I. Mental activity during sleep. *Sleep Med Rev* 2002; 6(4): 307–20.
6 Nielsen TA, Kuiken D, Alain G, Stenstrom P, Powell RA. Immediate and delayed incorporations of events into dreams: further replication and implications for dream function. *J Sleep Res* 2004; 13; 327–36.
7 Martin RJ, Banks-Schlegel S. Chronobiology of asthma. *Am J Respir Crit Care Med* 1998; 158: 1002–7.
8 Nielsen TA. Chronobiological features of dream production. *Sleep Med Rev* 2004; 8: 403–24.
9 Raymond I, Nielsen TA, Lavigne G, Choiniere M. Incorporation of pain in dreams of hospitalized burn victims. *Sleep* 2002; 25(7): 765–70.
10 Blagrove M, Farmer L, Williams E. The relationship of nightmare frequency and nightmare distress to well-being. *J Sleep Res* 2004; 13: 129–36.

11 Nomura T, Inoue Y, Mitani H, Kawahara R, Miyake M, Nakashima K. Visual hallucinations as REM sleep behavior disorders in patients with Parkinson's disease. *Mov Disord* 2003; 18: 812–17.

12 Woodward SH, Leskin GA, Sheikh JI. Movement during sleep: associations with posttraumatic stress disorder, nightmares, and comorbid panic disorder. *Sleep* 2002; 25(6): 681–8.

13 Pace-Schott EF, Gersh T, Silvestri R, Stickgold R, Salzman C, Hobson JA. SSRI treatment suppresses dream recall frequency but increases subjective dream intensity in normal subjects. *J Sleep Res* 2001; 10: 129–42.

9 Motor Disorders

Introduction

The presenting feature of behavioural or motor abnormalities in sleep is usually the report of the abnormal behaviour by the patient or more usually the partner, other members of the family, a friend or a carer. Occasionally, the patient or partner may be injured during the episode. Excessive daytime sleepiness and insomnia are unusual, except in periodic limb movements in sleep, epilepsy and REM sleep behaviour disorder. Excessive daytime sleepiness with snoring is a feature of motor abnormalities of the upper airway and of the respiratory pump, which are discussed in Chapters 10 and 11.

The term 'parasomnia' is commonly used to describe most of these types of events during sleep. They are conventionally defined as unusual, undesirable and episodic events which are not due to disorders of the sleep or wake mechanisms themselves. This definition is unsatisfactory for several reasons. First, inclusion of an undesirable element leads to a subjective assessment of what is, or is not, a parasomnia. Secondly, the sleep–wake mechanisms interact in a complex manner with the abnormal behavioural events during sleep, and cannot be clearly differentiated from them. Thirdly, the range of unusual events occurring during sleep is so diverse that the concept of a parasomnia has little value in understanding their nature or in guiding their management in clinical practice. Fourthly, many of the parasomnias are so common at certain ages that they merge into normality and should perhaps not be regarded as disorders of sleep.

A complex, and often inconsistent, classification of descriptive syndromes has been built up around the concept of parasomnias without sufficient regard for the underlying pathophysiological processes. In addition the distinction between sleep and wakefulness is not always clear cut. Features of both may coexist in mixed sleep–wake states, for instance during sleep paralysis when REM sleep intrudes into wakefulness. The transitions between sleep stages are also associated with various mixtures of the features of these two states, and underlie conditions such as sleep walking. In these episodes awareness of the environment and of activities may be suppressed, while movements take place which are often complex.

The organization of motor activity during sleep is very different from during wakefulness. The higher centres are active, particularly in REM sleep, but there is greater inhibition of lower motor neurone activity, especially in the postural muscles in REM sleep. As a result there is less movement during sleep with a reduction in muscle tone and in reflex responses, despite the activity of the higher centres. Motor activity can, however, break through either if the central activity increases or if its inhibition fails, even transiently.

The central activity may be intense and pathological as in an epileptic seizure, or more subtle and normal, or near normal, e.g. motor inhibition may be lost in young children in whom the sleep regulation systems are immature, in the elderly and in patients with degenerative neurological disorders, in whom sleep control also degenerates. There are fewer motor disorders in REM sleep than in NREM sleep because of the intense motor inhibition, but an exception is the REM sleep behaviour disorder in which release of motor inhibition allows complex movements, reflecting the content of vivid dreams, to be enacted. An abnormality of motor control which is present in both NREM and REM sleep probably underlies the occasional association of abnormal behaviour during both these sleep states, such as the combination of sleep walking and REM sleep behaviour disorder (parasomnia overlap syndrome).

The location of the abnormalities or the release of motor control within the central nervous system varies between different disorders. Complex behaviours can be organized without cortical input by control systems between the midbrain and the medulla, and the central pattern generator of the spinal cord can also produce complex stepping and similar actions.

Table 9.1 Sleep-state transition disorders.

Wake–REM sleep	Wake–NREM sleep
Cataplexy	Hypnic jerks
Sleep paralysis	Benign neonatal and fragmentary myoclonus
	Rhythmic movement disorder
REM sleep–wake	NREM sleep–wake
Sleep paralysis	Confusional arousal
Post-traumatic stress disorder	Sleep terror
	Sleep walking
	Sleep talking
	Sleep eating and drinking
	Panic attack
	Nocturnal cramp

NREM, non-rapid eye movement; REM, rapid eye movement.

Table 9.2 Sleep-state specific disorders.

NREM sleep	REM sleep
Epilepsy	REM sleep behaviour disorder
Sleep bruxism	Status dissociatus
RLS	
PLMS	

NREM, non-rapid eye movement; RLS, restless legs syndrome; PLMS, periodic limb movements in sleep; REM, rapid eye movement.

There are numerous classifications of the motor disorders during sleep, but in this chapter they will be classified primarily according to which stage of sleep they arise in and whether they are associated with a transition into or out of this sleep stage (Tables 9.1, 9.2). Movement disorders which are present during wakefulness but which are affected by sleep will be discussed last.

Assessment

History

A careful history is essential to accurately assess motor disorders during sleep (see Chapter 3). The issues that should be considered are as follows.

1 What is the nature of the movements? Do these affect the whole body or are they localized to one part, such as the limbs in periodic limb movements in sleep, or jaw movements as in sleep bruxism? Is there a sequence of movements as in Jacksonian epilepsy? Is the type of movement repetitive and what is its frequency and amplitude? Are the movements simple or complex and is violence a feature, either spontaneously or if restraint is attempted?

2 Are there any associated features such as sensory symptoms, dreams, autonomic activation or incontinence?

3 What is the mental state during the episode? Is the patient responsive to questions or commands? Is there any recall of the events and do any of the activities appear to be premeditated? Are there signs of anxiety? What happens after the event? Can the patient fall asleep readily or are there any abnormal behaviours?

4 How does the event relate to sleep, wakefulness or the transition between the two? Do similar episodes occur during wakefulness during the daytime? The age of the subject, the time of the events during the night and the presence of a family or previous history of similar types of sleep disorder may suggest a relationship of the episodes to sleep, wakefulness or the transition between the two.

5 What is the cause of the events? Are they precipitated by sleep deprivation, poor sleep hygiene, drug intake, including alcohol or its withdrawal, or caffeine? Is there any underlying neurological disorder such as dementia or Parkinsonism?

Physical examination

Physical examination may reveal signs of injury or effects of the abnormal movements such as ground-down teeth from sleep bruxism. Neurological examination may be required, but is usually of limited value, except in REM sleep behaviour disorder, epilepsy and movement disorders that are present during wakefulness.

Investigations

The history may suggest a diagnosis with a sufficient degree of certainty for management to be planned without the need for further investigation. This is usually so with sleep walking, sleep talking, rhythmic movement disorder and sleep bruxism. In most other situations, particularly when the movements are complex, potentially dangerous to the patient or to others, troublesome to the partner or carer, or if their nature is uncertain, referral to a specialist centre for more detailed assessment and investigation is needed. Investigations are directed to ascertaining the following.

Nature of the attacks

Polysomnography with video and audio recording is important in establishing the nature of the events, their relationship to the stage of sleep or to wakefulness, and the presence of other factors which may contribute to the clinical picture.

Cause of the attacks

This may be established by the following methods.
1 Blood tests, e.g. ferritin, urea and electrolyte estimation in restless legs syndrome.
2 Electro-encephalogram (EEG) in wakefulness to assist the diagnosis of epilepsy.
3 Brain imaging techniques, e.g. computerized tomography (CT) and magnetic resonance imaging (MRI) scans of the head, particularly to investigate REM sleep behaviour disorder, nocturnal frontal lobe epilepsy and involuntary movement disorders which are worse during wakefulness than during sleep.

Principles of treatment

The aims of treatment are as follows.
1 Explain the nature of the disorder to the subject and reassure when appropriate.
2 Sleep hygiene advice. This minimizes the risk of sleep deprivation which may precipitate motor disorders during sleep, and can also be directed to reduce the risk of arousal which is important in preventing sleep–wake transition disorders. Changes in the use of any drugs that may be adversely affecting the sleep–wake patterns should be considered.
3 Treat the underlying disorder, e.g. by treating the cause of iron loss and replacing iron in restless legs syndrome, prescription of anticonvulsants for epilepsy, dopamine agonists for restless legs syndrome and Parkinsonism, and benzodiazepines in REM sleep behaviour disorder.

4 Modification of sleep–wake patterns by drugs, e.g. use of benzodiazepines to consolidate stage 2 NREM sleep and thereby reduce the risk of sleep–wake transition disorders; tricyclic antidepressants to reduce the duration of REM sleep to minimize, for instance, sleep paralysis; or avoiding stimulants such as caffeine to reduce the risk of arousal and of sleep–wake transition disorders.
5 Protection. This may be required for the patient in the form of a helmet, locking the windows and bedroom door, or constructing a stair gate. Localized movement disorders need specific equipment, such as a gum shield for sleep bruxism. Protection for the partner usually takes the form of sleeping in a separate bed or bedroom, if necessary with the door locked.
6 Lifestyle advice. This may be required to cope both with any stress which may be contributing to the disorder and with its impact. Psychotherapy is occasionally needed.

Sleep violence

Causes

There are several observations that make it more or less probable that a violent act was carried out as a result of a sleep disorder (Table 9.3). Polysomnography may not show any specific features of some of the causes, such as an arousal disorder, but may indicate the presence of others such as the REM sleep behaviour disorder. The most important types of sleep disorder are as follows.

Arousal disorders

Violence may occur abruptly towards the end of an episode of sleep walking, especially if the sleep walker is restrained. It also occurs occasionally in confusional arousals when it erupts within a few seconds if the subject perceives that he or she is being threatened. The subject then often rapidly calms and apologizes for the actions that have been carried out. In both conditions the subject may appear to be in a panic, and to have enormous strength, and may carry out repeated actions, such as stabbings.

Post-traumatic stress disorder

The subject may wake suddenly from sleep, leap out of the bed and behave violently as part of a re-enactment of the traumatic experience.

REM sleep behaviour disorder

Extreme violence may occur, but this is not specifically

Table 9.3 Violence and sleep disorders.

Sleep disorder likely	Sleep disorder unlikely
Previous history of sleep walking or family history of sleep walking	Premeditation
Senseless crime	Highly complex actions or series of actions
Amnesia for event	Recall of events
Perplexed and horrified reaction after the event	
No attempt to conceal the crime	

aimed at the victim unless he or she is misinterpreted by the subject as an assailant.

Status dissociatus

This causes similar activities to the REM sleep behaviour disorder.

Narcolepsy

Violence is rare unless there is a hypnagogic hallucination in which the subject feels that aggression should be directed to the victim.

Obstructive sleep apnoeas

Violence may occur, usually in association with hallucinations, if severe sleep apnoeas cause REM sleep fragmentation or rebound. Obstructive sleep apnoeas also lead to confusional arousals which may be associated with violent behaviour quite separately from any REM sleep-related violence.

Epilepsy

This is an uncommon cause of nocturnal violence, but this is seen occasionally in nocturnal frontal lobe epilepsy or temporal epilepsy.

Psychogenic causes

Dissociative disorders are associated with violence during sleep. These episodes occur after 30–90 s of wakefulness during which the subject appears behaviourally to be asleep. Occasionally wandering from the bed and re-enactment of previous abuse situations form part of the violence.

Legal aspects

Violent acts during sleep may lead to prosecution which is usually defended on the basis of 'automatism'. This defence may be successful even if it is admitted that the violent act occurred and that the accused carried it out if it can be shown that the subject was completely unaware of his or her actions. An automatism is any movement of the limbs or body which is not controlled by the mind. This includes not only violence during sleep, but also driving a motor vehicle, sexual activity or indecent exposure. An automatism implies absence of mental function and not just clouding of consciousness and it implies that the subject did not know the nature of the act or that it was wrong.

Automatism is not accepted purely because of a lack of memory of the episode, or because the accused states he or she could not control the impulse to carry out the act. Even impaired or partial awareness is sufficient for the act to be regarded legally as under the control of the patient's mind.

If the act was carried out as an automatism it needs to be established whether this was either a 'sane automatism' or an 'insane automatism'.

Sane automatism

This term implies that there was a trigger factor for the actions which was external to the subject, and not due to any disease of the mind. This might include, for instance, a head injury, drugs or an animal sting, which initiated the action. The defence of a drug-induced sane automatism only succeeds if the drug was taken for medical purposes and not for the purpose of pleasure or intoxication.

If a sane automatism is accepted the subject is found not guilty of the offence and discharged. Sleep walking is regarded as a sane automatism, unless the subject carried out an act such as drinking excessive alcohol which he or she knew from past experience might have triggered the episode.

Insane automatism

This implies that there is an internal cause for the action. It may for instance be epilepsy, diabetes or a psychiatric disorder such as schizophrenia or depression.

If this is accepted by the court the subject may be sentenced to detention in a mental hospital for custodial care and treatment.

Wakefulness–NREM sleep transition movements

Propriospinal myoclonus

These irregular jerking movements occur in the supine position during relaxed wakefulness before sleep and are inhibited by sleep [1]. Each jerk lasts 150–300 ms and involves large muscles, including those of the neck, chest and abdomen. They appear to be generated by a spreading wave of activity in the propriospinal system in the spinal cord due to loss of brainstem or higher centre inhibition.

They are commoner in males, usually have no clinical significance, but may lead to insomnia. They can be confused with hypnic jerks, although these only occur during sleep, and with periodic limb movements. They respond to clonazepam or anticonvulsants.

Hypnic jerks (sleep starts, hypnic myoclonus)

Overview

Hypnic jerks are brief twitching movements that occur only at the onset of sleep. They may be associated with vivid sensations, particularly a feeling of falling.

Occurrence

They are very common, occurring occasionally in 60–70% of normal adults. They are equally frequent in males and females.

Pathogenesis

They are due to momentary failure of inhibition of lower motor neurone activity during the unstable phase of sleep onset. Hypnic jerks may be provoked by central nervous system stimulants such as caffeine, sleep deprivation and stress.

Clinical features

Hypnic jerks are usually single, although occasionally a few jerks may follow in quick succession. They involve especially the legs, are usually bilateral, but can occasionally be asymmetrical. The jerks last less than 1 s and occur at or soon after the onset of sleep. They arise from stages 1 or 2 NREM sleep. They may be evoked by external stimuli, and are followed by a brief arousal to wakefulness with EEG features of arousal, including K-complexes. Occasionally there is a brief cry or autonomic changes, including an increase in heart or respiratory rate, and sweating.

They fluctuate in their severity and frequency, and can lead to a fear of falling asleep.

The sensations that often accompany hypnic jerks are described on page 190.

Investigations

None are usually needed.

Differential diagnosis

1 Periodic limb movements in sleep. These are repetitive, of longer duration and affect predominantly the legs.
2 Fragmentary myoclonus.
3 Myoclonic epilepsy. Epileptiform discharges are detectable on polysomnography.
4 Startle disease (hyperekplexia). This is a rare and often familial and autosomally inherited disorder of motor control causing an exaggerated response to stimuli, often with loss of balance and falls. There is no loss of consciousness, but injuries are common since the arms are held stiffly during the fall. Repetitive jerky movements of the limbs occur at night and hyper-reflexia is present. Clonazepam and sodium valproate may be effective.

Problems

Occasional sleep-onset insomnia due to either fear of falling asleep or repeated awakenings, and anxiety regarding the nature of the symptoms.

Treatment

1 Reassurance.
2 Sleep hygiene advice, especially to avoid sleep deprivation.
3 Avoid stimulants such as caffeine.
4 Benzodiazepines, such as clonazepam or temazepam, are occasionally required.

Benign neonatal myoclonus

Benign neonatal myoclonus is often familial and is seen soon after birth, especially in premature infants. It may last for a few months and is characterized by symmetrical but irregular twitching of the fingers, toes and face during the lighter stages of NREM sleep. It should be distinguished from myoclonic epilepsy.

Fragmentary myoclonus (partial myoclonus)

This is similar to benign neonatal myoclonus, but often asymmetrical, with small-amplitude focal jerks of the limbs and occasionally of the face. They last for less than 150 ms, are associated with K-complexes and occur usually at sleep onset or during NREM sleep. They are uncommon and more frequent in males and can lead to sufficient sleep fragmentation to cause excessive daytime sleepiness. Like benign neonatal myoclonus, they represent either an increase in higher centre activation which overcomes a normal level of motor inhibition or, more probably, a transient recurrent failure of the latter.

Rhythmic movement disorder (head banging, jactatio capitis nocturna)

Overview
This disorder is characterized by repetitive movements of large muscle groups before and soon after the onset of sleep. Head banging is the best recognized pattern.

Occurrence and aetiology
This is three to four times more common in males than in females. Body rocking usually appears at around 6 months and head banging and head rolling at around 9 months. These movements often disappear by around 18 months of age and are uncommon after the age of 4 years. They can persist into adult life, particularly if there are abnormalities such as mental retardation or autism, or following a head injury, but also occasionally in otherwise normal subjects. Daytime head banging is a separate entity which is usually suppressed during sleep. It is a transient phase in young children, but in adults is associated with learning disabilities, autism and psychotic states.

Pathogenesis
Little is known about the cause of this disorder. It is not usually associated with any other abnormality in children. The movements may assist development of vestibular function.

Clinical features
The repetitive stereotyped movements usually begin during drowsiness and persist into light NREM sleep, often for 10–15 min. They appear to be pleasurable, possibly because of the vestibular stimulation that they provide, and may promote the onset of sleep. The usual frequency of the movements is 0.5–2/s. Head banging against a pillow, the framework of the bed or a wall is the most common pattern, but head rolling from side to side and rocking or rolling of the entire body with flexion and extension or lateral body movements may be seen. The child may squat on his hands and knees or rock in a sitting position, and there may be repetitive vocalizations or humming. Scalp lacerations and even subdural haematomas can occur, but other injuries are uncommon.

Investigations
Polysomnography is rarely required but shows rhythmic movement artefacts during drowsiness and in stages 1 and 2 NREM sleep. There are no EEG features of arousal from sleep by the rocking movements. Video recordings confirm the nature of the movements.

Differential diagnosis
1 Epilepsy, e.g. infantile spasms.
2 Periodic limb movements in sleep.
3 Bruxism.

Problems
1 Parental anxiety and insomnia.
2 Occasional injury such as subdural haematoma.

Treatment
1 Explanation and reassurance to the family, and treatment of any psychological cause.
2 Protection of the child, e.g. by padding the bed-head or provision of a protective helmet.
3 Benzodiazepines, tricyclic antidepressants, e.g. imipramine, or gabapentin may occasionally be required, but the response is variable.

NREM sleep–wakefulness transition movements (arousal disorders)

Quiet awakenings from stages 3 and 4 NREM sleep are common normal events. The subject may briefly sit up and then lie back and fall asleep again or make gross body movements. These postural movements are associated with a slight elevation of heart rate and blood pressure and the eyes may open briefly. There is no recall of the brief arousal and sleep is soon re-entered. These events usually occur at sleep onset, during stages 1 and 2 NREM sleep, or at the start or end of a REM sleep episode. They are most common in the second half of the night and often occur three to four times per hour.

In contrast, arousal disorders represent an abnormality of the transition from stages 3 and 4 NREM sleep to wakefulness in which both the behaviour and level

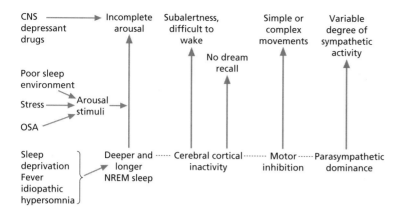

Fig. 9.1 Arousal disorders.

of alertness reflect an intermediate state between these two conditions. These disorders all have the following features in common (Fig. 9.1).

1 The movements may be simple and repetitive, or complex (automatic behaviour).

2 There is no dream content and little or no recall of the event (retrograde amnesia). There may be a vague recollection of a frightening image or of an imminent catastrophe.

3 There is a misperception and reduced or even absence of awareness of the surroundings. The subject is unresponsive, or virtually so, to contact with other people. This loss of awareness is probably analogous to sleep inertia, but much more marked.

4 There is a variable degree of autonomic activation. Parasympathetic activity usually predominates over sympathetic activity during sleep, but at the time of these arousals sympathetic activity may be marked, especially in sleep terrors.

5 It is difficult to wake the subject from the attacks, but if challenged he or she may become angry, startled and violent.

6 These episodes do not cause insomnia or excessive daytime sleepiness.

7 They tend to occur during the first third of the night and particularly around 1 h after sleep onset, when NREM sleep, especially stages 3 and 4, is most prolonged. They usually arise at the end of the first or second NREM sleep cycle, and although the macrostructure of sleep is normal, the events probably begin at moments when the cyclic alternating pattern favours arousal.

8 They are commonest in childhood, especially between the ages of 3 and 10 years.

9 There is often a family history, probably reflecting a similarity in the neurodevelopmental problems responsible for the manifestation of the disorder. Several of these disorders often coexist either in the same individual or in the same family. Inheritance is probably polygenic and it is the cumulative effect of many genes which determines the phenotype of the arousal disorder.

Pathogenesis

These disorders arise from stages 3 and 4 NREM sleep so that they are particularly frequent in any situation in which these stages are increased or in which there is a tendency to arouse.

1 Causes of increase in stages 3 and 4 NREM sleep with incomplete arousal.

  (a) Age. In childhood the duration and intensity of stages 3 and 4 NREM sleep are increased and the immaturity of the sleep regulating mechanisms predisposes to incomplete arousals.

  (b) Central nervous system depressant drugs, e.g. hypnotics, antipsychotics, tricyclic antidepressants and alcohol.

  (c) Sleep deprivation. This increases the duration of stages 3 and 4 NREM sleep.

  (d) Fever

  (e) Idiopathic hypersomnia.

2 Causes of frequent arousals.

  (a) Environmental factors. These include noise and forced awakenings by a parent or carer.

  (b) Sleep disorders. Sleep fragmentation may be due to obstructive sleep apnoeas or the restless legs syndrome or periodic limb movements in sleep.

  (c) Other factors, e.g. pain, stress, drugs, including alcohol.

Confusional arousal (sleep drunkenness)

Overview

Confusional arousals occur at the transition from stages 3 and 4 NREM sleep to wakefulness when the attainment of full alertness is delayed. The subject appears confused and carries out inappropriate actions (automatic behaviour).

Occurrence

Confusional arousals are equally common in males and females, and are almost universal in children under the age of 5 years if they are woken from stages 3 and 4 NREM sleep. They occur in around 1% of susceptible adults, particularly when they are sleep deprived, and are less common in the elderly because of the reduction in duration of stages 3 and 4 NREM sleep.

Pathogenesis

Confusional arousals are the manifestation of a delayed and partial reorganization of cortical activity at the transition from stages 3 and 4 NREM sleep to wakefulness. They are more common when these sleep stages are enhanced, as in, for instance, idiopathic hypersomnia, and following sleep deprivation, shift work, alcohol and obstructive sleep apnoeas which may all lead to rebound NREM sleep. They are also more common with hypnotics and in disorders that reduce the normal level of alertness, such as hepatic and renal encephalopathy and narcolepsy. Confusional arousals can, rarely, be associated with lesions in the diencephalon and periventricular grey matter in the brainstem.

Clinical features

Confusional arousals occur most frequently during the first third of the night. They may arise spontaneously or in response to external stimuli or forced awakening. Sleep is not re-entered after arousal but a period of subalertness manifested by confusion follows. Disorientation in time and space with slow and inappropriate responses to questions and commands is common.

Confusional arousals are an exaggerated form of sleep inertia but the state of subalertness and confusion is combined with abnormal and often complex motor activity (Table 9.4). Children may cry, call out, or roll around the bed. Adults may carry out activities such as picking up a glass instead of the telephone or putting sugar into the kettle. The subject appears confused and disorientated, and speech is often unintelligible. Restraint is resisted, often aggressively, but violence is never premeditated.

Confusional arousals may last for several minutes and afterwards full alertness is regained.

There is little recall of the event in children, but in adults there may be brief flashbacks of what has

Table 9.4 Differential diagnosis of complex activities in sleep and on arousal.

Confusional arousal
Frontal lobe epilepsy
Temporal lobe epilepsy
REM sleep behaviour disorder
Sleep walking
Panic attack
Sundowning syndrome

REM, rapid eye movement.

happened. There is no dream content, anxiety or autonomic activation. If there is more than one confusional arousal per night the earlier episodes are usually the more intense.

The features of confusional arousals may also merge into the end of a sleep terror or episode of sleep walking, following which the subject then falls asleep readily.

Investigations

Polysomnography is only occasionally required in children, to distinguish confusional arousals from other conditions, if there are atypical features. It is more often indicated in adults, particularly if the episodes have caused injury, or if the diagnosis is unclear.

Polysomnography is often normal but may show frequent arousals from stages 3 and 4 NREM sleep even when confusional arousals are not apparent. These sleep stages may be more evenly distributed during the night than normal and hypersynchronous delta waves may be detected before the events. During the arousal there may be some residual delta waves combined with alpha and theta, suggesting that electrophysiological aspects of both wakefulness and sleep are present simultaneously. The presence of alpha waves does not indicate a psychogenic origin of the episodes. Video recordings may clarify the nature of the activities carried out during these episodes.

Differential diagnosis

1 Sleep terrors.
2 Sleep walking.
3 Sleep talking.
4 Epilepsy.
5 Episodic nocturnal wanderings.
6 REM sleep behaviour disorder.
7 Nightmares.
8 Fugue states.

Problems

There is danger both to the subject and to the partner or witnesses.

Treatment

1 Explanation and reassurance.
2 Advice not to restrain the subject.
3 Reduce any tendency to excessive stages 3 and 4 NREM sleep, e.g. sleep hygiene advice.
4 Minimize the risk of arousals during the first third of the night, especially in children.
5 Promotion of attainment of full alertness, e.g. discontinue hypnotics.
6 Treat the cause of subalertness, e.g. narcolepsy, hepatic failure and obstructive sleep apnoeas.

Sleep terrors (night terrors, pavor nocturnus, pavor incubus)

Overview

Sleep terrors are sudden and brief episodes which occur especially in children and which are characterized by panic and confusion with intense autonomic activation.

Occurrence

They are more common in males than in females, they are often familial, and there is a familial association with confusional arousals and sleep walking. They occur from the age of around 1 year, are most common between 5 and 7 years, and arise in around 3% of children aged 4–12 years, but they then become increasingly uncommon. If they persist after the age of 20 there is often associated psychopathology such as anxiety, depression or phobias. It is very uncommon for sleep terrors to either appear in or persist into old age, in which stages 3 and 4 NREM sleep are much reduced. They are common in those who sleep walk or sleep talk and also in Tourette's syndrome.

Pathogenesis and aetiology

Sleep terrors are due to incomplete arousal from stages 3 and 4 NREM sleep and the same factors that predispose to confusional arousals can provoke them. Fever is an additional risk factor, possibly through predisposing to arousal from stages 3 and 4 NREM sleep, or by impairing the arousal process itself. Episodes are often precipitated by stress.

Clinical features

Sleep terrors appear especially during the first half of the night, mainly in the first NREM sleep cycle, and

Table 9.5 Differential diagnosis of autonomic activation in sleep and on arousal.

Sleep terror
Nightmare
REM sleep behaviour disorder
Panic attack
Post-traumatic stress disorder

REM, rapid eye movement.

may occur more than once per night. The episodes may last for only a few seconds, or for up to 10–20 min which is longer than most epileptic seizures. The child suddenly appears to waken with a gasp, loud scream or cry and with the appearance of extreme fear, agitation and panic (Table 9.5). Sweating, dilated pupils, rapid respiratory and heart rates and an increase in muscle tone are characteristic and enuresis occasionally occurs. The child may sit up or leap out of bed, utter meaningless speech, and occasionally run wildly around the room. This is more common in adolescence than in younger children, but there may be injuries through, for instance, running out of doors or jumping through windows. The child is unresponsive to questions or commands and resists restraint, often causing harm to both the patient and others. The sleep terrors may be followed by an awakening with confusion and incoherent speech, and behaviour which is identical to a confusional arousal. Sleep is then re-entered promptly.

There is no detailed recall of the event or of any dream content but there may be a sensation of intense fear as if the subject is coming out of a faint or a frightening near-death situation. This is similar to what is experienced in nocturnal frontal lobe epilepsy. Recall of this type is more common if alertness is attained before the subsidence of autonomic activation.

Investigations

Polysomnography is only occasionally needed but shows abrupt arousal from stages 3 or 4 NREM sleep usually within 1–4 h of sleep onset at the onset of a sleep terror. There are also frequent transitions to lighter stages of NREM sleep at other times which are not associated with sleep terrors. Video recordings show the details of the episode.

Differential diagnosis

1 Confusional arousals.

2 Sleep walking.
3 Sleep talking.
4 Epilepsy.
5 Episodic nocturnal wanderings.
6 REM sleep behaviour disorder.
7 Nightmares.
8 Nocturnal panic attacks.
9 Post-traumatic stress disorder.

Problems

1 Sleep disruption and anxiety for the parents.
2 Embarrassment for the child.
3 Occasional injury to the child or others.

Treatment

1 Reassurance and explanation. This may be sufficient if the attacks are infrequent.
2 Sleep hygiene advice and in particular avoidance of sleep deprivation and caffeine.
3 Scheduled awakenings 15–30 min before the usual time of the sleep terror.
4 Benzodiazepines.
5 Beta blockers such as propranolol may reduce the autonomic effects.
6 Measures to prevent injury to the child, e.g. remove any breakable objects and if necessary lock doors and windows of the bedroom.
7 Explore any psychological causes of anxiety or stress which might precipitate the attacks.

Sleep walking (somnambulism)

Overview

Sleep walking is a common manifestation of incomplete arousal from stages 3 and 4 NREM sleep in children and young adults.

Occurrence

This is equally common in males and females and is often familial. It only occurs after the ability to walk has been attained, but similar episodes occur in infancy in which the child may simply crawl around. Its onset is usually after around 18 months and it is most common between the ages of 4 and 8 years. It affects around 10% of children and, while it becomes less common after adolescence, around 20% of children who sleep walk continue to do so as adults. Around 1–2% of adults sleep walk, but if it begins in adult life there is usually a readily detectable cause or significant psychopathology. It may be associated with other

arousal disorders, such as confusional arousals and sleep terrors, but is rare in the elderly.

Pathogenesis and aetiology

Any factor which promotes stages 3 and 4 NREM sleep or arousal from sleep will increase the likelihood of sleep walking in a susceptible subject. Factors such as a noisy sleep environment, a distended bladder, pain, stress, fever or obstructive sleep apnoeas may all precipitate sleep walking or other arousal disorders.

Sleep walking is said to be more common in those with migraines, suggesting that an abnormality of 5HT transmission may be linked to both these conditions. It is also common in Tourette's syndrome.

Clinical features

Sleep walking usually occurs during the first third of the night. The subject may sit up in bed, open the eyes, pick at the bedclothes, move around semipurposefully and attempt to leave the bed (Table 9.6). Children may walk into their parents' bedroom and enter their bed and make simple responses to questions and commands. Micturition occasionally occurs. The subject may try to dress and then walk around the bedroom indecisively, but often avoiding obstacles. A few words may be spoken and the subject may climb stairs, handle kitchen utensils and attempt to prepare a meal, open the front door of the home, walk considerable distances and even drive a motor vehicle. Injuries may result from falling down stairs or through windows, or after walking outside the home.

The subject usually allows him- or herself to be put back to bed without resistance, but attempts to restrain or waken the sleep walker should be avoided. They can cause a confusional arousal with disorientation, anxiety and a desire to escape which may evoke sudden violence [2]. There is no autonomic activation

Table 9.6 Differential diagnosis of walking during sleep.

Sleep walking
Sleep terror
Frontal lobe epilepsy
Temporal lobe epilepsy
REM sleep behaviour disorder
Confusional arousal
Sundowning syndrome
Psychogenic fugue
Malingering

REM, rapid eye movement.

or dream content during sleep walking and no recall of the event. Sleep is readily entered afterwards.

Investigations

Polysomnography may be required to differentiate sleep walking from other behavioural abnormalities in sleep. It often shows hypersynchronous (high-voltage) delta waves for a few seconds on a background of stages 1 and 2 NREM sleep without any epileptic features before the sleep walking, as well as frequent arousals directly from stages 3 and 4 NREM sleep to wakefulness may be unassociated with episodes of sleep walking. Video recording will show the pattern of activity.

Differential diagnosis

1 Confusional arousals.
2 Sleep terrors.
3 Epilepsy.
4 Episodic nocturnal wanderings.
5 REM sleep behaviour disorder.
6 Psychogenic fugues.
7 Malingering.

Problems

1 Embarrassment.
2 Risk of injury such as falling down stairs or out of a window, and occasionally to others through resisting restraint.

Treatment

Treatment is usually not required, but if the attacks are frequent or if the subject is at risk of injury the following measures should be considered.
1 Attention to sleep hygiene.
2 Reduction of stress and sleep deprivation.
3 Scheduled awakenings 15–30 min before the usual time of the sleep walking.
4 Benzodiazepines, such as clonazepam 0.25–2 mg or diazepam, prevent arousals and consolidate stages 1 and 2 NREM sleep, although they are usually used only intermittently.
5 Environmental protection. This includes closing and locking windows, locking stairs with a stair gate, putting bells on the bedroom door to alert the parents, sleeping in a low bed, avoiding an upper bunk, moving sharp or breakable objects from the bedroom, and staying in ground floor accommodation, for instance in hotels.
6 Psychotherapy may be of help in adults if the episodes are potentially dangerous.
7 Antidepressants may occasionally be of help.

NREM sleep related disorders

Sleep eating and drinking (sleep-related eating disorder)

Clinical features

Children

Sleep-related eating is common in children, particularly if there is parentally induced poor sleep hygiene and overfeeding during the day. This combination leads to alterations in the circadian rhythms, particularly of endocrine function.

Adults

This is probably an arousal disorder related to confusional arousals and sleep walking and is most common between the ages of 20 and 40 years; 65–90% of subjects are female.

It is characterized by recurrent, often nightly, episodes of eating, drinking and preparing food during sleep. These episodes usually occur in the first 2–3 h of sleep and may arise during partial arousals from stages 3 and 4 NREM sleep. They are not prevented by eating a large meal before going to sleep. There is little awareness or recall of the activities. No specific food preference has been observed, but high calorie food is often eaten. Alcohol is rarely drunk. Subjects occasionally choke while eating and there is also a risk of fire from the cooker being left on after the episode of eating or preparing food. There is no evidence of any eating disorder during wakefulness, but considerable weight may be gained.

This condition is often familial and there is frequently a history of sleep walking. It is occasionally associated with obstructive sleep apnoeas or the restless legs syndrome and periodic limb movements in sleep which may contribute to arousals from sleep. It is not usually related to any daytime eating disorder.

Differential diagnosis

These disorders should be distinguished from the following [3].

Night eating

This occurs in adults during wakefulness before the initiation of sleep and during awakenings from sleep. It is commonest in the difficulty in initiating sleep type of insomnia and is associated with anxiety states and stress. Carbohydrate-containing food is often preferred. The serum melatonin levels are low during sleep, predisposing to wakefulness, and the level of leptin, which suppresses appetite, is also reduced.

Bulimia nervosa

Binge eating at night is uncommon but if it does occur it is usually associated with similar episodes during the day, self-induced vomiting and difficulty in initiating sleep [4]. Nocturnal eating tends to occur when daytime symptoms are most marked and there is often a history of an arousal disorder such as sleep walking.

Narcolepsy

Awakenings during sleep are often associated with eating, particularly carbohydrates.

Kleine–Levin syndrome

Intermittent episodes of excessive daytime sleepiness occur in conjunction with a voracious appetite (megaphagia).

Awakenings from other sleep disorders

Eating at night often occurs during awakenings from, for instance, periodic limb movements and, less frequently, obstructive sleep apnoeas. There is no food preference.

Treatment

Treatment of sleep eating and drinking due to partial arousals from NREM sleep is unsatisfactory. Benzodiazepines such as clonazepam or L-dopa or a dopamine agonist either alone or with codeine may be effective. Food which the subject might be allergic to should be locked away or removed from the accommodation.

Sexual activity in sleep

This is a rarely reported disorder which is much commoner in males and usually appears in early adult life.

Clinical features

Sexual intercourse is usually attempted and often achieved. There may also be prolonged masturbation and sexual activity with children, which may lead to the allegation of sexual abuse or assault. There is no recollection of the event but afterwards there may be a feeling of guilt, shame or embarrassment.

There is usually a history of other behavioural disorders in sleep, especially sleep walking, and often a family history of these conditions. The events may be triggered by sleep deprivation, or sleep fragmentation due to, for instance, obstructive sleep apnoeas, alcohol and stress.

Differential diagnosis

This disorder should be distinguished from the following.
1 Sexual approaches during wakefulness but with no recall admitted subsequently. This is almost always carried out by males rather than females.
2 Dissociative states in which complex movements take place during wakefulness as demonstrated electrophysiologically. These states are associated with severe psychopathology and there is amnesia for the activity.
3 Kleine–Levin syndrome. Increased sexual activity is commonly associated with episodes of hypersomnia.
4 REM sleep behaviour disorder. This only very rarely leads to sexual activity in sleep.

Treatment

Benzodiazepines such as clonazepam are effective, but treatment of the precipitating factors may be sufficient.

Legal aspects

The defence of automatism (page 197) has been used to counter allegations of sexual activity during sleep and indecent exposure. The same legal criteria apply as with sleep violence. Unaccustomed homosexual activities may take place either during confusional arousals or in the Kleine–Levin syndrome.

Indecent exposure is common in sleep walkers who sleep in the nude. If an erection is observed during apparent sleep walking the episode is unlikely to represent an arousal disorder such as sleep walking or a confusional arousal, since erections are not a feature of NREM sleep. The REM sleep behaviour disorder does not lead to dreams of a sexual nature and erections are not a feature of this condition. They are more likely to indicate that the subject was awake at the time of the event rather than asleep.

Panic attacks

Panic attacks are commoner in adolescents and young adults and two to three times more frequent in females than in males. They occur during wakefulness, usually in the morning but also in sleep, particularly during the first third of the night and usually at the time of NREM sleep transition from stage 2 to 3 or 3 to 4. They are not associated with dreams and the patient awakens fully, often with a sensation of intense fear, choking, breathlessness, palpitations, tremor and hyperarousal which prevents subsequent sleep. There is no tendency towards aggression or violence, but recall of the fear experienced during the event is retained. Panic attacks may lead to a fear of falling asleep.

Differential diagnosis
1 Hyperventilation.
2 Gastro-oesophageal reflux.
3 Obstructive sleep apnoeas.
4 Vocal cord adduction.
5 Left ventricular failure.

Treatment
1 Reassurance.
2 Treatment of the cause.
3 Psychotherapy or anxiolytics may be indicated.

Sleep talking (somniloquy)

Overview
This common disorder is characterized by speech which may be incoherent and which does not significantly contribute to communication to others.

Occurrence
It is equally common in males and females in childhood, but is more frequent in males in adult life. It is occasionally familial and becomes less common during adolescence. Most adults who sleep talk have done so since childhood, but in those in whom the age of onset is over around 25 years there is usually significant psychopathology.

Pathogenesis
Sleep talking is associated with brief arousals from stages 1 and 2 NREM sleep, and while it may occur without any external stimulation, it may be triggered by factors that cause arousal from sleep.

Clinical features
Sleep talking usually occurs during the first third of the night and only lasts for a few minutes. Speech is usually incoherent or unintelligible, and often has little meaning (Table 9.7). Words are spoken in short sentences and usually without emotion, although occasionally long tirades are delivered which are related to a preoccupation of the sleep talker. The speech may be in any language that the subject is capable of speaking. There is no autonomic activation or recall of the events. Sleep talking may be followed by a confusional arousal and can be associated with sleep walking.

Table 9.7 Differential diagnosis of sleep vocalization.

Sleep talking
Sleep terror
Frontal lobe epilepsy
REM sleep behaviour disorder
Confusional arousal

REM, rapid eye movement.

Investigations
Polysomnography may be required, especially in adults, to distinguish sleep talking from other disorders that lead to vocalization. It shows brief arousals from stages 1 and 2 NREM sleep in most subjects.

Differential diagnosis
1 REM sleep behaviour disorder. Sleep talking occurs in REM sleep and is associated with aggressive dream content.
2 Confusional arousals.
3 Sleep terrors.
4 Talking during brief spells of wakefulness which occur between sleep episodes.
5 Epilepsy.
6 Fugue states.

Problems
Annoyance to bed partner, especially if the sleep talking occurs frequently.

Treatment
1 Reassurance and explanation.
2 Advice on sleep hygiene, especially avoidance of sleep deprivation, and of any factors that may cause arousal from sleep.
3 Benzodiazepines, such as clonazepam, used intermittently or in short courses may help to consolidate stage 2 NREM sleep.

Sleep bruxism (tooth grinding or crunching)

Overview
The repetitive movements of sleep bruxism are confined to the muscles moving the lower jaw and they cause a range of dental and jaw problems.

Occurrence
Sleep bruxism is equally common in males and females and occurs occasionally in up to 50% of children and frequently in 5–20%. It is familial in 50% of subjects.

The prevalence decreases linearly with age. It is most frequent between the ages of 3 and 12 years but occurs in only 2–5% of young adults and around 1% of the elderly.

Pathogenesis

Sleep bruxism is due to contraction of the masseter, temporalis and pterygoid muscles, more frequently, repetitively and with more force than is normal. It may represent a disorder of dopaminergic movement control. In adults it may be precipitated by oral problems and dental conditions such as malocclusion, mandibular or maxillary disorders, as well as anxiety, sleep deprivation, L-dopa, SSRI antidepressants, alcohol and possibly gastro-oesophageal reflux. If it occurs during wakefulness as well as sleep it usually has a different aetiology and is associated with diffuse brain damage, mental retardation or cerebral palsy.

Clinical features

Sleep bruxism is manifested by repetitive rhythmic chewing movements leading to grinding or crunching of the teeth and an increase in production of saliva. It varies in severity, but there are often hundreds of episodes each night. They usually occur at a frequency of around 1 Hz and in runs of 5–10. The noise is usually felt to be unpleasant and the movements cause grinding down of the teeth, dental decay, periodontal damage, increased tooth mobility and temporo-mandibular joint dysfunction, with pain which is usually worst on waking.

Investigations

Polysomnography is rarely needed to establish the diagnosis but may be required to establish whether any other sleep disorder is present and exacerbating bruxism. It shows masseter and temporalis muscle activity as an artefact, especially during stage 2 NREM sleep and occasionally stage 1 NREM or REM sleep. It can also occur during stages 3 and 4 NREM sleep, and the bruxism often leads to brief arousals.

Differential diagnosis

Epilepsy with rhythmic jaw movements.

Problems

1 Dental and temporo-mandibular joint disorders.
2 Insomnia for the partner.

Treatment

1 Sleep hygiene, especially avoiding sleep deprivation and relevant drugs.

2 Correction of any dental malocclusion or other oral disorders.
3 Dental moulds and mouth guards which protect the teeth from damage from friction.
4 Relief of anxiety.

Nocturnal cramps

Overview

These are painful episodes due to sudden muscle tension which usually cause arousal from sleep.

Occurrence

They are most common in elderly subjects, in pregnancy and in those on diuretics, or glucocorticoids, in Parkinson's disease and in peripheral neuropathies due to, for example, diabetes mellitus.

Pathogenesis

The cramps are due to sudden contraction of skeletal muscles. Their cause is obscure, but they represent a sudden localized loss of motor inhibition. They occur during NREM sleep and usually cause arousal to wakefulness. They are not a feature of REM sleep, probably because of the more intense motor inhibition.

Clinical features

The cramps cause intermittent episodes of localized tightness and pain in the muscles, particularly of the calves and feet, and there may be soreness of the muscles afterwards. The frequency of the cramps fluctuates. They often occur on most nights for several days or weeks and then go into remission. There is no dream recall on arousal with the cramp.

Investigations

None are required.

Differential diagnosis

Periodic limb movements in sleep.

Problems

1 Leg pain.
2 Early morning wakening.

Treatment

1 Stretch muscles, e.g. by dorsiflexion of foot.
2 Quinine sulphate 200–300 mg nocte is usually effective but clonazepam, carbamazepine, verapamil and vitamin E have been used.

Sleep-related neurogenic tachypnoea

This rare condition is characterized by a rapid respiratory frequency on entering NREM sleep without any pulmonary cause for this. It is seen in multiple sclerosis, the lateral medullary syndrome and benign intracranial hypertension.

Sleep related expiratory groaning (catathrenia)

This rare condition is characterised by prolonged expiratory groaning, which is often loud and disruptive. The groaning appears to arise at laryngeal level. Its onset is in adolescence and it may persist throughout life. There may be a family history, but there is no association with any psychological or medical disorder. Polysomnography shows that the abnormal respiration occurs particularly in stages 1 and 2 NREM sleep, although occasionally in REM sleep, and is often associated with brief episodes of hyperventilation or central apnoeas. There is no effective treatment.

REM sleep related disorders

Only a few movements normally prevail over the intense motor inhibition of REM sleep. The saccadic rapid eye movements and movements of the middle ear muscles, posterior crico-arytenoids, diaphragm and parasternal intercostal muscles are well recognized. Irregular jerky movements of the facial and distal limb muscles lasting less than 1 s also occur, especially with rapid eye movements.

The most important abnormalities of movement in REM sleep are as follows.

Sleep paralysis

Overview

Sleep paralysis is the inability to move at the onset or end of sleep while the subject is awake. It is the converse of the REM sleep behaviour disorder in which muscle tone is preserved, but sleep persists.

Occurrence

The onset of sleep paralysis is usually between the ages of 15 and 35 years. It occurs in three situations.

Sporadic

This is the commonest type and males and females are equally frequently affected. Up to 50% of normal subjects have one or more episodes of sleep paralysis,

and it occurs regularly in up to 6%. It usually appears in adolescence, becomes less frequent in adult life and returns around the age of 60 years. It is often triggered by sleep deprivation, and time zone changes when travelling from east to west, which induce sleep-onset REM sleep. It is commoner on awakening than before falling asleep.

Familial

This is rare, but the tendency can be inherited as a dominant X chromosome-linked condition. It usually affects women, and recurrent episodes, usually at sleep onset, are characteristic.

Narcolepsy

Sleep paralysis, often at sleep onset, occurs in 60% of narcoleptics with cataplexy. Narcolepsy is the most likely diagnosis if sleep paralysis occurs frequently.

Pathogenesis

Sleep paralysis occurs when the motor inhibition of REM sleep persists despite alertness being regained. Dissociation of these two major aspects of REM sleep is a feature of narcolepsy.

Clinical features

Sleep paralysis is often triggered by sleep deprivation, irregular sleep–wake schedules, such as shift work, or psychological stress. The subject is almost invariably supine and there is an inability to move, although respiration, predominantly due to diaphragmatic activity, continues. Some eye movements may still be possible as in REM sleep. The episode usually lasts from a few seconds to several minutes. There is awareness of the situation which is usually frightening, although occasionally it is felt to be enjoyably relaxing. Hypnagogic and hypnopompic hallucinations occur in narcolepsy and contribute to the sensation of fear. The episode either terminates spontaneously through intense efforts to move, or is terminated by a noise or, more commonly, by a touch from the bed partner.

Investigations

Polysomnography is rarely needed but may confirm that these episodes occur at the transition into and out of REM sleep.

Differential diagnosis

1 Periodic hypokalaemic paralysis. This occurs at rest while awake as well as on awakening, especially in adolescent males after alcohol or a large carbohydrate

meal. A low serum potassium is detectable during the attacks.

2 Epilepsy (atonic seizures).
3 Hysteria.
4 Drop attacks.
5 Faints.

Problems
Anxiety for the subject.

Treatment
1 Sleep hygiene advice.
2 Tricyclic antidepressants, e.g. clomipramine, if the episodes are a recurrent problem.
3 Sodium oxybate is of benefit when sleep paralysis is a manifestation of narcolepsy.

REM sleep behaviour disorder (RBD)

Overview
The essential features are vivid, aggressive dreams associated with abnormal movements in REM sleep ranging from twitches to complex and often violent actions. These are due to abnormal REM sleep generation in the pons and loss of the normal atonia of REM sleep.

Occurrence
This is occasionally seen in children, where it may be due to narcolepsy or occasionally autism or may occur in association with arousal disorders such as sleep walking. It also occurs in young adults, but is much commoner over the age of 50 years. Ninety per cent of patients are male. It is occasionally familial.

Pathogenesis
The characteristic feature of REM sleep behaviour disorder is the failure of motor inhibition during REM sleep so that muscle tone returns and movements related to cortical activities and dream mentation take place. The abnormality is probably located in the pons or medulla in the areas that are responsible for inhibition of muscle activity during REM sleep. There may be pontine tegmental lesions close to the LDT/PPT which disturb the medullary inhibition of motor activity that normally occurs in REM sleep. Lesions of the substantia nigra, which is an important inhibitor of the mesencephalic locomotor system, may also contribute. The exact location and extent of the lesions determine the type and severity of the clinical features.

Aetiology

Acute
REM sleep behaviour disorder may be due to acute drug intoxication, e.g. alcohol, or to acute withdrawal of REM sleep suppressant drugs leading to REM sleep rebound. This reaction is seen with amphetamines and related drugs, including cocaine and selegiline, anticholinergic agents, monoamine oxidase inhibitors, tricyclic antidepressants, selective serotonin re-uptake inhibitors, venlafaxine and caffeine.

Chronic
Idiopathic. No cause is found in around 40% of subjects with REM sleep behaviour disorder.

Alpha synucleinopathies.
1 Parkinsonism. Approximately one-third of those with idiopathic Parkinsonism have REM sleep behaviour disorder [5]. This may appear up to 10–15 years before any other features of Parkinsonism are apparent [6].
2 Multiple system atrophy. REM sleep behaviour disorder is present in around 90% of subjects.
3 Lewy body disease. Twenty-five per cent of subjects have REM sleep behaviour disorder. The visual hallucinations of this condition are a separate feature.

Tauopathies
1 Alzheimer's disease. REM sleep behaviour disorder is only occasionally associated with this condition.
2 Progressive supranuclear palsy (PSP). Ten per cent of subjects develop the REM sleep behaviour disorder.

Prionopathies. Both fatal familial insomnia and Creutzfeld–Jakob disease are associated with REM sleep behaviour disorder.

Narcolepsy. REM sleep behaviour disorder is more common in narcolepsy than in normal subjects.

Disorders that increase REM sleep drive. Any situation in which there is REM sleep deprivation or fragmentation, e.g. severe obstructive sleep apnoeas in REM sleep, may trigger this condition.

NREM sleep motor disorders. There may be an overlap between some NREM and REM sleep motor disorders. Periodic limb movements in NREM sleep are seen in two-thirds of subjects with REM sleep behaviour disorder in which non-periodic limb movements are also common in NREM sleep. These phenomena, which probably represent failure to inhibit motor activity in NREM sleep, are more frequent when the REM sleep behaviour disorder is due to a neurodegenerative disorder.

Other neurological conditions. There is a possible association with cerebrovascular disease, brain injury, brainstem tumours and multiple sclerosis.

Drugs. Chronic administration of antidepressants, particularly venlafaxine, but also tricyclic and selective serotonin re-uptake inhibitor antidepressants, and even gradual withdrawal of amphetamines and cocaine may cause REM sleep behaviour disorder.

Clinical features

Dreams are often, but not invariably, recalled, but there is no recollection of the movements during sleep [7]. The vivid dreams and abnormal movements can occur during any REM sleep cycle but are most common during the first. This is usually around 90 min after sleep onset and symptoms tend to recur at around 90-min intervals during the night (Table 9.8). In around 25% of subjects there may be limb and trunk movements for several years which may represent an exaggeration of the normal irregular muscle twitches or jerks that can be seen in REM sleep, as well as periodic limb movements.

As the condition becomes more severe, complex, organized actions, including flailing of the arms, hand waving, finger pointing, punching, laughing, talking, shouting, often intelligible commands, screaming, swearing, sitting up, kicking, getting out or diving out of bed, walking, running and jumping, may be seen.

The movements appear to represent exploratory or aggressive behaviour. These actions may injure either the subject or the bed partner. The subject resists restraint and can be violent and appears to feel intense emotion, but there are no sexual or feeding activities.

If awakened during the episode, a vivid intense dream with an unpleasant or aggressive and violent content is reported. Dreams are often repetitive, and involve being threatened, persecuted or confronted either by unfamiliar people or by animals, leading the subject to react by fleeing or fighting back. There is a close linkage between dream content and the type of physical activity. Fear, but not anger, is experienced. Similar dreams may be recalled between the episodes of movements. Ordinary dreams are not enacted physically, but in severe cases there may be recall only of abnormal dreams. In 10% of subjects, however, particularly those with neurodegenerative disorders, there is no dream recall.

The arousals from sleep cause excessive daytime sleepiness in around 20% of subjects due to sleep fragmentation.

Investigations

Polysomnography
This is important in establishing the diagnosis and excluding other disorders. It shows normal sleep architecture, except for an occasional increase in REM sleep duration and density, and slightly prolonged stages 3 and 4 NREM sleep. Muscle tone is maintained during some or all of REM sleep and there is an increase in phasic motor activity, particularly limb twitching, and generalized restlessness in REM sleep.

Table 9.8 Confusional arousal, frontal lobe epilepsy and REM sleep behaviour disorder.

Characteristic	Confusional arousal	Frontal lobe epilepsy	REM sleep behaviour disorder
Age	Especially children	Adults	> 50 years
Gender	M = F	M > F	M > F
Family history	Common	Occasional	Occasional
Time during night	First third	Any	Last third
Sleep stage	3 and 4 NREM	2, 3 and 4 NREM	REM
Dream content	Nil	Nil	Vivid
Recall	Nil	Nil	Intense
Behaviour	Slow complex activity, aggressive if restrained	Screams with repetitive movements	Simple and complex movements
Autonomic activation	Nil	Nil	Variable

F, female; M, male; NREM, non-rapid eye movement; REM, rapid eye movement.

Periodic limb movements may be seen in both REM and NREM sleep. There are no epileptic features. Video recordings show the pattern of activity. There is little variation between nights in these findings and a single night polysomnography is usually sufficient to confirm the diagnosis.

Magnetic resonance imaging or computerized tomography head scans
These may be required to diagnose the cause of the REM sleep behaviour disorder.

Differential diagnosis
1 Nightmares.
2 Confusional arousals.
3 Sleep terrors.
4 Sleep walking.
5 Post-traumatic stress disorder.
6 Epilepsy, especially temporal lobe epilepsy.
7 Episodic nocturnal wanderings.
8 Sudden arousals from REM sleep in obstructive sleep apnoeas.
9 Panic attacks.
10 Nocturnal psychogenic dissociative states in which the subject awakens and after 30–60 s enacts what is perceived as a dream, which is usually related to previous abuse.
11 Malingering.

Problems
Danger to patient and partner.

Treatment
1 Protection of the patient and partner if violence appears likely. Implements that can be used aggressively should be removed from the sleeping area. Placing a mattress on the floor with pillows around it may reduce the risk of injury. Physical restraint may cause serious injuries and should be avoided.
2 Gradual withdrawal of contributory drugs, e.g. venlafaxine and SSRI antidepressants.
3 Benzodiazepines, e.g. clonazepam 0.5–4 mg. These reduce muscle tone and are promptly effective in around 90% of subjects. They suppress phasic REM sleep activity, but have no action on REM sleep atonia between episodes, and therefore do not appear to act directly on the motor abnormality in the brainstem. Tolerance and addiction are rarely seen with long-term treatment.
4 Melatonin 3–15 mg nocte. This reduces tonic motor activity in REM sleep and can be used in combination with benzodiazepines.

5 Other drugs, e.g. clonidine 0.1–0.3 mg nocte, gabapentin, carbamazepine, clozapine, donepezil and quetiapine. Tricyclic antidepressants are of little benefit, except possibly dothiepin in Lewy body dementia. Buprobion, is the only antidepressant which does not exacerbate REM sleep behaviour disorder. Dopaminergic agents have little effect.

Status dissociatus
This rare disorder may represent a severe form of the REM sleep behaviour disorder. EEG recordings show continuous dissociation of NREM and REM sleep features with rapid oscillation of sleep states, and features of wakefulness [8]. Sleep is characterized by frequent muscle twitches, gross body movements, vocalizations, and vivid dreams, which are identical in nature to those of the REM sleep behaviour disorder. Sleep is refreshing and patients do not complain of excessive daytime sleepiness.

Status dissociatus may be caused by degenerative disorders such as multiple system atrophy, and fatal familial insomnia, but may also be due to narcolepsy and withdrawal from alcohol after protracted abuse. Clonazepam is often effective.

Restless legs syndrome (RLS, Ekbom's syndrome) and periodic limb movements in sleep (PLMS) (nocturnal myoclonus)

Overview
The restless legs syndrome is characterized by abnormal sensations in the legs with an urge to move them, restlessness of the legs and involuntary jerks. These symptoms are all worse at rest, relieved by exercise and worse in the evening and at night. The limb movements may be present during sleep and are virtually identical to the periodic limb movements which can occur in other situations without any symptoms of the restless legs syndrome.

In 60% of subjects the restless legs syndrome is primary, and although there is no detectable cause is often a family history. In 40% it is secondary, in which case it is usually sporadic and a cause can be found.

Occurrence
The restless legs syndrome is thought to occur in around 10% of the adult population and in around 3–5% it causes symptoms on most nights of the week [9]. It is approximately three times more common at the age of 65 than at age 30 years. Eighty per cent of

Table 9.9 Age and behavioural abnormalities in sleep; REM, rapid eye movement.

Neonatal	Childhood	Adolescence	Young and middle-aged adults	Old age
Benign neonatal myoclonus				
		Confusional arousal		
	Sleep terror			
		Sleep walking		
		Sleep talking		
		Sleep eating		
		Panic attacks		
				Nocturnal cramps
		Hypnic jerks		
	Rhythmic movement disorder			
		Cataplexy		
		Sleep paralysis		
		Post-traumatic stress disorder		
		Restless legs syndrome		
		Epilepsy		
	Sleep bruxism			
			REM sleep behaviour disorder	
			Status dissociatus	

those with RLS have PLMS and around 35% of those with PLMS have RLS. The prevalence of PLMS is uncertain, but may be around 5% between the ages of 30 and 50 years, 30% between 50 and 65 years, and 45% in the population over the age of 65. The severity of PLMS fluctuates, but overall usually worsens with age.

Forty per cent of adults with RLS and PLMS date the onset of their symptoms to before the age of 20. In children the symptoms may be mild and difficult to diagnose (Table 9.9). PLMS symptoms are often more prominent than RLS symptoms, which the child may find hard to describe They may be diagnosed as 'growing pains' and there is often a family history of 'growing pains', RLS or PLMS. The sleep fragmentation due to PLMS may cause irritability and troublesome behaviour similar to that in obstructive sleep apnoeas. Twenty per cent of children diagnosed with ADHD have PLMS. In this group treating the PLMS often improves the symptoms of ADHD. PLMS are also common in autism and childhood REM sleep behaviour disorder.

The restless legs syndrome is slightly more common in females than in males, but this difference is largely due to the increased prevalence in pregnancy.

There is a family history of RLS in over one-third of subjects overall and in up to 60% of those with primary RLS. There is a fivefold increased risk of RLS in first-degree relatives of those with RLS compared to normal subjects, and a threefold increased risk in second-degree relatives. In those with a positive family history RLS occurs at a younger age. It deteriorates more during pregnancy, is slowly progressive and has little relationship to iron status. In contrast, those without a family history have a more rapid progression of symptoms and are often iron deficient.

Pathogenesis

The pathogenesis of RLS probably involves cortical mechanisms [10] and sensory processing as well as subcortical abnormalities. The increasing frequency of RLS in the elderly may be due to degenerative processes within the central nervous system which facilitate the expression of the movements or sensations, or fail to suppress or control their generation.

There is a regular periodicity of PLMS of around 15–40 s which suggests that there is a central nervous system oscillator which is able to overcome the motor inhibition of stages 1 and 2 NREM sleep. Periodic limb movements in sleep are less common in stages 3 and

4 NREM and REM sleep, probably because motor inhibition is more intense [11]. This periodicity is similar to that of the cyclic alternating pattern (CAP) and the oscillations in the heart rate and blood pressure (Mayer waves) which represent fluctuations in sympathetic activity.

The location of the oscillator is uncertain, but it probably has functional connections with the basal ganglia, particularly the caudate and putamen which are closely connected with the substantia nigra in the midbrain. The red nucleus may also be involved in generating PLMS and subcortical sensory processing disorders may involve the thalamus.

Dopamine is a neurotransmitter in most of these nuclei and abnormalities of its function probably underlie both RLS and PLMS. The plasma dopamine level falls at night like that of noradrenaline and adrenaline. PET and SPECT scans have indicated abnormalities in D2 receptor binding in the basal ganglia. Mu opioid receptor function in the cerebellum may also be impaired in RLS, and naloxone, an opiate antagonist, worsens RLS.

RLS and PLMS can occur even with complete spinal cord transection or during spinal cord anaesthesia, suggesting that loss of inhibition from higher motor centres may be an important factor. Dysfunction of the pyramidal tract and reticulospinal tract probably contributes to the motor features, and the latter may also be responsible for the sensory symptoms through its influence on the dorsal horns in the spinal cord.

The spinal flexor response, which leads to withdrawal of the limb and which is an anti-nociceptive reflex, is released from higher centre inhibition and has a lower threshold. The limb movements may be finally generated by the propriospinal system in the spinal cord which spreads activity to adjacent spinal segments. The flexor muscles are characteristically activated in PLMS without RLS, but when this is present a wider range of muscles is involved. In both situations the anterior tibialis and extensor digitorum brevis are most commonly activated.

The oscillator or generator of PLMS appears to have a circadian influence as well as a sleep-related mechanism. PLMS tend to occur early during sleep when they are associated with RLS, but otherwise they occur later in the night. These timings may be related to reduction in ferritin or dopamine production during sleep.

Aetiology of periodic limb movements

Periodic limb movements are common in normal subjects, especially the elderly. A PLMI of less than 5/h is usually considered to be normal, but this cut-off point may be too low in older subjects. When PLMS occur with other features of the restless legs syndrome, they are conventionally considered to be part of this, rather than a separate disorder. They are equally frequent in primary and secondary RLS.

Periodic limb movements in sleep also occur in the following situations.

1 Synucleinopathies, e.g. Parkinson's disease, multiple system atrophy, Lewy body disease.
2 REM sleep disorders, e.g. narcolepsy, REM sleep behaviour disorder.
3 Huntington's disease.
4 Tourette's syndrome.
5 Obstructive sleep apnoeas. The relationship of PLMS to obstructive sleep apnoeas is complex. The diagnosis of PLMS may be difficult in the presence of obstructive sleep apnoeas because arousal from the apnoeas often causes a limb movement indistinguishable from a PLM. The sleep fragmentation due to obstructive sleep apnoeas may also induce PLMS. Treatment of sleep apnoeas with, for instance, nasal continuous positive airway pressure may clarify the situation by abolishing the limb movements, but equally it may lead to more consolidated sleep and increase the number of PLMS.
6 Drugs. PLMS like RLS can be precipitated by a wide range of drugs (see page 215).

The periodic limb movement disorder (PLMD) is defined as the presence of an abnormal number of PLMS for the subject's age in the absence of RLS or any other disorder or drug that causes PLMS and with symptoms, particularly insomnia or excessive daytime sleepiness, due to the limb movements (Table 9.10). PLMD can be graded as mild (PLMI 5–24), moderate (PLMI 25–49) or severe (PLMI 50 or more or a PLMAI of 25 or more per hour).

Aetiology of restless legs syndrome

Genetic factors

The mode of inheritance is heterogeneous, but usually autosomal dominant with age-dependent penetrance which is complete by around the age of 60 years. Anticipation, in which successive generations have more severe features, is common, and in other disorders this is due to expanded trinucleotide repeat genes. Abnormalities of genes on chromosome 12q close to the circadian rhythm genes and chromosome 14q and 9p have been detected. The latter is particularly associated with a younger onset of symptoms.

Table 9.10 Periodic limb movements definitions.

PLMS	Periodic limb movements in sleep	These are defined as movements of 0.5–5 s duration occurring in clusters of 4 or more. The interval between movements is 5–90 s
PLMW	Periodic limb movements in wakefulness occurring between the onset and termination of sleep	The duration of the limb movements occurring during wakefulness is conventionally defined as 0.5–10 s
PLMI	Periodic limb movement index	The number of PLMS per hour of sleep
PLMAI	Periodic limb movement arousal index	The number of periodic limb movements causing microarousals per hour of sleep
PLMD	Periodic limb movement disorder	This is the presence of more than the normal number of PLMS per hour for age, plus a complaint of insomnia or excessive daytime sleepiness, provided that the PLMS are not due to any other disorder such as RLS or REM sleep behaviour disorder or drug induced

REM, rapid eye movement; RLS, restless legs syndrome.

Iron deficiency

RLS is common in iron deficiency, for instance during pregnancy and in rheumatoid arthritis, and it may be the first sign of iron deficiency. The serum ferritin level is inversely proportional to the severity of RLS symptoms and sleep efficiency as shown by polysomnography. Both RLS and PLMS can be improved by iron supplementation even when the serum ferritin is within the generally accepted normal range, but below 45–50 µg/l.

RLS may be due not only to iron deficiency but also to a defect in its availability within the basal ganglia and related structures. Iron is normally present in the brain particularly in the substantia nigra, striatum, deep cerebellar nuclei and the red nucleus in which dopamine is a prominent neurotransmitter. MRI studies have shown less iron in the substantia nigra and putamen in RLS than in normal subjects.

Iron absorption in the gut is controlled by the body stores [12]. Iron is mobilized as transferrin which crosses the blood–brain barrier, and an abnormality of transferrin receptors has been proposed in primary RLS. Iron is stored as ferritin. The serum ferritin level drops by 30–50% at night. It may be normal despite a low cerebrospinal fluid ferritin level, suggesting a blood–brain barrier abnormality with reduced iron availability to the brain.

L-dopa is synthesized from tyrosine by tyrosine hydroxylase which requires ferrous ions to be activated. L-dopa is then converted by dopa decarboxylase to dopamine. The iron-dependent synthesis of L-dopa can be the rate-limiting step in the production of dopamine. There is no evidence for iron deficiency altering the function of the iron-containing D2 receptors.

Iron overload

RLS is common in haemochromatosis, presumably because of a lack of availability of iron despite the increased iron stores. RLS may be the first feature of haemochromatosis, particularly in post-menopausal women and men receiving iron supplementation.

Magnesium deficiency

This may contribute to RLS. Magnesium shares with iron the same protein for assisting transfer of the ion into cells.

Pregnancy and menstruation

RLS is often worse premenstrually and occurs in around 20% of pregnancies, usually in the second and third trimesters. It is uncertain whether or not this is purely due to iron deficiency, but in 90% of subjects it resolves within around four weeks after delivery.

Renal failure

This causes anaemia, which is often partly due to iron deficiency. RLS and PLMS occur in up to 70% of those with renal failure and are not relieved either by peritoneal dialysis or haemodialysis. The frequency of PLMS is a marker of survival in end stage renal failure. Renal transplantation may relieve both RLS and PLMS.

Chronic neurological disorders

Parkinsonism. RLS is present in around 20% of those with untreated Parkinsonism and PLMS may be even more frequent. Both these conditions may precede other Parkinsonian features. They are usually more prominent on the side of the worse motor symptoms. Iron deficiency is common in those with RLS and PLMS and the symptoms may respond to iron supplementation as well as dopaminergic agents.

REM sleep behaviour disorder. Periodic limb movements may be seen in both REM and NREM sleep.

Narcolepsy. Symptoms of the restless legs syndrome may occur but are less frequent than PLMS, which may be present in both REM and NREM sleep.

Huntington's disease. This causes both RLS and PLMS.

Tourette's syndrome.

Spinal cord lesions
Spinal cord lesions such as syringomyelia or transection may be associated with RLS and PLMS. These conditions are also present in spinocerebellar ataxia type 3.

Peripheral neuropathies
RLS is associated with some types of peripheral neuropathy, particularly axonal neuropathies, which presumably modify the sensory input to the spinal cord and brainstem. It is a feature of Charcot Marie Tooth type 2 polyneuropathy, amyloid and familial (axonal) neuropathy as well as diabetes mellitus. RLS often appears in older subjects with an acute onset and rapid progression, and may be associated with neuropathic pain.

Drugs
Most central nervous system stimulants and dopamine antagonists worsen RLS and PLMS. The most important drugs are shown in Table 9.11. There is some evidence that RLS and PLMS are worsened by chronic alcohol consumption and smoking.

Clinical features
RLS causes disagreeable sensory and motor symptoms in the evenings and at night, difficulty in initiating sleep because of these problems and excessive day-

Table 9.11 Drugs which worsen RLS and PLMS.

Caffeine
Glucocorticoids
Monoamine oxidase inhibitors
Tricyclic and probably selective serotonin re-uptake inhibitor antidepressants
Lithium
Antipsychotics, e.g. phenothiazines
Antihistamines
Calcium channel blockers
Dopamine antagonists, e.g. metoclopramide
Withdrawal from anticonvulsants and hypnotics

time sleepiness if sleep restriction or fragmentation is significant. These symptoms may be intermittent and mild, or they may be distressful and have a significant impact on the quality of life [13, 14].

Sensory symptoms
The sensations within the limbs are hard to describe, but the terms usually used by patients are listed in Table 9.12. The sensations are felt deep within the legs, particularly around the knees, but also in the thighs, calves, and even the buttocks and lower back, but only occasionally in the feet, arms or hands. It is usually bilateral.

The sensations only occur at rest, for instance while sitting in a seat, as a car or train passenger, in an aeroplane, cinema, theatre or lecture. They are relieved by movements such as walking or stretching the limb. Massage of the muscle, but not isometric contraction, may relieve the unpleasant sensation. Cooling the legs, or occasionally warming them, may give relief. It is possible to distract the subject from the unpleasant sensations if they are mild, but not once they become severe. They are relieved by sleep, even if

Table 9.12 Terms used to describe limb sensations.

Unpleasant	Tired
Uncomfortable	Tingling
Creeping	Pins and needles
Crawling	Electric
Alive	Burning
Irritating	Aching
Pulling	Itching
Stretching	Painful
Heavy	Like insects or worms inside the legs

this is a brief nap, but are not helped simply by lying down.

These sensations may be seasonal, usually worse in the summer, may improve temporarily during a fever, but are almost invariably worse in the evening and early in the night. When they are severe, they spread earlier into the day, but are least severe on waking in the mornings. They may prevent sleep onset and maintenance of sleep and can occur even if the limb has been amputated (phantom RLS).

Limb movements while awake

Voluntary 'fidgety' movements are characteristic of RLS. The subject has an urge to move the legs which may be irresistible and he or she frequently walks around and often attempts to cool the legs. The unpleasant limb sensations also lead to involuntary jerks which cannot be consciously suppressed. They involve extension of the big toe and flexion of the ankle, knee and hip. The limb movements can be reduced by adopting a flexed position. They tend to coincide with the most intense limb sensations. Limb movements while awake are less regular in their periodicity than PLMS.

Periodic limb movements also occur during wakefulness (PLMW) at night. They are a major complaint in 10–15% of RLS patients. PLMW occur at intervals of 10–15 s, and are more prolonged than limb movements during sleep.

Periodic limb movements in sleep

The periodic limb movements in sleep are characterized by sudden movements of the limbs, usually the legs. They are not as brief as myoclonic jerks and the muscles usually take longer to relax than to contract [15]. The movements last from 0.5–5 s, but usually 1.5–2.5 s. They are usually bilateral and symmetrical, but can be unilateral or asynchronous. The movements occur in clusters with intervals of 5–90 s, but usually 15–40 s between movements. The intervals are often constant in any one sleep stage during a single night in an individual patient. They are most frequent in stages 1 and 2 NREM sleep, less frequent in stages 3 and 4 and almost absent in REM sleep in which motor inhibition is maximal. There is considerable variation in the number from night to night.

There may be more than one type of movement in any individual, but each type occurs repetitively. The most common is extension of the big toe with ankle dorsiflexion and knee and hip flexion. If the arms are affected, the movements characteristically involve extension, particularly of the fingers. They are uncommon unless there are also severe leg symptoms and paraesthesiae in the arms. Occasionally the movements are so severe that the whole body moves relentlessly for several hours and unusual positions are adopted to obtain temporary relief.

Insomnia

Periodic limb movements are most frequent shortly after sleep onset when stages 1 and 2 NREM sleep are developing. They cause brief arousals or prolonged awakenings during the night. The patient may become distressed about the need to move the legs and to keep them cool. He or she may be aware of difficulty in initiating sleep, and may be unable to fall asleep readily once the movements have caused an awakening. Protruding the feet from the bedclothes to cool them or leaving the bed to walk about is often helpful.

Excessive daytime sleepiness

Excessive daytime sleepiness is probably due to the prolonged episodes of wakefulness which lead to sleep restriction, as well as to microarousals from the PLMS. It is unknown which properties of the limb movements lead to microarousals. The frequency of the movements, a change in their frequency, the amplitude of movement or the termination of a cluster of PLMS have all been proposed as arousal stimuli. Arousal may, however, occur before the limb movement is detectable, which suggests that it is not the movement, but the neurological activity that it represents, which causes arousal.

Excessive sleepiness may be felt throughout the day, but it may be impossible to re-establish sleep because of the sensory symptoms and restlessness. The degree of daytime sleepiness is, however, very variable. If it is intense it may lead to accidents and injuries through falling during microsleeps as well as during episodes of automatic behaviour.

Investigations

Self reported rating scales

The International Restless Legs Study Group developed a self-reported rating scale (Appendix 9) to evaluate the severity and frequency of RLS symptoms, but the questions only cover some aspects of the condition and may not be readily understood. The impact on quality of life can also be assessed by questionnaire (Appendix 10).

Blood tests

The serum ferritin should be estimated in all patients with suspected RLS since it may be the first manifestation of iron deficiency. The haemoglobin concentration may also be useful and urea and electrolytes should be checked if there is any suspicion of renal failure.

Actigraphy

Detection of PLMS by acceleration monitors can be performed without polysomnography. This is suitable for outpatient and serial use, for instance to monitor the effects of treatment. The frequency and type of limb movements can be quantified.

Polysomnography

PLMS can be detected using anterior tibial electromyogram electrodes. Video recordings reveal the type and frequency of the movements, but they may be obscured by the bedclothes if they are of small amplitude or are out of the field of view of the video. The frequency of the PLMS and PLMW can be assessed as well as the sleep stage during which the movements occur. Their effects on sleep architecture, the frequency of arousals and the presence of other factors contributing to sleep disruption can all be demonstrated. Polysomnography usually shows that the movements are most common in stages 1 and 2 NREM sleep, but, particularly in the REM sleep behaviour disorder and narcolepsy, they may appear in REM sleep.

PLMS are conventionally recorded as the number of movements per hour of sleep (PLMI). The PLMI is usually less than around 5 per hour, but increases in normal subjects with age. The frequency of arousals per hour of sleep associated with the PLMS (PLMAI) can also be calculated. Prolonged awakenings are not recognized by either of these scoring systems, which also ignore the limb movements occurring during wakefulness at night (PLMW).

Polysomnography is not necessary to diagnose RLS if the clinical picture is characteristic, but its indications are as follows.
1 In children.
2 If the diagnosis is uncertain.
3 If other conditions such as obstructive sleep apnoeas may be contributing.
4 When RLS or PLMS may be a feature of a separate disorder such as narcolepsy.
5 If symptoms fail to respond to drug therapy.

Forced immobilization test

The time for which the subject can remain still until a leg movement occurs is measured. This test causes discomfort and does not discriminate well between patients and normal controls.

Suggested immobilization test

The subject is asked to sit at an angle of 45° on the bed with the legs stretched out and is instructed to relax and not to tighten the muscles in the legs or to move them. The number of movements detected by actigraphy or EMG during 1 h, usually before nocturnal polysomnography is carried out, is recorded and the subject completes a 1–5 visual analogue scale of the severity of the sensory symptoms every 5 min. This test gives an indication of the urge to move the legs during wakefulness, but is not a direct measure of other sensory aspects of RLS or of periodic limb movements during sleep.

Differential diagnosis

The diagnosis of restless legs syndrome and periodic limb movements during sleep is often delayed and it is estimated that currently only around 10% of subjects have the correct diagnosis in the UK and 30% in the USA. The delay in diagnosis is partly due to the subject being unaware that their symptoms represent a treatable disorder, difficulties in the patient expressing the nature of their symptoms in a way that healthcare professionals recognize, and a lack of awareness of the condition and that effective treatments are available.

The most important differential diagnoses are as follows.

Restless legs syndrome

Paraesthesia due to peripheral neuropathies. The sensations tend to be more constant throughout the day and, unlike RLS, there are often neurological abnormalities on examination.

Akathisia. This is usually due to antipsychotic, antidepressant or dopamine agonist drugs or their withdrawal, or to idiopathic Parkinsonism. There is an urge to move the whole body, especially the legs, in response to a general inner feeling of restlessness, but there are no specific sensory symptoms. Akathisia is not related to any particular time of the day or night. It is not worsened by immobility and may involve persistent repetitive movements of large muscle groups, leading to body rocking and walking. It often responds to withdrawal of the antipsychotic drug, or administration of benzodiazepines or propranolol.

Table 9.13 Differential diagnosis of limb jerking.

Hypnic jerks
Fragmentary myoclonus
Startle disease
PLMS
REM sleep behaviour disorder
Epilepsy, e.g. frontal lobe epilepsy
Arousals due to, for example, OSA

OSA, obstructive sleep apnoeas; PLMS, periodic limb movements in sleep; REM, rapid eye movement.

Attention deficit hyperactivity disorder (ADHD). Both RLS and ADHD may cause restlessness and poor concentration [16]. Around 20% of children with ADHD have RLS. While these two conditions may be separate they may both be due to a dopaminergic abnormality.

Nocturnal cramps. These cause localized pain which can usually be easily distinguished from the more diffuse sensations of RLS.

Ischaemic leg pain. This is not relieved by movement or confined to the evening and night.

Neuropathic pain. This is not relieved by movement.

Periodic limb movements in sleep
1 Hypnic jerks. These are usually single and occur at the onset of sleep.
2 Epilepsy.
3 Leg movements due to arousals from, for instance, obstructive sleep apnoeas.
4 Other causes of limb movements (Table 9.13).

Problems

Restless legs syndrome
1 Unpleasant sensations in the legs which may lead to social limitations, such as the inability to travel as a car passenger or sit in a cinema.
2 Difficulty in initiating and also maintaining sleep.
3 Excessive daytime sleepiness.

Periodic limb movements in sleep
1 Insomnia or excessive daytime sleepiness.
2 Sleep disturbance of the bed partner.

Treatment

The treatment of RLS and PLMS is similar (Fig. 9.2). The following steps should be followed.
1 Explanation and reassurance.
2 Sleep hygiene advice, especially if sleep deprivation is a factor. Reduction in alcohol consumption and tobacco smoking may be of help. It is important to minimize caffeine intake, particularly in the evenings since RLS symptoms are worst in the evenings. Patients often prefer to go to bed later, after their leg symptoms have subsided, because it is then easier to initiate sleep. They also wake up later and this pattern simulates the delayed sleep phase syndrome.
3 Symptomatic measures, e.g. keeping the feet cold, through for instance wearing loose footwear, keeping the feet out of the bedclothes, or having a fan in the bedroom at night. Advice to maintain mental alertness may help since this appears to reduce RLS symptoms.
4 Treat the cause, such as iron deficiency. Iron is better absorbed in the ferrous state and the addition of vitamin C 200 mg bd or tds, which keeps it reduced, helps absorption. Ferrous sulphate 200 mg bd or tds is usually required, but if it is not possible to increase the serum ferritin to greater than 45–50 μg/l despite oral iron supplementation and if the symptoms of restless legs and periodic limb movements persist despite addition of first-line drugs, improvement may then be obtained with intravenous iron therapy. This increases the iron stores and bypasses the limitation on absorption in the gut. The risk of allergic reactions to intravenous iron is, however, significant. Iron supplementation is particularly valuable in children and in pregnancy when other treatments are relatively contraindicated.
5 Avoid causative drugs, e.g. tricyclic antidepressants, caffeine. Bupropion is the only antidepressant which has not been demonstrated to worsen RLS.
6 Drug treatment. This is often effective, but should be avoided wherever possible in children because of the unknown long-term toxicity. The drugs that have been most commonly used in children, apart from iron supplementation, are codeine, clonazepam and gabapentin. Drugs, with the exception of iron replacement, should also be avoided if possible during pregnancy. Most of the effective treatments cross the placenta, enter breast milk, and can cause sedation of the infant. Dopamine agonists also reduce prolactin release and inhibit lactation.

Whichever drug is chosen should be used initially in a low dose and timed to be given before the onset of symptoms. It is often necessary for the first dose to be

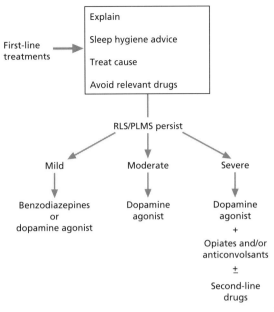

Fig. 9.2 Treatment of restless legs syndrome and periodic limb movements in sleep.

given at around 6.00 PM before the evening symptoms begin, and for a second, usually larger, dose to be given before going to bed. The dose of the drugs should be gradually increased until the symptoms are adequately controlled.

First-line drugs
Dopaminergic agents are the most effective drug treatment for RLS and PLMS and are usually prescribed initially. If they are poorly tolerated or ineffective, benzodiazepines, opiates or gabapentin can be used either alone or in combination.

L-dopa and dopamine agonists
L-dopa is usually given with a dopa decarboxylase inhibitor such as carbidopa or benserazide, which prevents peripheral metabolism to dopamine, but does not itself cross the blood–brain barrier. Entacapone, which blocks peripheral conversion of L-dopa to inactive metabolites, has also been used. These combinations increase the dopamine level in the central nervous system and reduce peripheral side-effects. 100–400 mg L-dopa can be given 30 min before sleep and a second similar dose repeated during the night if the patient wakes, unless a slow release preparation is used before sleep. L-dopa can also be used half an hour before a situation, such as air travel, in which it is important that symptoms are well controlled.

Only around 50% of patients continue with L-dopa in the long term, because of rebound and augmentation. Rebound symptoms occur in around 20% of subjects late in the night or early in the morning because of the short duration of action of the L-dopa preparations. Augmentation, which is the worsening of symptoms during the day often despite adequate control of the evening and night-time symptoms, arises in around 75% of those taking L-dopa. This augmentation worsens if the dose is increased at night or if it is taken progressively earlier in the day before the onset of symptoms.

The risk of augmentation is greater in dopaminergic agents which have a short duration of action. Augmentation is dose related and may take several months to appear. If it has occurred with one drug it is more likely to develop with a second drug. It occurs in 10–15% of patients with ropinirole, pergolide and pramipexole, but is very unusual with cabergoline, or with opiates, or gabapentin.

Dopaminergic agents are preferable to other drugs in most situations if regular treatment is required, but should be avoided in angle closure glaucoma. They often cause nausea, which can be treated with domperidone 10 mg tds. They have been implicated, particularly ropinirole and pramipexole, as the cause of sleep attacks in Parkinson's disease, but these are unlikely to occur with the small doses used at night in RLS. Their effects on dopamine receptor function in the long term are uncertain. They could theoretically lead to an akinetic state, although this has not been documented. The ergot-derived dopamine receptor agonists such as pergolide, lisuride, cabergoline, and bromocriptine can cause fibrosis of the lungs and pleura, retroperitoneum and tricuspid and other cardiac valves. Dopaminergic agents have a teratogenic potential in children.

Apomorphine 18–48 mg by subcutaneous infusion overnight with domperidone to relieve nausea has been used in severe RLS which is resistant to other treatments.

Benzodiazepines
Long-acting drugs such as diazepam should be avoided because of the risk of sedation, but clonazepam and temazepam are useful. They consolidate stage 2 NREM sleep and reduce sleep-stage transitions and arousals from sleep, but only partially relieve the movements through their muscle relaxant effect. The patient therefore obtains more benefit than the partner. They are best if the condition is mild, and especially when

insomnia is a problem, but may worsen other associated disorders, e.g. obstructive sleep apnoeas. They can be used intermittently in short courses. Dependency and tolerance are rare.

Opiates

These may be useful, especially in severe RLS. Codeine 30–60 mg nocte, dextropropoxyphene 65 mg nocte, tramadol 50–150 mg nocte, morphine 5–15 mg nocte or methadone, which has a longer half-life, 5–10 mg nocte are effective. Tolerance to and dependency on these drugs rarely occur, although there is a risk of respiratory depression.

Anticonvulsants

Gabapentin is the most effective. The initial dose of around 300 mg nocte should be increased by 100 mg nocte at 1–2 week intervals to around 1800 mg nocte if necessary. It is particularly effective if RLS is experienced as pain, and during haemodialysis. It may cause drowsiness if given in the evenings and before sleep, and ataxia at night, as well as weight gain. Carbamazepine 100–600 mg daily, sodium valproate 125–600 mg daily and lamotrigine 100 mg daily are alternatives.

Second-line drugs

These may be required if symptoms are severe or resistant to first-line drugs. They are usually used in addition to one or more of the first-line drugs.

Baclofen. 20–40 mg daily. This is occasionally helpful. It reduces the amplitude of the movements and the number of arousals, but not the frequency of the movements.

Beta blockers. Propranolol, 40–80 mg nocte.

Clonidine. 0.15–0.9 mg. This may be particularly effective in relieving sensory rather than motor symptoms, and if RLS and PLMS are due to renal failure.

Melatonin. This may reduce the frequency of PLMS, possibly by modifying any underlying circadian rhythm disorder.

Epilepsy

Overview

The wide variety of clinical manifestations of epilepsy are all due to a synchronized and excessive electrical discharge in various regions of the brain. Sleep and the transition to wakefulness affect the threshold for these discharges to arise and propagate.

Pathogenesis

Intermittent synchronized excessive generalized or focal electrical discharges may arise either in a central core of malfunctioning neurones, which lead directly to the epileptic seizure, or in neurones which provide an abnormal influence on healthy neurones and predispose them to initiate the seizure. The site and spread of the electrical discharge determine the clinical features, which, particularly with temporal and frontal lobe epilepsy, may include complex motor activities.

The influences of NREM and REM sleep on epilepsy are very different. The diffuse cortical synchronization of NREM sleep due to the thalamocortical projections predisposes towards rhythmic bursts of neuronal activity and facilitates propagation of an epileptic discharge. The maintenance of muscle tone allows this to be manifested whereas the atonia of REM sleep hides any motor activity and the asynchronous divergent synaptic activity does not augment any propagation.

Any factor which increases NREM sleep will tend to precipitate epilepsy. This includes sleep deprivation and NREM sleep rebound. Epileptic seizures occur particularly at the moment of arousal or during a sleep-stage transition, often related to the cyclic alternating pattern (CAP) or to arousals from sleep disorders such as obstructive sleep apnoeas. Even allowing for the different durations of sleep stages, epileptiform discharges are most common in stage 2 NREM sleep and often coincide with K-complexes or sleep spindles.

Clinical features

There is a bimodal time distribution of nocturnal epilepsy. Seizures tend to occur either early in the night, particularly in stages 1 and 2 NREM sleep [17], or 1–2 h before or after the transition from sleep to wakefulness in the morning.

Nocturnal seizures disorganize sleep architecture during the episode and tend to reduce sleep efficiency, increase sleep fragmentation, increase the REM sleep latency and reduce REM sleep duration. The usual complaint by the partner, parent or carer is of frightening or disturbing movements during sleep (Table 9.13). The seizures rarely lead to a complaint of insomnia despite the events interrupting sleep. Excessive daytime sleepiness may result from frequent nocturnal seizures and interictal epileptic discharges as well as postictal sleepiness from seizures during the day and the effects of anticonvulsant drugs.

Nocturnal epilepsy may be difficult to distinguish from other movement disorders during sleep, but the episodes are more stereotyped. Innate patterns of motor behaviour may emerge, such as uttering non-intelligible noises, walking and grasping movements. The pattern depends on the site of the epileptic focus and the regions to which it spreads. Tonic posturing early in the episode is characteristic of epilepsy, and nocturnal choking in children is often due to epilepsy rather than gastro-oesophageal reflux. Seizures may be precipitated by sleep deprivation, stress and alcohol withdrawal.

Obstructive sleep apnoeas may lower the threshold for epilepsy by inducing sleep deprivation through fragmentation of sleep. Commonly, however, the twitching movements associated with an arousal at the end of an apnoea are mistaken for epileptic seizures. Treatment of obstructive sleep apnoeas may improve epileptic control, but conversely, treatment for presumed epilepsy usually worsens obstructive sleep apnoeas and makes the nocturnal arousal movements more frequent. Any of the sedative anticonvulsants can have this effect and phenytoin also leads to hypertrophy of the tissue of the upper airway which predisposes to obstructive sleep apnoeas.

Sudden, unexpected death in epileptics usually occurs during sleep. Its cause is uncertain but it is more frequent in males aged between 20 and 50 years, particularly if their epilepsy is poorly controlled. It often occurs after a single fit rather than in status epilepticus, and may result from a cardiac dysrhythmia due to sleep-related excessive sympathetic activation or to metabolic changes, such as a transient increase in serum potassium after the seizure. It may also be caused by central apnoeas caused by a failure of the respiratory centres to generate any respiratory movements, or alternatively by persistent tonic activity of the chest wall muscles preventing effective inspiration and leading to hypoxia.

Treatment of any condition which causes sleep deprivation or fragmentation may improve the control of nocturnal epilepsy. The effectiveness of anticonvulsant drugs on seizures during sleep cannot be precisely predicted directly from their effects during wakefulness, since they have different tendencies to promote or abolish NREM sleep (page 101). They may also induce conditions such as obstructive sleep apnoeas, which lead to sleep fragmentation. In general, however, if they improve the control of epilepsy, the subjective perception of the quality of sleep also improves.

Types of epilepsy

The most important types of epilepsy that are related to sleep are as follows.

Infantile spasms (West's syndrome)

These occur particularly between the ages of 3 and 9 months. The child briefly flexes the neck, lumbar spine and often the knees and elbows ('salaam spasms'). These events occur particularly when the child is drowsy or soon after waking, but rarely during sleep, although the EEG pattern of hypsarrhythmia (irregular high-voltage slow waves with spikes or sharp waves) may only be seen during sleep.

Lennox–Gastaut syndrome

This appears between the ages of 3 and 6 years and one-third of children present with the features of infantile spasms. The EEG shows bursts of 8–26 Hz spikes during NREM sleep. A variety of types of seizure appear, but during NREM sleep these are usually of the tonic type. Mental retardation is characteristic and the prognosis is poor.

Febrile convulsions

These occur in 3% of children, especially between the ages of 6 months and 5 years, and are usually associated with a temperature over 38°C. Fifty per cent of febrile convulsions occur either close to the start or close to the end of sleep, and a further 25% soon after wakening.

Landau–Kleffner syndrome

This usually appears before the age of 7 years and is characterized by multifocal spikes detectable on the EEG. Seventy per cent of children have generalized or partial seizures and there is an acquired dysphasia and auditory inattention.

Electrical status epilepticus of sleep

This condition is defined by the EEG appearances of continuous 2–2.5 Hz spike and wave activity occupying more than 85% of NREM sleep. The EEG is usually normal in REM sleep. The condition is equally common in males and females and arises between the ages of 5 and 15 years. Nocturnal seizures may be present, but the EEG abnormality often improves after a few years despite persistence of learning difficulties and behavioural abnormalities.

Absence seizures (petit mal epilepsy)

These sudden episodes of loss of muscle tone usually cause brief episodes of blinking or staring and occur most frequently soon after waking and during drowsiness. Spike and wave discharges of 3 Hz are common, especially in stages 2–4 NREM sleep.

Benign rolandic epilepsy (benign epilepsy with centrotemporal spikes, sylvian seizures)

These seizures occur more frequently in males than in females and usually between the ages of 2 and 12 years. They are the most common simple partial seizures in childhood and represent 25% of childhood epilepsy. Twitching of the face, lips and tongue associated with dysarthria, difficulty in swallowing and drooling are characteristic. There may also be dysarthria after the episodes. Seventy-five per cent of subjects only have these seizures during sleep and in a further 15% they are seen both during sleep and during wakefulness. They occur particularly in stages 1 and 2 NREM sleep. This condition may be confused with bruxism. The prognosis is good.

Juvenile myoclonic epilepsy (Janz syndrome)

This is equally frequent in males and females and usually occurs between the ages of 10 and 25 years. The synchronized bilateral myoclonic jerks of the limbs, particularly the arms, usually appear within 1 h of waking, and are commoner if the subject is sleep deprived or is woken from NREM sleep. The subject may appear clumsy and drop objects. There may be confusion but no loss of consciousness. The EEG shows synchronized frontal bilateral spike and wave or polyspike and wave discharges at a frequency of 4–6 Hz during the episode, at sleep onset, or on awakening.

Myoclonic seizures

These occur in adults, especially at sleep onset and on awakening, and are associated with a brief loss of consciousness.

Generalized seizures

Generalized tonic–clonic seizures usually occur soon after falling asleep or on awakening. They occur during sleep in up to 25% of subjects and daytime seizures are unlikely to develop if they have not appeared within 2 years of the onset of the nocturnal episodes.

Parietal and occipital lobe epilepsy

The seizures rarely occur in sleep.

Temporal lobe epilepsy (complex partial seizures, psychomotor epilepsy, limbic epilepsy)

The seizures are mainly diurnal and it is rare for them to be exclusively nocturnal. The aura may wake the subject from sleep who may then be motionless or carry out a range of activities, and occasionally there may be catastrophic rage leading to violence. Inappropriate complex behaviour patterns (automatisms), such as picking at clothing, smacking the lips or wandering around the room, are common [18]. There may be hallucinations, particularly of smells and taste, illusions of familiarity with strange environments and intense feelings of anxiety and fear. There is no tonic posturing or hyperkinetic activity.

The episodes usually occur soon after sleep onset, or just before waking. There is often a history of temporal lobe epilepsy in wakefulness as a child, and recurrence with nocturnal episodes after an interval of 10–20 years is common. There is rarely a family history.

Temporal lobe seizures are associated with a low sleep efficiency due to frequent or prolonged awakenings which are mainly unrelated to nocturnal seizures. The duration of REM sleep is reduced, but there is a variable effect on stages 3 and 4 NREM sleep. The seizures themselves have been thought to be related to the start or end of REM sleep episodes but are much more common in NREM sleep.

Longer lasting epileptic fugues with less change in the level of consciousness, complex behaviour patterns and a tendency to wander should be distinguished from the more protracted hysterical fugues and from postictal sleepiness with automatic behaviour.

Frontal lobe seizures (paroxysmal arousal, nocturnal paroxysmal dystonia and episodic nocturnal wandering)

Frontal lobe seizures can be either focal motor seizures with unilateral movements of the limbs, head and neck, or complex partial seizures. They have in the past been differentiated on clinical grounds into paroxysmal arousals, nocturnal paroxysmal dystonias and episodic nocturnal wanderings [19] but these are only different clinical manifestations of the same fundamental type of seizure.

Occurrence

They are three to five times as frequent in males as in females and usually appear around the age of 10–12 years. They are familial in 20–40% of patients in whom they are inherited autosomal dominantly, although there is genetic heterogeneity. The mutations appear to cause abnormalities of cation channels. The clinical pattern of epilepsy is identical in sporadic and familial cases but in the latter there is an increased prevalence of other types of epileptic seizures.

Pathogenesis
Most of these episodes represent the effects of epileptic discharges in the anterior and medial (orbitomedial) regions of the frontal lobes. This may be triggered by changes in ascending input from the thalamus which affects particularly the cholinergic systems within the frontal lobes.

These seizures arise suddenly from NREM sleep, usually stage 2, but also stages 3 and 4.

Clinical features
Paroxysmal arousals are brief and only last for a few seconds or occasionally up to a few minutes [20]. They occur up to 20 times per night and on most nights. They usually continue for many years unless they are treated, but remit spontaneously in around 5% of subjects. Nocturnal paroxysmal dystonias are more prolonged and episodic nocturnal wanderings may last for several minutes. Unlike temporal lobe seizures, these attacks usually occur only during sleep.

Each subject may have two to three patterns of activity, but these are stereotyped for each individual and they are usually frenetic. The first manifestation is usually a brief scream, moan or howl associated with opening of the eyes and an expression of fright or surprise. There may also be initial brief dystonic or athetoid posturing or semipurposeful limb movements with signs of autonomic activation such as a tachycardia. Grimacing, dystonic posturing of the head, trunk and limbs and choreoathetoid movements may be marked and may even lead to opisthotonus. The episode may terminate with repetitive, often ballistic, limb movements such as grasping, punching, flailing, shaking, running, jumping, cycling or kicking. Occasionally pelvic thrusting, genital manipulation or tonic posturing is seen. The patient may leave the bed and resist restraint with violence. There is no dream content, a rapid resumption of consciousness, and little or no recall of the episode with no tongue biting or incontinence. In all three of these disorders the episode terminates with a return to sleep.

Investigations
1 Polysomnography. This shows movement artefact at the onset of the episode and no detectable epileptic discharges, probably because the focus is deep in the frontal lobe. Video recording reveals the types of movements.
2 Interictal EEG. This may show abnormalities indicative of epilepsy, but is often normal.
3 MRI scans of the brain are normal.

Differential diagnosis
1 Other epileptic episodes, especially temporal lobe epilepsy.
2 Fugue states in which global amnesia is associated with wandering, although the subjects are awake and in touch with the environment.
3 Periodic limb movements in sleep.
4 Sleep terrors.
5 REM sleep behaviour disorder.
6 Panic attacks.
7 Hypoglycaemia.
8 Transient cerebral ischaemic attacks.
9 Rhythmic movement disorders.
10 Nocturnal pseudo-seizures. These are characterized by large amplitude motor activities, such as cycling movements, but are not stereotyped. They are commonest in adolescents and may occur during the day as well as at night, but always during wakefulness. The subject may believe that the episodes are arising from sleep, but may have recall of events during the episode, which is usually followed by pseudo-sleep in which the EEG shows alpha activity.
11 Psychogenic dissociative states. These are due to severe psychiatric disease. The activities occur while the subject is awake, but are reported by the subject as if he or she is acting out a dream.

Investigations

Electroencephalogram
High-amplitude abnormal electrical activity, particularly spikes (less than 70 ms) or waves (70–120 ms), may be detected between or during seizures, especially in NREM sleep. Synchronized depolarization causes the spikes and hyperpolarization causes the waves. A standard full montage EEG during wakefulness may be sufficient to detect electrical epileptic activity, especially with hyperventilation or photic stimulation.

A sleep EEG is indicated if epilepsy is suspected and if the EEG while awake is non-diagnostic, especially if seizures are mainly nocturnal or infrequent. Sleep may be entered during the day following sleep deprivation on the previous night, or if sedation is given, although this will not induce a physiological sleep state. Sleep deprivation is usually induced by asking the subject to go to bed 2 h later and to wake up 2 h earlier than usual on the night before the EEG. Epileptic features may be detected even if only stages 1 and 2 NREM sleep occur, as is common with daytime sleep EEGs. The alternative is to carry out an EEG examination during overnight sleep. A full montage EEG is preferable to the standard polysomnography EEG montage since more of the cerebral cortex is sampled. A 24-h or even longer 'ambulatory' recording may be required, but the signals are often of poor quality, artefacts are common and fewer electrodes can be used than with a standard EEG. Absence of abnormalities between seizures with any of these techniques does not exclude epilepsy.

Polysomnography

This is insensitive at detecting epileptic discharges, but if they do occur they make any further sleep staging during the seizure impossible. Video recordings show the nature of the movement disorder which in epilepsy is more repetitive and stereotyped than in most other motor disorders. Polysomnography only occasionally demonstrates frontal lobe epilepsy, and rarely confirms a diagnosis of temporal lobe epilepsy, but is of most value in demonstrating non-epileptic behavioural abnormalities during sleep.

Computerized tomography and magnetic resonance imaging scans

These may reveal the presence of the cause of the epilepsy, such as a space occupying lesion or cerebrovascular disease. Computerized tomography and MRI scans are usually normal in frontal lobe epilepsy.

Differential diagnosis

This includes faints, panic attacks, hyperventilation, hypoglycaemia, transient cerebral ischaemic attacks, drop attacks, periodic limb movements in sleep, REM sleep behaviour disorder and rhythmic movement disorders. These can usually be distinguished since epileptic seizures are repetitive, often complex and the subject is uncontactable during the episode, and often sleepy afterwards with little recall of the event.

Problems

1 Insomnia, which may occur if the episodes are frequent.
2 Physical injuries.
3 Disrupted sleep for the bed partner.
4 Excessive daytime sleepiness.

Treatment

Treatment of any condition causing sleep deprivation or fragmentation may improve the control of nocturnal epilepsy.

Frontal lobe seizures usually respond to anticonvulsant therapy, particularly sodium valproate, carbamazepine, phenytoin and clonazepam.

Sleep and movement disorders of wakefulness

Effects of sleep on movement disorders

Movement disorders which are most prominent during wakefulness persist to a variable degree during sleep. The extent of the influence of sleep on these movements depends on their origin.

Psychogenic movement disorders

These disappear during sleep, except perhaps in stage 1 NREM sleep, but reappear during arousals from sleep.

Upper motor neurone movement disorders

These movement disorders, such as Parkinsonism and Huntington's disease, are subject to the generalized motor inhibition of NREM and REM sleep. They are most suppressed in stages 3 and 4 NREM sleep, less prominent in REM sleep and most marked in stages 1 and 2 NREM sleep and particularly at times of arousal from sleep. This indicates that they are selectively suppressed by NREM sleep since normal muscle activity is at its least in REM rather than NREM sleep.

Lower motor neurone movement disorders

These conditions, such as palatal myoclonus, hemifacial spasm and fasciculations, usually persist during sleep, probably because the disorder causing the movement at least partially disrupts the supraspinal inhibition of the lower motor neurones.

Effects of movement disorders on sleep

Movement disorders frequently fragment sleep sufficiently to cause excessive daytime sleepiness, but also have important indirect effects on sleep, which need to be treated appropriately. The ways in which these movement disorders influence sleep are described below.

1 Degenerative disorders disrupt sleep in a similar way to the normal changes seen in the elderly. Sleep efficiency and total sleep time are reduced with an increase in the number of arousals and sleep-stage transitions. Stages 3 and 4 NREM sleep are shortened.

These abnormalities may improve with drug treatment of the movement disorder.

2 There may be associated sleep disorders. Huntington's disease, for instance, is associated with periodic limb movements in sleep and RLS, and multiple system atrophy is associated with the REM sleep behaviour disorder. Children with tics are predisposed to sleep walk and talk.

3 Some disorders, particularly the degenerative ones, are associated with respiratory abnormalities such as obstructive or central sleep apnoeas which cause sleep fragmentation.

4 There may be indirect effects on sleep due to, for instance, dementia which alters the regulation of sleep. Changes in environmental stimuli such as a reduction in exposure to light may also affect sleep control, and other factors such as depression and sleep fragmentation due to discomfort and pain are features of many of these conditions, particularly Parkinsonism.

5 Drugs used therapeutically may help to relieve the movement disorder, but may induce other sleep disorders.

Chorea

In this disorder there are frequent irregular movements which migrate from one part of the body to another and affect particularly the face and limbs. The movements are worse with activity. In Sydenham's chorea the movements can persist during REM sleep, but little is known about the other types of chorea except for that seen in Huntington's disease. This causes dementia, depression, psychosis and personality changes as well as chorea. It is steadily progressive and is due to widespread cerebral degeneration. The initial complaint is insomnia, but as the disease progresses sleep becomes increasingly fragmented with loss of sleep efficiency, increased sleep latency, an increased number of arousals, and a reduction in duration of stages 3 and 4 NREM and REM sleep. The density and amplitude of sleep spindles are increased, in contrast to Parkinsonism, possibly because of increased dopamine levels within the brain. The chorea is most prominent in stages 1 and 2 NREM sleep and during arousals, and least prominent in stages 3 and 4 NREM sleep. Periodic limb movements and the restless legs syndrome may be present.

Unilateral chorea (hemiballism) is usually due to contralateral damage to the subthalamic nucleus or its connections, most often because of ischaemia. These movements persist in stages 1 and 2 NREM sleep and REM sleep, although both this and stages 3 and 4 NREM sleep are reduced in duration.

Myoclonus

This diverse group of conditions is characterized by abrupt jerking movements separated by a longer pause than in chorea, but the degree of sleep disruption that they cause and the effect of sleep on the movements depend on where they are generated.

Cerebral cortex
The movements are not detectable during sleep.

Basal ganglia
These movements are partially suppressed in sleep, as in Huntington's disease.

Brainstem and spinal cord
Movements such as spinal myoclonus and palatal myoclonus persist, although their amplitude and frequency may be reduced during sleep. This suggests that some higher inhibitory control persists over the largely autonomous oscillators which are responsible for these movements, which in palatal myoclonus probably arises in the region of the dentate nucleus. The myoclonic jerks of Startle disease (hyperekplaxia syndrome) are less intense than during wakefulness, but persist even during stages 3 and 4 NREM sleep in response to minor stimuli. The repetitive twitches of one side of the face in hemifacial spasm, which is due to damage to the facial nerve nucleus, persist, but are reduced in frequency in both stages 3 and 4 NREM sleep and REM sleep.

Torsion dystonias

This is a heterogeneous group of disorders which cause sustained distorting or twisting postures and movements, but do not appear to impair the motor inhibition of sleep. They usually persist in stages 1 and 2 NREM and REM sleep, but with a reduced frequency and amplitude of movement, and then become less marked in stages 3 and 4 NREM sleep. As they become more severe they tend to increase the fragmentation of sleep, with a low sleep efficiency, long sleep latency and loss of stages 3 and 4 NREM and REM sleep, and in some patients exaggerated sleep spindles are seen.

Tics

These are rapid, repetitive twitching movements which may be simple or complex.

Tourette's syndrome, which arises in childhood and adolescence, is characterized by multiple tics with vocalizations, including grunting and squealing noises and often obscenities, as well as obsessive and compulsive thoughts and behaviours. It is due to genetically determined disinhibition of corticostriatal and thalamic circuits leading to poor impulse control, obsessive–compulsive behaviour and symptoms similar to the attention deficit hyperactivity disorder.

The tics are most pronounced in stages 1 and 2 NREM sleep and less obvious in REM and stages 3 and 4 NREM sleep, but the larger body movements are most frequent in REM sleep. The restless legs syndrome and periodic limb movements in sleep are common. Sleep becomes fragmented with loss of both NREM and REM sleep. Insomnia may gradually improve but sleep terrors and sleep walking are common. Treatment with neuroleptic drugs is often effective.

Parkinsonism

This is due to degeneration and loss of dopamine in the basal ganglia and causes bradykinesia, tremor and rigidity. There are two main forms which are discussed below.

Idiopathic Parkinsonism (Parkinson's disease)
This is due to degeneration in the basal ganglia and related structures. The substantia nigra in the midbrain has close relationships with the LDT/PPT in the pons which controls REM sleep, and with the raphe nuclei and locus coeruleus which are involved with NREM sleep. The initial degeneration probably occurs in the pons, which may explain the frequency of postural hypotension and the appearance of the REM sleep behaviour disorder often several years before other features of Parkinsonism appear. As the disease advances it may extend into the dorsolateral prefrontal cerebral cortex.

Several sleep abnormalities are associated with idiopathic Parkinsonism.
1 Excessive daytime sleepiness (page 158).
2 Insomnia (page 182).
3 Hallucinations and vivid dreams (page 191).
4 Motor abnormalities.

The Parkinsonian tremor is most prominent at the moment of arousal from sleep, or at transitions from a deeper to a lighter stage of sleep, and in stages 1 and 2 NREM sleep. In 10–25% of subjects the dyskinesias improve initially after sleep for between 30 min and 3 h ('sleep benefit') and then deteriorate during the day [21]. The mechanism whereby sleep may be beneficial is uncertain.

Periodic limb movements are rarely seen once treatment with dopaminergic agents has been initiated,

but in untreated subjects they are frequent and often associated with the symptoms of the restless legs syndrome. Iron deficiency is often present and iron supplementation, as well as dopaminergic agents, may be of help.

Obstructive sleep apnoeas are said to be more frequent in Parkinsonism than in normal subjects, but there is no evidence to support this. The REM sleep behaviour disorder is, however, a frequent association. It occurs in around one-third of those with idiopathic Parkinsonism and often appears many years before other features of Parkinsonism. This is probably due to degeneration of the LDT/PPT and the locus subcoeruleus, leading to failure of normal motor inhibition during REM sleep. Dopaminergic treatment is ineffective, suggesting that there may be degeneration in noradrenergic or cholinergic mechanisms. Interestingly the vigorous physical enactment of dreams during REM sleep behaviour disorder is not impaired by any bradykinesia, tremor or other motor abnormality present in wakefulness.

Polysomnography characteristically shows a reduction in total sleep time and in sleep efficiency, an increase in wakefulness after sleep onset and sleep fragmentation. There is often a reduction in amplitude and frequency of sleep spindles, which can be reversed by L-dopa therapy. Sleep-onset REM sleep is common both during overnight polysomnography and during naps in the day. Muscle tone is increased in REM sleep in those with the REM sleep behaviour disorder, and REM sleep-onset blepharospasm is recognized. Periodic limb movements and sleep apnoeas may be seen.

Secondary Parkinsonism
Patients with these disorders, such as multiple system atrophy and Lewy body disease, have the same difficulties with sleep as those with idiopathic Parkinsonism, but with additional problems specific to their condition. The effects of post-encephalitic Parkinsonism are described in Chapter 6.

Multiple system atrophy. In this condition there is widespread CNS degeneration with loss of control of the autonomic nervous system. Insomnia occurs with frequent awakenings, reduction in stages 3 and 4 NREM sleep and, especially in the olivopontocerebellar atrophy variant, loss of REM sleep duration and density, and prolonged episodes which are difficult to classify either as NREM or as REM sleep.

REM sleep behaviour disorder may appear early in its natural history and precede other features by as long as 2–3 years, and eventually appears in around 90% of subjects.

Involvement of the nucleus ambiguus impairs control of the vocal cords and leads to episodes of adduction associated with stridor and choking, often at night, but also occasionally during the day. These respond to a proton pump inhibitor since they are triggered by occult gastro-oesophageal reflux. They cause obstructive sleep apnoeas and occasionally a tracheostomy may be required. An irregular respiratory pattern with prolonged central apnoeas also develops.

Lewy body disease. This degenerative disorder is associated with Parkinsonism, progressive cognitive defects and visual hallucinations. The REM sleep behaviour disorder is present in around 25% of subjects.

Progressive supranuclear palsy (PSP). In this condition Parkinsonism is combined with dementia, dystonic gait, a disturbance of axial rigidity and a vertical voluntary gaze palsy. Degeneration develops in the core (tegmentum) of the pons and midbrain, particularly in the region of the locus coeruleus.

The sleep disturbance is proportional to the degree of motor abnormalities and can be severe. Depression, nocturia and discomfort due to immobility may all contribute to the sleep disruption. There is difficulty in maintaining sleep and early morning awakening. The REM sleep behaviour disorder occurs in 10% of subjects. Dream recall is reduced or absent due to damage to the REM sleep generating mechanisms, and there is little response of the sleep disturbances to L-dopa or dopamine receptor agonists. The main symptoms are difficulty maintaining wakefulness and early morning waking.

Polysomnography shows a reduction in total sleep time, increased sleep latency, frequent awakenings, reduction of sleep spindles, fewer REM sleep episodes and a shortened total duration of REM sleep, and there may be loss of muscle atonia during REM sleep [22].

Insomnia is more marked than in other dementias, such as Alzheimer's disease or idiopathic Parkinsonism, and is related to the severity of the disorder.

References

1 Vetrugno R, Provini F, Meletti S, Plazzi G, Liguori R, Cortelli P, Lugaresi E, Montagna P. Propriospinal myoclonus at the sleep–wake transition: a new type of parasomnia. *Sleep* 2001; 24(7): 835–43.

2 Kavey NB, Whyte J, Resor SR, Gidro-Frank S. Somnambulism in adults. *Neurology* 1990; 40: 749–52.

3 Schenck CH, Mahowald MW. Review of nocturnal sleep-related eating disorders. *Int J Eat Disord* 1994; 15: 343–56.

4 Lauer CJ, Krieg J-C. Sleep in eating disorders. *Sleep Med Rev* 2004; 8: 109–18.

5 Schenck CH, Bundlie SR, Mahowald MW. Delayed emergence of a parkinsonian disorder in 38% of 29 older men initially diagnosed with idiopathic rapid eye movement sleep behavior disorder. *Neurology* 1996; 46: 388–93.

6 Sforza E, Krieger J, Petiau C. REM sleep behavior disorder: clinical and physiopathological findings. *Sleep Med Rev* 1997; 1: 57–6.

7 Schenck CH, Mahowald MW. REM sleep behavior disorder: clinical, developmental, and neuroscience perspectives 16 years after its formal identification in sleep. *Sleep* 2002; 25(2): 120–38.

8 Mahowald MW, Schenck CH. Status dissociatus – a perspective on states of being. *Sleep* 1991; 14: 69–79.

9 Hening W, Walters AS, Allen RP, Montplaisir J, Myers A, Ferini-Strambi L. Impact, diagnosis and treatment of restless legs syndrome (RLS) in a primary care population: the REST (RLS epidemiology, symptoms, and treatment) primary care study. *Sleep Med* 2004; 5: 237–46.

10 Iriarte J, Urresarazu E, Alegre M, Valencia M, Artieda J. Oscillatory cortical changes during periodic limb movements. *Sleep* 2004; 27(8): 1493–8.

11 Pollmacher T, Schulz H. Periodic leg movements (PLM): their relationship to sleep stages. *Sleep* 1993; 16: 572–7.

12 Krieger J, Schroeder C. Iron, brain and restless legs syndrome. *Sleep Med Rev* 2001; 5(4): 277–86.

13 Bassetti CL, Mauerhofer D, Gugger M, Mathis J, Hess CW. Restless legs syndrome: a clinical study of 55 patients. *Eur Neurol* 2001; 45: 67–74.

14 Abetz L, Allen R, Follet A, Washburn T, Earley C, Kirsch J, Knight H. Evaluating the quality of life of patients with restless legs syndrome. *Clin Ther* 2004; 26: 925–35.

15 Coleman RM, Pollak CP, Weitzman ED. Periodic movements in sleep (nocturnal myoclonus): relation to sleep disorders. *Ann Neurol* 1980; 8: 416–21.

16 Wagner ML, Walters AS, Fisher B. Symptoms of attention-deficit/hyperactivity disorder in adults with restless legs syndrome. *Sleep* 2004; 27(8): 1499–504.

17 Minecan D, Natarajan A, Marzec M, Malow B. Relationshiop of epileptic seizures to sleep stage and sleep depth. *Sleep* 2002; 25(8): 899–904.

18 Nobili L, Francione S, Cardinale F, Russo GL. Epileptic nocturnal wanderings with a temporal lobe origin: a stereo-electroencephalographic study. *Sleep* 2002; 25(6): 669–71.

19 Meierkord H, Fish DR, Smith SJM, Scott CA, Shorvon SD, Marsden CD. Is nocturnal paroxysmal dystonia a form of frontal lobe epilepsy? *Mov Disord* 1992; 7: 38–42.

20 Crespel A, Baldy-Moulinier M, Coubes P. The relationship between sleep and epilepsy in frontal and temporal lobe epilepsies. *Epilepsia* 1998; 39: 150–7.

21 Bateman DE, Levett K, Marsden CD. Sleep benefit in Parkinson's disease. *J Neurol Neurosurg Psychiatry* 1999; 67: 384–5.

22 Aldrich MS, Foster NL, White RF, Bluemlein L, Prokopowicz G. Sleep abnormalities in progressive supranuclear palsy. *Ann Neurol* 1989; 25: 577–81.

10 Obstructive Sleep Apnoeas and Snoring

Introduction

Obstructive sleep apnoeas (OSA) are due to transient closure of the upper airway during sleep. Air is prevented from entering the lungs and this interrupts the continuous gas exchange in the alveoli (Fig. 3.7). Obstructive sleep apnoeas are common and form a continuous spectrum ranging from normality with a few obstructions to a life-threatening state which may present with respiratory, cardiovascular or sleep-related complications.

The term obstructive sleep apnoea syndrome (OSAS) refers to the combination of symptoms and the presence of apnoeas [1]. An identical clinical picture may result from hypopnoeas (obstructive sleep apnoea hypopnoea syndrome, OSAHS). There is, however, only a moderate correlation between the objective findings of apnoeas and hypopnoeas during sleep and the severity of symptoms. The latter are also determined by physiological changes during sleep which are not identified accurately by simply counting the apnoeas or hypopnoeas, as well as other factors such as shift work and individual vulnerability to the sleep fragmentation from the apnoeas.

Prevalence

Approximately 2–4% of middle-aged men and 1–2% of middle-aged women have clinically significant OSAs [2]. In obese males around 3–4% have more than 5 OSAs per hour, 1% more than 10 per hour and 0.3% more than 20 per hour. This prevalence is likely to increase as obesity becomes more common. Symptomatic OSA is probably at least twice as frequent in the USA as in the UK because of this factor, although in some ethnic groups such as Polynesians, Chinese and those of other Far Eastern countries, OSA is less closely related to obesity. Obesity is also less of a risk factor in children and in the elderly.

Obstructive sleep apnoeas most commonly occur in children around the age of 2–6 years and then become less frequent as the tonsils and adenoids involute. In adults they become progressively more frequent with age and the odds ratio of developing OSA doubles every 10 years until around the age of 60. Beyond this age OSA continues to become more frequent, although it may become less clinically significant.

There is a familial tendency to develop sleep apnoeas. The risk is doubled if a sibling or parent has OSA and this relationship is apparent even in the elderly. If there is more than one relative with OSA there is a greater chance of the subject having a higher apnoea–hypopnoea index and requiring a greater level of continuous positive airway pressure (CPAP) to control the apnoeas, even when the body mass index (BMI) is adjusted for. Inheritance is probably polygenic and may determine the shape or size of the upper airway by determining the formation of both the bones and soft tissues [3]. There may also be a genetically directed pattern of respiratory and upper airway control which predisposes to apnoeas. The familial tendency to obesity may be partly inherited, but is also partly acquired through common eating habits within a family. These or genetic factors may also determine other behavioural factors, such as taking exercise or a tendency to smoke or drink alcohol.

Upper airway resistance syndrome (UARS)

The concept of the upper airway resistance syndrome is based on the idea that identical clinical and physiological effects can result from narrowing without closure of the upper airway [4]. Neither apnoeas nor hypopnoeas may be detectable and the oxygen saturation may remain normal. Airflow may be reduced or compensated for by increased inspiratory muscle activity. This increased respiratory effort is responsible for the arousals from sleep which lead to sleep fragmentation and other physiological consequences.

There has been considerable debate as to whether this syndrome exists or whether it is an artefact due to insensitivity of the available sensors for detecting changes in airflow and therefore the establishment of whether apnoeas and hypopnoeas are present. The syndrome may be due to an abnormally low arousal threshold so that arousal results from relatively little increase in inspiratory muscle effort and before changes in airflow are apparent. This syndrome in effect avoids airway closure at the expense of increasing sleep fragmentation.

The UARS affects males and females equally frequently. UARS is more frequent in the non-obese than OSA and it is uncertain whether it is simply a phase which occurs between simple snoring and the appearance of sleep apnoeas or whether it is a separate 'variant' of abnormal upper airway behaviour which does not change despite, for instance, increasing age or weight.

Initiation and termination of apnoeas

The pharyngeal airway becomes progressively smaller during each of the breaths leading up to airway closure. During the apnoea the airway may open temporarily during expiration to allow some gas to leave the lungs, and in the upper airway resistance syndrome the airway narrows, but does not completely close.

Closure of the airway depends primarily on the relationship between the pressure in the tissues around it and the intraluminal pressure. The bulk of adipose and muscle tissue around the airway is the main factor determining the tissue pressure. Increasing activity of the inspiratory muscles with successive breaths as the airway narrows or closes reduces the intraluminal pressure to a certain level but, since the airway functions as a Starling resistor, there is a limit to this effect. Narrowing of the airway from any cause increases the inspiratory effort needed to overcome this and lowers the airway pressure proximally. By Laplace's law it

also increases the positive pressure within the lumen which is required to open or enlarge the airway.

The pharyngeal airway tends to become smaller during expiration and if this is prolonged, as in for instance a central sleep apnoea, or if there is an instability of respiratory control, it tends to close [5]. Once the airway is closed, surface forces may hold the mucosae of the airway walls together and increase the force required to open the airway. During each apnoea the section of the airway that is closed spreads progressively proximally.

Termination of the OSA requires arousal from a deeper to a lighter stage of sleep or wakefulness (Table 10.1). The increase in the intensity of inspiratory muscle effort as the respiratory drive increases during the OSA is the main factor causing arousal. Intrapleural pressures of up to -80 cmH20 may be reached, although in normal subjects a pressure around -15 cmH20 is usually sufficient to lead to arousal.

The respiratory stimulant effects of hypoxia and to a lesser extent hypercapnia also contribute to the moment when arousal occurs, although the responses to these biochemical stimuli are less during sleep than wakefulness. They probably cause arousal both by increasing the inspiratory muscle force and more directly by impulses from the respiratory centres stimulating the ascending reticular arousal system.

The threshold for arousal is lowest in stages 1 and 2 NREM sleep, higher in stages 3 and 4 and greatest in REM sleep in which the longest apnoeas are seen.

At the moment of arousal the activity of the upper airway dilator muscles returns and the upper airway resistance falls. The airway often opens suddenly with a loud snoring noise and following this there is compensatory hyperventilation with a reduction in $P\text{CO}_2$ and return of the $P\text{O}_2$ to normal. The respiratory effort then wanes and the subject returns to sleep at which time the upper airway dilator muscles become

Table 10.1 Maintenance and termination of an obstructive sleep apnoea.

	Onset of apnoea	Maintenance of apnoea	Apnoea termination point	Post apnoea
Upper airway dilator muscle activity	−	−	++	+
Surface forces	−	+	−	−
Respiratory drive	+	++	+++	++
Inspiratory chest wall muscle force	+	++	+++	++
Arousal	−	−	+	+
Airflow	−	−	−	++

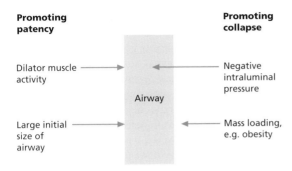

Fig. 10.1 Control of upper airway patency.

less active again and the cycle is repeated. This process may recur up to 500 times per night.

Pathophysiology

The patency of the upper airway depends on the balance of forces across it and on its compliance [6] (Fig. 10.1). The airway between the oropharynx and the larynx is a single muscular tube which conducts air in and out of the lungs, and food, drink and upper airway secretions into the oesophagus. Above the oropharynx two airways (the nasal and oral) are in parallel so that obstruction of either does not cause airflow to cease. Below the larynx the airway is supported by cartilaginous rings which prevent its collapse. Any factor which narrows the upper airway, increases the pressure around it, reduces the pressure within it, or increases its compliance, will predispose towards OSA.

The site of obstruction varies between individuals (Fig. 10.2). The soft palate may be drawn like a wedge between the posterior aspect of the tongue and the posterior pharyngeal wall. Posterior displacement of the tongue, particularly due to loss of genioglossus activity and the effect of gravity, will close the airway at pharyngeal level. This is more common in adults than in children. Laryngeal abnormalities, which may be organic lesions or due to disorders of their innervation, may cause OSA and localized anatomical variations or pathological lesions within the airway may cause obstruction at other levels.

The most important factors which determine whether or not OSA develop are as follows.

Small size of upper airway

The size, and probably the shape, of the upper airway influence whether it is likely to close during sleep. The pharyngeal airway is narrowed laterally in OSA compared to normal subjects but the causes and

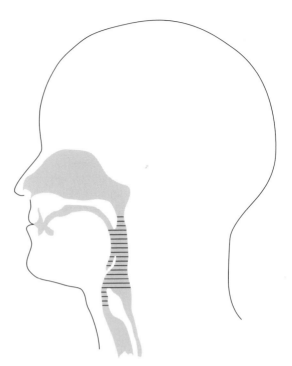

Fig. 10.2 Sites of upper airway obstruction. The hatched area shows the usual area of occlusion of the airway during obstructive sleep apnoeas.

significance of this are uncertain. The smaller airway is more vulnerable because of the following.

1 By Laplace's law, the narrower the airway the greater the expanding force that is required to generate sufficient wall tension to maintain its patency.

2 If the airway is smaller it takes less change for it to close.

3 A narrow airway increases the resistance to flow and a more negative pressure is required proximally to compensate for this. This tends to cause the airway walls to be sucked together at that point.

Upper airway compliance

The upper airway is more collapsible in OSA than in normal subjects because of a combination of mechanical and neurological factors. Vibration trauma to the soft palate and pharyngeal walls due to their rapid fluttering within each breath and repetitive closure and opening lead to tissue damage and oedema which probably increase as the severity of the OSA progresses.

The other important factor is the activity of the pharyngeal dilator and constrictor muscles. Tonic activity in both these muscle groups is less during sleep, especially REM sleep, than during wakefulness.

Airway obstruction is due to a failure of the dilator muscles to counteract the physical forces tending to close the airway, rather than to an increase in constrictor muscle activity.

The changes in dilator muscle contraction vary between the individual muscles. The genioglossus, which protrudes the tongue, and the geniohyoid, which pulls the hyoid forwards, are both upper airway dilators with mainly phasic inspiratory activity which is largely retained at the onset of NREM sleep. In contrast, the tensor palatini, which retracts the soft palate, has mainly tonic activity and this is lost in NREM sleep. The loss of this tonic muscle activity is largely responsible for the increase in upper airway resistance which is seen during normal sleep. Relaxation of the medial and lateral pterygoid muscles lessens the degree of mandibular protrusion, so that the base of the tongue becomes more posterior, the mouth falls open and the pharyngeal airway becomes smaller.

The neurophysiological basis for these changes is uncertain. They may be mediated in part through 5HT release by neurones from the dorsal raphe nuclei projecting to the respiratory centres and lower cranial nerve nuclei in the medulla.

The main neurological factors which determine whether or not the airway is likely to close are as follows.
1 The upper airway diameter falls through a reflex mechanism as the lung volume, and in particular the functional residual capacity, decreases.
2 A negative pressure within the upper airway normally generates activity in the upper airway muscles which prevents airway closure. This reflex may be reduced or absent in individuals with OSA.
3 The normal sequence of activation of respiratory muscles during each inspiration, beginning with the alae nasi, followed by other upper airway muscles and ending with activation of the diaphragm, may be lost. This failure to stabilize the upper airway before the chest wall muscles contract and reduce the pressure within it promotes airway obstruction. It is also seen in certain types of ventilatory support during sleep, particularly in negative pressure ventilation used in the control mode and in phrenic nerve stimulation.
4 Upper airway obstruction may be due to an increase in the force of the chest wall muscles relative to that of the upper airway dilators so that the negative pressure in the airway overcomes the stabilizing effect of dilator muscle activity.
5 The proportion of Type II fast twitch fatiguable muscle fibres in the genioglossus is increased in OSA, which may predispose to a loss of dilator muscle force during sleep. These changes and abnormal muscle fibre

morphology and remodelling of the upper airway muscles may all be the result of vibration trauma from the OSA [7]. Neuropathic changes have also been reported, probably due to trauma, and may contribute to dilator muscle dysfunction. Diabetics with an autonomic neuropathy appear to have a higher incidence of OSA, possibly due to neuropathic changes within the upper airway muscles.

These changes in the sequence or relative force of contraction in the upper airway and chest wall muscles vary according to, for instance, the P_{CO_2}, stage of sleep, and the individual response to factors such as sleep deprivation, the nasal cycle, and changes in position. There is also breath-to-breath variability within REM sleep which may predispose to apnoeas developing intermittently.

Chest wall muscle activity

The pressure within the upper airway is determined by the activity of the chest wall muscles and the extent to which this is transmitted to the upper airway. During NREM sleep, the diaphragm, intercostal and accessory respiratory muscles are all active, but in REM sleep the diaphragm alone is responsible for inspiration. The pressure that these muscles generate in the upper airway depends on their contractility, mass, length, rate of shortening and mechanical advantage as well as the compliance and resistance of the lungs and chest wall.

Causes of obstructive sleep apnoea

The most important causes of OSA are as follows (Table 10.2).

Small size of upper airway

The causes of this may be diffuse, as in obesity, or focal as in tonsillar enlargement. The most important individual causes are as follows.

Obesity

Obesity is one of the major risk factors for OSA in Caucasian and Afro-American adults, but to a lesser extent in children and the elderly and in Polynesians, Chinese and those from other Far Eastern countries. The adipose tissue that is most relevant is that which is deposited within the neck rather than elsewhere in the body. The fat is located not within the wall of the airway but around it, and when the muscle tone is reduced during sleep the fatty tissue, in effect, mass-loads the airway and tends to collapse it.

Obesity also predisposes to OSA by reducing the functional residual capacity and thereby reflexly reducing

Table 10.2 Factors predisposing to obstructive sleep apnoea.

Factors	Causes	Examples
Small upper airway	Obesity Tobacco smoking Hormonal factors	Menopause Acromegaly Hypothyroidism
	Supine position Upper airway lesions	Nose: polyps, rhinitis Pharynx: tonsils and adenoids, cysts and tumours Larynx: congenital webs and cysts Crico-arytenoid arthritis Congenital and traumatic abnormalities Retrognathia
	Skeletal abnormality	
Loss of upper airway dilator muscle activity	Sleep deprivation and fragmentation Benzodiazepines Alcohol Neurological disorders	Diffuse, e.g. poliomyelitis, Duchenne's muscular dystrophy Focal, e.g. Arnold–Chiari malformation, strokes
	General anaesthetic Ventilatory support	Nasal and negative pressure ventilation, phrenic nerve pacemakers
Increased chest wall muscle force		

the upper airway dimensions. It causes ventilation–perfusion mismatching with hypoxia, mass-loads the chest wall muscles, stretches the diaphragm beyond its optimal length and probably impairs muscle contractility. All these factors may contribute to the obesity hypoventilation syndrome.

Obstructive sleep apnoeas also predispose to obesity (page 14) and this may be secondary to other sleep disorders, particularly the Prader–Willi and Kleine–Levin syndromes, sleep eating or narcolepsy, all of which can therefore be complicated by OSA.

Neck muscle hypertrophy
Hypertrophy of the muscles within the neck can act in a similar way to obesity and compress the upper airway. This is usually seen in those engaged in competitive sports which require strong neck muscles, and following regular physical training.

Tobacco
Tobacco smoking is associated with an increased risk of OSA, probably because it causes a diffuse mucositis, affecting the oral and pharyngeal airway, including the soft palate. Nicotine in tobacco may also alter

respiratory control. Its pharmacological effects are discussed in Chapter 4.

Sleeping position
In the supine position, the weight of the tongue and mandible is unopposed by tonic muscle activity in the upper airway and they fall back into the pharynx, narrowing it. This is more marked in REM sleep than in NREM sleep where muscle relaxation is greater. The functional residual capacity also falls in the supine position and this reflexly reduces the upper airway dimensions.

The effect of position on OSA is most apparent in younger adults with mild or moderately severe OSA. It is less important in obesity, presumably because the excess fatty tissue surrounds the airway and causes apnoeas in any position. Neck flexion and opening of the mouth also increase the upper airway resistance and contribute to apnoeas and snoring.

Nasal obstruction
Complete nasal obstruction leads to mouth breathing which may predispose to OSA, and the lack of stimulation of nasal pressure and flow receptors may reduce the

stability of the upper airway. Partial nasal obstruction leads to a more negative pharyngeal pressure during inspiration to overcome it and this predisposes to OSA.

The most important causes are nasal polyps, rhinitis and a deviated nasal septum.

Tonsil and adenoid enlargement

Enlargement of the tonsils, adenoids or both contributes to OSA, particularly in children. This enlargement may be temporary during infections, and respond to antibiotics, but chronic enlargement is more important.

Laryngeal obstruction

Organic disorders of the larynx may cause OSA. These may be congenital webs or cysts, thickening of the laryngeal tissues as in acromegaly and hypothyroidism, or crico-arytenoid arthritis due to rheumatoid arthritis in which abduction of the vocal cords is limited.

Craniofacial causes

No obvious anatomical abnormality is found in most subjects with OSA, although imaging techniques have shown that the pharyngeal airway is smaller than in those without apnoeas. This is probably mainly due to variations in skeletal and soft tissue morphology which are probably at least partly genetically determined, but also vary with age. A long soft palate with a margin which falls below the level of the tongue may wedge between this and the posterior pharyngeal wall. Oedema due to trauma from the apnoeas may exacerbate this, but can be relieved by effective treatment of OSA. A slightly short mandible, or a more inferior hyoid, may also predispose to OSA.

Marfan's syndrome causes a high arched hard palate which is associated with a small pharyngeal airway, as well as increased laxity of the pharyngeal airway, which predispose to OSA. A large tongue is a feature of amyloidosis as well as acromegaly.

Craniofacial trauma may cause OSA but there are several specific congenital disorders that may also lead to this. These fall into the following categories.

Mandibular hypoplasia (micrognathia)

Hypoplasia (micrognathia) or a posteriorly positioned (retrognathia) mandible lead to a dental overbite and may induce OSA, particularly in the supine position when the tongue tends to fall back into the pharyngeal airway.

Pierre Robin sequence. In this syndrome there is micrognathia with posterior displacement of the tongue and soft palate, which is often cleft. There may also be other malformations of the upper respiratory tract. Obstructive sleep apnoeas are often severe neonatally, but improve as the mandible grows. They can be overcome initially with a nasopharyngeal tube rather than a tracheostomy. Sleep apnoeas may present later in life, at which time an adenotonsillectomy may be at least partially effective. Nasal CPAP is an alternative.

Treacher–Collins syndrome. Mandibular hypoplasia is associated with other abnormalities such as conduction deafness. Obstructive sleep apnoeas are common and usually respond to mandibular advancement surgery or nasal CPAP.

Mid-face hypoplasia

Craniosynostes. The three commonest syndromes are Apert's, Crouzon's and Pfeiffer's syndromes in which different cranial sutures become prematurely fused. They lead to failure of growth of the maxilla with posterior displacement of the tongue. They are often associated with cleft palate and mental retardation. Obstructive sleep apnoeas gradually worsen as the tonsils and adenoids and soft palate enlarge, since the maxilla fails to grow. The apnoeas usually respond to surgical advancement of the mid-face, but nasal CPAP is an alternative.

Achondroplasia. Mid-face hypoplasia is associated with a wide range of other anatomical abnormalities including a triangular foramen magnum. This may lead to hydrocephalus and brainstem and spinal cord compression, causing central sleep apnoeas. Decompression of the foramen magnum may be required. Obstructive apnoeas are, however, more common and are usually due to the mid-face hypoplasia. Adenotonsillectomy is often effective, but nasal CPAP may be required.

Down's syndrome. Mid-face hypoplasia is associated with a narrowed nasal airway, enlargement of the adenoids and tonsils, macroglossia and a hypotonic upper airway. Abnormalities of respiratory control may lead to central sleep apnoeas, but obstructive apnoeas are more common. The ventilatory responses to carbon dioxide and oxygen are reduced, and hypercapnia may appear. There is a significant risk of pulmonary hypertension to which congenital heart defects may contribute, but there may be an abnormal sensitivity of the pulmonary microcirculation to hypoxia. There is usually a long sleep latency and REM sleep latency with reduction in the frequency of sleep spindles and an increased arousal index.

The obstructive apnoeas partially respond to adenotonsillectomy, but in view of their multifactorial origin nasal CPAP is often required as well. Treatment of OSA should be initiated early in order to prevent pulmonary hypertension, and if neither adenotonsillectomy nor CPAP are feasible, nocturnal oxygen should be considered, unless it causes carbon dioxide retention.

Smith–Magenis syndrome. In this condition there is mid-face hypoplasia which leads to obstructive sleep apnoeas as well as abnormalities of the circadian rhythms and reduction in duration of REM sleep.

Mucopolysaccharidoses

In the Hunter, Hurler and Scheie syndromes acid mucopolysaccharides are deposited in the upper airway, particularly the tonsils, adenoids and epiglottis. There is diffuse pharyngeal thickening, macroglossia and coarse facial features. Obstructive sleep apnoeas are frequent. Adenotonsillectomy is usually ineffective because of the diffuse abnormalities, but the apnoeas respond either to nasal CPAP or to bone marrow transplantation.

Hormonal factors

Endocrine differences between males and females contribute to the difference in prevalence of OSA in men and women (page 243), and endocrine abnormalities [8] also contribute to OSA in the following situations.

Acromegaly

OSA is present in 20–75% of those with acromegaly, especially if the growth hormone level is markedly raised, in older subjects, and in those with an increased neck circumference. OSA is not closely related to obesity or findings on examination of the nose and pharynx. The increase in growth hormone alters the craniofacial skeletal dimensions and leads to enlargement of the tongue and diffuse thickening of the upper airway including the larynx.

OSA persists in around 20% of subjects after treatment of acromegaly, especially if the growth hormone or IGF-1 remains raised, in older subjects, or if the neck circumference remains increased. Persistence of OSA may be due to failure of the skeletal or soft tissue changes to resolve or to irreversible changes in the reflex control of the upper airway.

Hypothyroidism

This characteristically leads to fatigue, but may also cause OSA because of a myopathy of the upper airway muscles and infiltration with 'oedema', as well as because of obesity. It is commoner if there is myxoedema. Abnormalities of respiratory control may also lead to central apnoeas.

Cushing's syndrome

Obesity and myopathy of the vocal cords predispose to OSA.

Diabetes mellitus

OSA is commoner in diabetes if there is an autonomic neuropathy, possibly because this may be associated with a neuropathy affecting the upper airway muscles. The relationship of diabetes to OSA is, however, complex since the effects of OSA can lead to diabetes and obesity is common to both conditions.

Loss of upper airway muscle activity

The increase in the compliance of the upper airway due to loss of dilator muscle activity during sleep may be caused by one or more of the following.

Sleep deprivation and sleep fragmentation

These reduce the respiratory drive and in particular the response of the chest wall muscles to upper airway obstruction, thereby delaying arousal from the apnoeas. This increase in the arousal threshold worsens the degree of oxygen desaturation and of hypercapnia during the apnoeas, and may also reduce the rate of resaturation after the apnoea and even prevent normal blood gases from being attained before the next apnoea begins. The ventilatory response to hypercapnia is reduced.

Benzodiazepines

These drugs reduce the ability to arouse from OSAs and also reduce muscle tone in the upper airway.

Alcohol

This has similar effects to benzodiazepines. The decrease in arousability prolongs the apnoeas and the reduction in upper airway dilator muscle activity impairs the post-apnoea hyperventilation so that the rate of oxygen resaturation is slower. Alcohol also increases the nasal airflow resistance by causing hyperaemia of the nasal mucosa.

Neuromuscular conditions

Disorders such as poliomyelitis, Duchenne's muscular dystrophy and myotonic dystrophy diffusely weaken the upper airway dilator muscles and lead to OSA.

Other conditions have a more focal effect. Unilateral or bilateral vocal cord adduction develops in achondroplasia, syringobulbia, Arnold–Chiari malformation, multiple system atrophy, and following neurosurgery and neck surgery. Unilateral weakness of the pharynx and larynx occurs in strokes affecting the posterior inferior cerebellar artery territory (lateral medullary syndrome).

Specific neurological conditions associated with OSA include the following.

Cerebral palsy

Cerebral palsy is due to a perinatal event which causes spasticity of the legs or of all four limbs. During sleep, there is hypotonia of the pharynx, probably due to abnormal respiratory control. Large tonsils and adenoids, micrognathia, macroglossia and backward prolapse of the tongue (glossoptosis) all contribute to OSA, although mixed and central apnoeas may also appear. Apnoeas may also follow epileptic seizures during sleep, and daytime sleepiness may be the result either of these medical problems or of sedation from anticonvulsants and other drugs, such as benzodiazepines.

Adenotonsillectomy usually gives partial relief of the apnoeas. Nasal CPAP may be required.

Arnold–Chiari malformation

In this condition there is herniation of the brainstem and cerebellum through the foramen magnum leading to lower cranial nerve palsies. These include damage to the 9th and 10th cranial nerves, causing vocal cord adduction, abnormal control of the pharyngeal muscles and changes in respiratory drive. Nasal CPAP may be required.

The brainstem compression also reduces the ventilatory response to oxygen and carbon dioxide, causing central sleep apnoeas, and these may improve with posterior fossa decompression.

Prader–Willi syndrome

In this disorder, obesity, hypogonadism and mental retardation are combined with hypotonia and hypothalamic abnormalities. Excessive daytime sleepiness is seen in around 70% of subjects. The sleepiness may be partly due to an intrinsic hypersomnia related to hypothalamic abnormalities, but obstructive sleep apnoeas are frequent and often contribute. They may lead to respiratory and right heart failure, and respond to weight loss and either nasal CPAP or bilevel pressure support ventilation. There is also a reduction in the ventilatory response to carbon dioxide which contributes to hypercapnia, which is initially seen during REM sleep at night and later during wakefulness.

General anaesthesia

Central control of the upper airway is altered so that the muscles lose their activity. Obstructive 'anaesthetic' apnoeas occur both during the anaesthetic and in the recovery phase.

Ventilatory support

Obstructive sleep apnoeas can be induced by loss of the normal sequence of muscle contraction, in which the upper airway muscles are activated before the chest wall muscles, in negative pressure ventilation using the control mode and with phrenic nerve stimulation. This can also be provoked by nasal positive pressure ventilation, possibly through a similar mechanism or through changes in airway pressure and flow causing passive closure of the airway, usually at laryngeal level.

Chest wall muscle activity

Obstructive sleep apnoeas can be accentuated by an increase in the chest wall muscle activity relative to that of the pharyngeal dilator muscles. This may contribute to OSA in certain situations, but there is little direct evidence for this.

Physiological effects

Oxygen saturation

The depth of oxygen desaturation during each apnoea depends on the following factors.

Prior oxygen saturation

The sigmoid shape of the oxyhaemoglobin dissociation curve dictates that at a normal Po_2 of around 13.3 kPa the oxygen saturation is above 95%, and a fall in the Po_2 of as much as 4 kPa will only reduce the saturation to around 90%. If, however, the initial Po_2 is 8 kPa, the oxygen saturation is around 90%, but will fall to as low as 60% when the Po_2 falls by 4 kPa. Patients with a lower initial Po_2 will have greater desaturation for any fall in Po_2 than those in whom initial oxygenation is normal. In REM sleep the impaired ventilation–perfusion matching reduces the baseline oxygen saturation and predisposes to deeper dips.

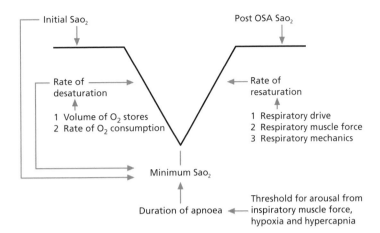

Fig. 10.3 Factors affecting oxygen desaturation in an obstructive sleep apnoea.

Rate of desaturation

The rate of desaturation is determined by the volume of oxygen stored in the body and the rate of oxygen consumption (Fig. 10.3). Oxygen stores are smaller in REM sleep than in NREM sleep because of the reduced lung volumes.

Duration of apnoea

Apnoea duration is related to the threshold for arousal from the increased inspiratory muscle force, although hypercapnia, and to a lesser extent hypoxia, also contribute to the break-point. Muscle relaxation is greater in REM sleep than in NREM sleep and arousal occurs later in the former. Sleep fragmentation reduces the arousability and prolongs apnoeas. This underlies the longer apnoeas seen later in the night.

Completeness of apnoea

The rate of resaturation after the apnoea is determined by the respiratory drive and the ability of the chest wall muscles to increase ventilation. This is impaired in neuromuscular disorders where there is a reduced respiratory pump capacity, and in gross obesity and chronic airflow obstruction where the work of breathing is increased. Sleep fragmentation caused by OSA reduces the ventilatory response to hypercapnia, prevents compensatory hypoventilation and predisposes to a rise in $P\text{CO}_2$ initially only at night, but later during wakefulness.

Intrapleural pressure swings

The increasingly strong respiratory efforts against the closed airway during an OSA generate large swings in intrapleural pressure. This may fall to as low as $-80 \text{ cmH}_2\text{O}$. This has cardiovascular effects and also

leads to large changes in the atrial dimensions as their transmural pressure alters. The repetitive stretching of the atria leads to increased secretion of atrial natriuretic peptide (ANP) which increases renal sodium and water loss resulting in nocturia and occasionally urinary incontinence.

Heart rate and dysrhythmias

The heart rate initially slows during an OSA and then rises towards the end of it and early in the postapnoea phase. This alternating bradycardia and tachycardia may be mistaken for the brady–tachy syndrome and pacemakers have been implanted unnecessarily on the basis of this erroneous diagnosis. Bradycardias can be profound with heart rates of less than 30 per minute and asystole lasting for more than 2.5 s. First and second degree atrioventricular heart block may appear in otherwise normal subjects, especially in REM sleep. Inspiratory efforts against a closed airway increase the parasympathetic activity and contribute to the bradycardias. The degree of the subsequent tachycardia is proportional to the fall in $P\text{O}_2$.

Systemic blood pressure

The swings in parasympathetic and sympathetic activity during and after each apnoea lead to a fall in blood pressure early in the apnoea followed by a rise of around 50% above the level seen between the apnoeas [9]. The rise of sympathetic activity is due mainly to the arousal, but also to hypoxia. The baroceptor reflex settings may also be altered.

The swings in intrapleural pressure also affect the blood pressure. A fall in intrapleural pressure reduces the pressure in the aorta, impairs left ventricular emptying and increases the left ventricular end systolic volume. The lower intrapleural and intrathoracic pressure increase the venous return to the right atrium and the right ventricular end diastolic volume. This shifts the interventricular septum to the left, reducing the compliance of the left ventricle and predisposing to left ventricular failure and a reduced cardiac output.

Pulmonary artery pressure

Arousal from sleep, for instance by a sleep apnoea, does not itself alter the pulmonary artery pressure, but hypoxia during each apnoea causes pulmonary vasoconstriction with the result that the pulmonary artery pressure rises towards the end of the apnoea and immediately afterwards [10]. This causes systolic right ventricular afterload which reduces the stroke volume. This reduction in stroke volume contrasts with the situation towards the start of the apnoea when the right ventricular output is reduced because of the bradycardia although the stroke volume is normal.

If the apnoeas cause severe oxygen desaturation and are frequent there will be insufficient time between the apnoeas for the arterial Po_2 to return to normal. The pulmonary artery pressure will then be raised not only during apnoeas but between them. This is seen particularly during REM sleep in which the arousal threshold is higher, apnoeas are more prolonged and pulmonary vascular reactivity to hypoxia may be more pronounced than in NREM sleep.

The greatly negative inspiratory intrathoracic pressure increases the venous return to the right atrium and ventricle which then increases the pulmonary artery pressure. The left ventricular compliance, filling and ejection fraction all fall and the left ventricular end diastolic pressure increases. During the expiratory phase the changes are reversed and left ventricular filling increases. At the end of the apnoea the sympathetic activity increases and the systemic blood pressure increases rapidly, particularly with the sympathetic induced vasoconstriction. Occasionally, the fall in left ventricular compliance and stroke volume is sufficient to cause pulmonary oedema, especially if there is pre-existing left ventricular dysfunction.

Autonomic effects

The onset of each apnoea is associated with an increase in parasympathetic activity leading to a bradycardia, but as the physiological stress builds up during the apnoea the sympathetic activity predominates. This peaks shortly after the moment of arousal at which time there is systemic vasoconstriction, hypertension and a tachycardia.

If OSAs are frequent, the increase in sympathetic activity is maintained during wakefulness as well as intermittently during sleep. This is probably due to a combination of frequent arousals and intermittent hypoxia.

Arousals

The increase in intensity of inspiratory muscle effort combined with hypoxia and hypercapnia leads to microarousals which may occur up to 500 times each night. They have the protective effect of enabling the respiratory system to come temporarily under the control mechanisms of wakefulness, which increase pharyngeal dilator muscle activity, and improve the blood gases. They have the disadvantage that they lead to sleep fragmentation, which reduces ventilatory drive and probably the strength and endurance of the respiratory muscles in the upper airway and chest wall. Frequent arousals eventually predispose to hypoventilation and hypoxia which, although it is initially a respiratory stimulus, can depress respiration if it is severe.

Arousals in OSA occur particularly in stages 1 and 2 NREM sleep and REM sleep. Once effective treatment is initiated there may be a transient REM sleep rebound with vivid dreams or nightmares.

Haematological changes

Chronic hypoxia may lead to polycythaemia, which increases blood viscosity and which not only predisposes to thrombosis, but also in effect increases the vascular resistance.

OSA may also induce a hypercoagulable state due primarily to an increase in fibrinogen levels [11]. Fibrinogen is an acute phase protein which promotes thrombus formation and also leads to platelet aggregation and smooth muscle proliferation. The increased fibrinogen level is mainly due to oxygen desaturations. It peaks in the mornings, is independent of obesity, but can be slightly reduced by CPAP treatment.

Inflammatory reaction

Vascular endothelial dysfunction is a feature of OSA. It is a pro-inflammatory state which triggers the increases in C-reactive protein, TNF-alpha and IL-6 that are seen in OSA [12]. It leads to proliferation of vascular smooth muscle cells, platelet aggregation and adhesion. Platelet activation increases neutrophil chemotaxis so that these cells reach the media and promote atheroma. Adhesion molecules are also liberated by endothelial cell damage and by white cells due to intermittent hypoxia, and increase monocyte adherence to the endothelium. Both monocytes and macrophagies migrate into the vascular wall, leading to lipid peroxidation [13] and the appearance of foam cells.

Endothelial dysfunction is triggered by a lack of nitric oxide availability which leads to vasoconstriction. Intermittent hypoxia and reoxygenation lead to the production of oxygen free radicals (reactive oxygen species) which increase the oxidative stress on the endothelium. Sleep fragmentation itself appears not to be a significant factor.

Hypoxia also increases the synthesis of plasma vascular endothelial growth factor (VEGF). This is a glycoprotein and angiogenic cytokine, which also modifies vascular tone. It is increased in OSA, both during the day and at night, but its levels fall if nocturnal hypoxia is relieved by CPAP.

Metabolic effects

Obstructive sleep apnoeas are associated with gout and an increased urinary secretion of uric acid which returns to normal with effective treatment of OSA. Cyclic adenosine monophosphate (AMP) increases and there is a reduction in adenosine triphosphate (ATP). This increases the production of purine nucleotides such as adenosine and xanthine, which are metabolized to uric acid.

Endocrine effects

Growth hormone

The fragmentation of NREM sleep by OSA reduces the pituitary response to GHRH and both growth hormone and IGF-1 production is reduced. The fall in growth hormone reduces the muscle mass, increases fat deposition, reduces bone density and affects sodium metabolism, but can be reversed by CPAP treatment.

Testosterone

Severe OSA reduces luteinizing hormone secretion, and thereby reduces testosterone production [14]. Together with excessive daytime sleepiness this may contribute to a fall in libido and to erectile dysfunction.

Insulin

Insulin secretion is increased in OSA and while this is partly due to the central obesity which is common in this condition, the levels are raised even when this is taken into account. This may be because of increased sympathetic stimulation of the beta cells in the pancreas.

Insulin resistance develops independently of the body mass index [15] and leads to an increase in low-density lipoproteins (LDL) and a fall in high-density lipoproteins (HDL). This combination taken with hypertension comprises the metabolic syndrome to which OSA appears to be a contributory factor [16].

Leptin

Leptin is increased in OSA, even when obesity is taken into account [17]. This suggests that OSA leads to leptin resistance. The increase in leptin in OSA may be due to increased sympathetic activity. Leptin reduces food intake, increases activity and energy expenditure and is also a respiratory stimulant, increasing the ventilatory response to carbon dioxide.

Leptin resistance may contribute to the obesity hypoventilation syndrome. Treatment with CPAP reduces the leptin level in OSA independently of any effect on the body mass index.

The increase in sympathetic activity probably increases the energy expenditure despite the reduction in physical activity that is seen in OSA during the day. At night there is increased energy expenditure due to the high work of breathing and frequent arousals, and the movements that these cause.

Complications of obstructive sleep apnoeas

Hypercapnic respiratory failure

Chronic hypercapnia during wakefulness is an infrequent, but well-recognized complication of OSA [18]. It may present with early morning headaches in addition to excessive daytime sleepiness and other features of OSA. It is often associated with right heart failure and this combination represents the clinical picture of what was in the past known as the 'Pickwickian syndrome' or obesity hypoventilation syndrome (OHS). This comprises obesity, which is a risk factor for OSA, with excessive daytime sleepiness and respiratory and right heart failure, which is due to pulmonary hypertension.

Hypercapnia in OSA occasionally occurs in those who live alone, in whom the lack of social contact delays their presentation until an advanced stage in the natural history has been reached. More commonly it is associated with one or more of the following.

Gross obesity

This causes narrowing and intermittent obstruction of the upper airway which increases the work of breathing, but other effects such as the mass-loading of the chest wall muscles by the fat around the rib cage and abdomen which reduces the compliance of the chest wall, decreased contractility of the chest wall muscles, overstretching of the diaphragm and impairment of ventilation–perfusion matching may all contribute to respiratory failure.

Chronic lung disease

Chronic lung disease, such as chronic bronchitis and emphysema (chronic obstructive pulmonary disease, COPD), may cause hypoventilation when it occurs with OSA. Hypercapnia rarely occurs if the FEV1 is greater than 1.01–1.5 l without OSA, but if this is also present the FEV1 may be reduced to only around 2.0 l.

Neuromuscular disorders

The weak chest wall muscles may be unable to compensate for the increased work of breathing through a narrow upper airway, so that hypoventilation and hypercapnia develop, particularly if the patient is also obese, takes sedative drugs or alcohol. Sleep fragmentation reduces the respiratory drive and respiratory muscle function, which may lead to failure to fully reverse any oxygen desaturation during an apnoea before the next apnoea begins. The most common neuromuscular disorders causing hypercapnia with OSA are congenital myopathies, muscular dystrophies, and previous poliomyelitis.

Cardiac dysrhythmias

The physiological dysrhythmias occurring during OSA have been described on page 237. Other dysrhythmias are uncommon unless there is pre-existing cardiac disease, usually ischaemic heart disease. They include atrial and ventricular ectopics, atrial fibrillation and ventricular tachycardia. These dysrhythmias are most common if the oxygen saturation falls below around 75% and during REM sleep. Relapse of paroxysmal atrial fibrillation is less common once CPAP is started.

Myocardial infarction

There is an epidemiological association between OSA and myocardial infarction. This may be partly because of common confounding factors such as obesity, hypertension, diabetes and alcohol consumption, but OSA probably is an independent risk factor for myocardial infarction. This may be related to the effects of OSA on endothelial dysfunction, inflammatory mediators and an increased fibrinogen level, as well as its tendency to lead to diabetes mellitus and hypertension.

Stroke

Epidemiological studies have shown an association between OSA and strokes. This may be partly due to common risk factors such as obesity, alcohol consumption, age, diabetes mellitus and hypertension, but the link is probably a direct one. Strokes occur most frequently at 6.00–8.00 AM, suggesting that they are associated with the process of awakening, but no link has been found between OSA and the risk of transient cerebral ischaemic attacks.

The hypertensive surges during each apnoea may contribute to the risk of stroke, but sustained daytime hypertension is probably more important, together with endothelial dysfunction, inflammatory changes and increased fibrinogen, which are all seen in OSA. There also appears to be an increased risk of paradoxical embolization through a patent foramen ovale associated with severe oxygen desaturations during sleep [19].

OSA may occur following any type of stroke [20], but particularly with those involving the posterior inferior cerebellar artery, leading to pharyngeal and palatal dysfunction. Obstructive sleep apnoeas after a stroke correlate with early neurological deterioration and increased disability at 6 months, possibly because the lability of the blood pressure during each apnoea increases the extent of the cerebral damage. Treatment with nasal CPAP is poorly tolerated with only around 50% using it acutely and 10% at 3 months. Nasal CPAP could also have harmful effects, such as reducing the $P\text{CO}_2$, which leads to cerebral vasoconstriction.

Hypertension

Chronic hypertension is associated with obstructive sleep apnoeas even when confounding factors such as obesity, alcohol intake, diabetes mellitus and inactivity are taken into account. It is mainly due to sustained increased sympathetic activity during the day as a result of intermittent hypoxia at night. The blood pressure usually rises by around 3–5 mmHg.

Hypertension has been thought to be associated even with mild obstructive sleep apnoeas but is probably only significant when the desaturation index is greater than around 20 per hour. Hypertension is most closely associated with OSA between the ages of 30 and 50, possibly because of a greater sympathetic reaction to hypoxia in this age range, and may be drug resistant, although it is reversible with CPAP treatment.

Pre-eclampsia appears to be more common in pregnant women with OSA, possibly because of the systemic vasoconstriction that OSA lead to. It improves slightly with CPAP treatment [21].

Pulmonary hypertension

The changes in pulmonary artery pressure during each apnoea are reversible, but in certain situations chronic pulmonary hypertension develops. This requires the presence of hypoxia during the daytime in addition to during the OSA at night, as a result of, for instance, coexisting chronic airflow obstruction, severe ventilation–perfusion mismatching due to gross obesity, or hypoventilation due to neuromuscular or skeletal disorders.

Right ventricular hypertrophy develops and the pulmonary hypertension, together with endocrine and metabolic responses to hypoxia and hypercapnia, leads to right heart failure, usually at the time that daytime hypercapnia develops.

The pulmonary artery pressure may only fall slightly with CPAP treatment, at least in the short term, because persistent pulmonary hypertension causes vascular remodelling and structural changes in the pulmonary microcirculation.

Clinical features in adults

Obstructive sleep apnoeas are often asymptomatic but if they become frequent or severe a variety of clinical manifestations may be seen. The most prominent features are discussed below.

Noisy breathing in sleep

Sleep apnoeas usually follow many years of loud snoring and are associated with a change in the pattern of the noise. At the end of the apnoea the airway snaps open with a loud snorting or similar noise. The variety of irregular snoring noises indicates how many different patterns of hypopnoea, apnoea and arousal can occur. Acoustic frequency analysis of these noises shows them to be distinct from simple snoring, and a stridor-like character suggests that the obstruction is arising at laryngeal level. Noisy breathing during sleep can be confused with asthma or stridor, and in children with grunting.

The noises of OSA during sleep are complained of by the partner rather than the patient. The lack of a sleeping partner may delay referral for medical assessment and the diagnosis of OSA.

Awakenings from sleep

The partner may report that the patient stops breathing at night, often with a description of starting again with a gasp and jerking movements. The subject may wake feeling startled and that he or she has woken suddenly for no obvious reason. If the arousal occurs slightly earlier, there may be an awareness of the noise generated by the OSA, and if arousal occurs even earlier there is a sensation of choking since the airway is still closed. These episodes of choking should be distinguished from vocal cord adduction, which is often due to gastro-oesophageal reflux, nocturnal asthma and left ventricular failure.

Restlessness during sleep

At the moment of arousal from an OSA the subject often jerks, jumps, or jolts either the limbs or the whole body. The patient is rarely aware of these movements, but the partner frequently complains of them. They should be distinguished from nocturnal epilepsy, periodic limb movements in sleep or other motor disorders of sleep.

Other symptoms during sleep

Nocturia

This is due to excessive secretion of ANP with reduction in renin and aldosterone secretion. The stimulus to ANP production is right atrial distension due to the increased venous return in response to the increased negative inspiratory intrathoracic pressure and to transient pulmonary hypertension during each apnoea. Nocturia only occurs if OSA is severe, but can be confused with nocturia due to other causes such as benign prostatic hypertrophy, and it may occasionally lead to incontinence.

Gastro-oesophageal reflux

This may result from the repetitive Mueller manoeuvres during OSAs.

Excessive sweating

This is related to sympathetic over-activity.

Confusional arousals

These are occasionally seen following an arousal from OSA, particularly from stages 3 and 4 NREM sleep.

Nocturnal angina

Coronary artery blood flow falls during apnoeas because of vasoconstriction and changes in left ventricular stroke volume, and nocturnal angina may develop. Ischaemic electrocardiogram changes appear if there is pre-existing coronary artery disease, and are more common in REM sleep, and during long apnoeas with deep oxygen desaturations.

Sleepiness

Excessive daytime sleepiness is a characteristic effect of OSA [22]. Its severity is mainly related to the number of arousals from sleep, particularly NREM sleep. There may be a minimum duration of an arousal which contributes to excessive daytime sleepiness, or of sleep between arousals, which protects against this. The degree of sleepiness is not closely related to any objective measure of severity of sleep apnoeas, such as the apnoea–hypopnoea index, and depends on other factors such as individual vulnerability, sleep fragmentation, the individual's sleep requirements, the presence of other sleep disorders, such as periodic limb movements during sleep, and whether or not the subject is a shift worker.

It is usual for patients to wake feeling unrefreshed after a night's sleep and, while alertness often improves during the morning, sleepiness usually returns during the afternoons, particularly during monotonous activities and in passive situations. Sleepiness may develop during driving and the risk of road traffic accidents is increased by around six times in those with OSA if this is severe [23].

Cognitive effects

The ability to maintain attention and to concentrate falls and short-term memory, verbal fluency and motor skills deteriorate [24, 25]. Alterations in mood, particularly irritability and occasionally depression, may develop. Episodes of automatic behaviour with little recall of the events are common.

These neuropsychological changes have important implications for the quality of life. Marital and occupational difficulties because of loss of productivity at work may arise. An inability to develop interpersonal relationships may lead to loss of social contacts and recreational activities with the risk of secondary anxiety and depression. Depression may occur in children as well as in adults and is often associated with a reduction in self-respect and a feeling of loss of control. There is often guilt about disturbing the sleep of the partner, who may become frustrated and angry at the impact of the sleep apnoeas on his or her sleep, as well as fearful about the consequences of the apnoeas for the patient. The noisy breathing and physical restlessness of the OSA subject often leads to the partner sleeping in a separate bed or separate bedroom, and to a deterioration in their relationship. All these changes are probably reversible with effective treatment of the OSA, although there is some evidence that subtle cognitive abnormalities may persist.

Other daytime symptoms

These include the following.

1 *Frontal headaches*. These occur on waking, possibly related to the increased intracranial pressure during OSA, particularly in REM sleep, and occasionally to hypercapnia.

2 *A sore throat*. A dry and sore throat on waking is usually due to mouth breathing due to nasal obstruction.

3 *Reduced libido and impotence*. This is partly due to EDS resulting from sleep fragmentation and partly to reduced testosterone levels due to a reduction in gonadotrophin secretion during sleep. There are also fewer penile erections during sleep because of REM sleep fragmentation.

Natural history of obstructive sleep apnoeas in adults

OSA is usually preceded by many years of stable snoring which then worsens gradually or sometimes quite rapidly before the symptoms of OSA become prominent. Weight gain may accelerate the deterioration at the time that OSA is evolving from simple snoring. Snoring which can be reliably dated to childhood and which is still a problem in adult life is often due to enlarged tonsils or a skeletal abnormality of the face or mandible. Occasionally, OSA arises suddenly in adult life, in which case it is usually due to an identifiable event such as a stroke or facial injury, or to the development of a contributory disorder such as hypothyroidism. Nocturia, early morning headaches due to hypercapnia, and features of right heart failure develop late in the natural history of OSA.

Life expectancy

The severity of OSA is related to the increased risk of death. This may be as high as 20% at 5 years and 35% at 8 years in middle-aged males when the apnoea–hypopnoea index exceeds 20 per hour [26]. Death may be due to accidents, for instance while driving or at work, especially while handling moving machinery, or may occur as a result of strokes, myocardial infarction, cardiac dysrhythmias and consequences of hypertension.

The life expectancy of women with OSA is shorter than that of men. The cause of this is uncertain, but it may be because of a delay in presentation, a gender-specific susceptibility to endothelial dysfunction in response to repeated episodes of hypoxia, the presence of more comorbidity or poorer compliance with CPAP (see below).

OSA is rarely a cause of death in children, unless it is severe and unrecognized and leads to respiratory and right heart failure. In the elderly its relationship to premature death is uncertain since it is usually only one of several factors contributing to a fatal event such as a stroke or myocardial infarction.

Obstructive sleep apnoeas and gender

Obstructive sleep apnoeas, upper airway resistance syndrome and snoring are all at least twice as common in men as in women. The risk in women is five times greater after the menopause and twice as great while taking hormone replacement treatment, compared to before the menopause.

Women tend to complain more of fatigue rather than excessive daytime sleepiness and of difficulty in initiating and maintaining sleep at night, and perhaps for these reasons are less likely to be diagnosed as having OSA until it is more advanced. The risk of road traffic accidents in men with OSA is greater than in women, probably because it causes more sleepiness. Survival is shorter in women than in men, even when adjusted for obesity. This may be partly because of delayed diagnosis or increased comorbidity, but women also appear to have greater endothelial dysfunction due to sleep apnoeas which may predispose to atheroma and cardiovascular complications [27]. Compliance with CPAP may also be less than in males.

The mechanisms underlying the gender differences in OSA [28] include the following.

Endocrine differences
There may be a protective effect of oestrogen or progesterone or both in premenopausal women mediated through differences in the respiratory drive, dimensions of the upper airway structures, or distribution of fat in the neck relative to the rest of the body [29] in postmenopausal women.

Fat deposition
At any body mass index women have fewer sleep apnoeas than men, probably because in males the fat is deposited more centrally, particularly in the neck and abdomen, which predisposes to airway obstruction [29].

Anatomical factors
The lateral pharynx is narrower in men than in women and men also have a longer and more collapsible pharynx. Sleep apnoeas in the supine position are more common in men than in women.

Physiological factors
Males have a higher apnoeic threshold than women. This predisposes to central sleep apnoeas during NREM sleep-stage transitions. The hyperventilation related to arousal at the end of sleep apnoeas lowers the $P\text{CO}_2$ and if this falls below the apnoeic threshold it will lead to a central sleep apnoea. The upper airway tends to occlude during the prolonged expiration of a central sleep apnoea, particularly if the $P\text{CO}_2$ is low.

This difference in apnoeic threshold is probably hormone related. Administration of testosterone to women raises it to the male level and anti-androgens in men shift it to the female level.

Obstructive sleep apnoeas in children

Sleep apnoeas are particularly common between the ages of 2 and 6 years when the size of the tonsils and adenoids relative to the airway diameter is greater, although abnormalities in the development of upper airway muscle control may also be important at these ages [30]. At this age around 10% of children snore and 1% have OSA. Sleep apnoeas are equally common in boys and girls and, except in conditions such as the Prader–Willi syndrome, obesity is often absent. In normal children the upper airway is less collapsible than in adults but this may not be the case in those with OSA. Children are less likely to arouse from sleep apnoeas than adults, probably because their sleep is more consolidated.

The most common clinical features are snoring-like noises during sleep associated with observation by the parents or carers that the child stops breathing and is a restless sleeper [31]. Unusual sleeping positions may be adopted and there may be enuresis. Excessive daytime sleepiness is unusual, but behavioural disturbances during the day are frequent, and include irritability, hyperactivity, aggression, poor school performance with problems with reading and visual attention, and rapid mood changes. Impulsivity may be sufficient to lead to an initial diagnosis of attention deficit hyperactivity disorder (ADHD). There is often developmental delay, and if OSA is severe there may be failure to thrive. Short stature is probably due to reduction in secretion of growth hormone through fragmentation of the initial episode of stages 3 and 4 NREM sleep at night. Mid-face hypoplasia and pectus excavatum may develop and if sleep apnoeas remain unrecognized right heart failure eventually occurs.

The common causes, apart from obesity, are as follows.
1 Enlarged tonsils and adenoids.
2 Retrognathia and micrognathia, e.g. Pierre–Robin sequence, Treacher–Collins syndrome.
3 Craniofacial abnormalities, especially micrognathia and mid-face hypoplasia, e.g. Down's, Apert's and Crouzon's syndromes.
4 Systemic disorders, e.g. Prader–Willi syndrome, achondroplasia, cerebral palsy, mucopolysaccharidoses, sickle cell disease and Down's syndrome.
5 Chronic neuromuscular disorders, e.g. Duchenne's muscular dystrophy. These cause a loss of pharyngeal muscle tone.
6 Nasal obstruction.

Investigations

Oximetry normally shows no desaturations in children, and even a desaturation index of 1 per hour may indicate significant obstructive sleep apnoeas. Oximetry alone may not, however, be sufficiently sensitive and a sleep study with a home video and ideally an audio recording in addition may be helpful. Polysomnography is rarely used and difficult to interpret because adult scoring criteria are not valid in young children and there are few normal values.

Treatment

Weight loss

Treatment of rhinitis
This should be treated wherever possible, for instance with inhaled nasal steroids.

Adenotonsillectomy
A tonsillectomy with adenoidectomy is the treatment of choice and should be performed in most children with OSA. Surgery should be considered even if the tonsils and adenoids are not markedly enlarged since it is not their absolute size, but their size relative to the airway diameter, that is important. Adenotonsillectomy is effective in around 90% of children, except in conditions such as Down's syndrome and craniofacial

abnormalities where other factors contribute to the OSA. The long-term effects on immunological function of adenotonsillectomy are unknown. If surgery is contraindicated, e.g. in Down's syndrome or in cerebral palsy, systemic steroids may be of help.

Nasopharyngeal tubes
These may be useful temporarily in micrognathia if mandibular growth is expected in the first few months of life, e.g. in Pierre–Robin sequence and occasionally in Apert's and Crouzon's syndromes.

Mandibular advancement devices
These are poorly tolerated in children and there is a risk of altering facial growth.

Palatal surgery
This should be avoided in children unless there are congenital palatal abnormalities, because of the risk of alterations of speech and swallowing.

Orthognathic surgery
The use of mandibular and maxillary surgery is largely confined to congenital craniofacial abnormalities in children, in whom it may be very effective.

Resection of tongue base
This may be useful in Down's syndrome.

Tracheostomy
This is rarely required, except occasionally in neuromuscular disorders.

Nasal CPAP and bilevel pressure support
These systems are effective in most situations and are usually indicated if weight loss and adenotonsillectomy fail.

Obstructive sleep apnoeas in the elderly

Snoring is less commonly reported in the elderly, possibly because of the partner's deteriorating hearing, because the partner is in a separate bed or bedroom, or because the snorer lives alone. Obstructive sleep apnoeas, however, appear to become progressively more common in older age, although over the age of 60 the gender difference between males and females is less than in younger adults and obesity is less important. The familial association of OSA persists into old age. In women there is an increased prevalence of OSA after the menopause.

The diagnosis of OSA is often delayed in the elderly because of other medical conditions which mask its effects. Age-related symptoms such as nocturia, impotence, the need for naps during the day, waking at night and fatigue may be readily confused with symptoms of OSA and delay its diagnosis. Central sleep apnoeas and Cheyne–Stokes respiration are also more common than in younger adults.

OSA has less direct impact on symptoms and the quality of life in the elderly than in younger subjects. Nevertheless obstructive sleep apnoeas probably have the same additional cardiovascular risk as in younger subjects and may present with drug resistance hypertension. They are also associated with heart failure. OSA are in effect a cofactor with other conditions which contribute to morbidity and mortality, and are usually only one of several risk factors for cerebrovascular and ischaemic heart disease in this age group.

Assessment

History

A careful history is essential to accurately assess disorders of the upper airway (Chapter 3, Table 10.3). The issues that should be considered are as follows.

1 What noise is generated? Enquiries regarding the duration, severity and type of noise, and whether it is becoming louder or more frequent, should be made.

2 What is the respiratory pattern while the noise is being generated? The partner may be aware of how breathing starts and stops, and what noises are associated with this. The patient is occasionally aware of waking suddenly for no apparent reason, or with the noise or with a sensation of choking.

3 Are there any other associated symptoms, e.g. physical restlessness during sleep, nocturia?

4 How severe is the EDS? Is the patient unrefreshed on waking in the morning and does he or she fall asleep only in situations requiring a passive role or in more active situations as well? What is the impact of EDS on the subject's lifestyle, particularly with regard to school or work performance and family, driving, social and recreational activity? Is an excessive quantity of caffeinated drinks taken in order to cope with EDS?

5 What is the cause of any upper airway obstruction? Has the subject gained weight or increased their collar size? Are there symptoms of nasal obstruction? Does the subject smoke, drink alcohol, take any medication and are there any problems with sleep hygiene leading to sleep deprivation? Is there any significant medical history, for instance, of facial or nasal injury, or of a neuromuscular disorder which might induce laryngeal obstruction? Has previous surgery for snoring been carried out on the upper airway?

Physical examination

These questions should be supplemented by physical examination, particularly with regard to weight, presence of obesity, any upper airway abnormalities, retrognathia and any abnormalities of the neck. A neurological or thoracic examination is only indicated if neuromuscular or lung diseases may be contributing to the symptoms of upper airway obstruction, but the blood pressure should be noted and signs of pulmonary hypertension and right heart failure sought if OSA is severe.

Observation of the patient during sleep reveals either noisy breathing or intermittent silences during the apnoeas followed by a snort or similar noise at their termination. During the apnoea the rib cage and abdomen move paradoxically. During inspiration the abdomen expands and the rib cage is drawn in, and in expiration the converse is seen. This contrasts with

Table 10.3 When to suspect obstructive sleep apnoeas from the symptoms.

Cardinal symptoms	Snoring and snorting at night, usually with observation of stopping breathing or struggling to breathe *plus* waking unrefreshed and falling asleep readily during the day
Supportive symptoms	Nocturnal choking or breathlessness Nocturia (if OSA severe) Nocturnal restlessness Poor memory and concentration Irritability

OSA, obstructive sleep apnoea.

Table 10.4 Sleep study techniques for obstructive sleep apnoea.

Technique	Physiological measurement	Abnormality detected
Nasal thermistor End-tidal P_{CO_2} Nasal pressure	Airflow	Apnoea
Plethysmography 　(inductance, impedance) Magnetometry	Rib cage and abdominal movement	Airflow obstruction
Oximeter	SaO_2	O_2 desaturation
Transcutaneous P_{CO_2}	Transcutaneous CO_2	Hypoventilation
EEG EOG EMG	Awake–asleep Sleep stage	Cortical and behavioural arousals
ECG Pulse transit time Finger plethysmography	Heart rate Blood pressure	Chest wall muscle activity and autonomic 　arousals
Microphone	Noises due to airflow through upper airway	Snoring and snorting
Oesophageal pressure	Intrapleural pressure	Chest wall muscle activity due to OSA
Actigraphy Video recording	Movements	'Behavioural' arousals and respiratory pattern

ECG, electrocardiogram; EEG, electro-encephalogram; EMG, electro-myogram; EOG, electro-oculogram; OSA, obstructive sleep apnoeas.

diaphragmatic weakness where there is inward movement of the abdomen during inspiration in the supine position.

Investigations

Initial investigations

Initial investigations include thyroid function tests if hypothyroidism is suspected, arterial blood gases and haemoglobin concentration if sleep apnoeas are severe and respiratory failure is possible, and an electrocardiogram and echocardiogram if there is a possibility of right ventricular complications. A chest X-ray and respiratory functions tests are only required if there is a coexisting respiratory disorder.

Assessment of daytime sleepiness

An estimate of daytime sleepiness, such as the Epworth Sleepiness Scale, is advisable. In certain situations, such as assessing fitness to drive heavy goods vehicles, further tests such as maintenance of wakefulness tests and multiple sleep latency tests, or performance tests, such as driving simulators, may be indicated.

Sleep study

The range of sleep study techniques for identifying the various manifestations of OSA have been described in Chapter 3 (Table 10.4). The criteria for selecting the most appropriate techniques have not been settled and a balance has to be struck between the costs and benefits of the different types of studies. The costs include the price of equipment, the need for the sleep study to be carried out in hospital, the time of technical and other staff in setting up the study and interpreting the results, and the failure rate of the test. The benefits are usually assessed as the frequency with which the criteria for the diagnosis of OSA are demonstrated or the certainty with which this diagnosis is excluded, but the real value of these tests is more difficult to define. They should record the frequency of apnoeas and arousals that these cause, but, equally importantly, they should assess the risk to the individual of adverse events if treatment is not provided and be able to predict the effectiveness of any intervention with treatment.

None of the available techniques, even polysomnography, has been adequately evaluated from these points of view. An additional factor is that the degree of certainty in the diagnosis that is required before recommending a simple treatment, such as weight loss, is less than what is needed before initiating complex treatments, such as CPAP, and this has implications for the type of sleep study that is required.

Half-night studies have been shown to be less sensitive than overnight studies, although they may be adequate if the OSA is severe. Nap studies during the day have the same problems, but are usually less costly. Occasionally, a second night study is needed, particularly if the patient shows the 'first night effect' and sleeps poorly during the test, or if no REM sleep or sleep in the supine position is obtained during the first night. In general, studies in the home provide less data than hospital studies, but sleep quality is often better, with more stages 3 and 4 NREM sleep.

These considerations suggest that different types of sleep study should be performed according to the pretest probabilities of each diagnosis and the treatment options [32, 33]. These situations include the following.

Population screening

A cheap, easily applied, sensitive, but not necessarily highly specific test is advisable. Oximetry is the most appropriate.

Low clinical probability for OSA

Excessive daytime sleepiness, but with no known snoring or risk factors such as obesity, is an example. A simple screening study such as oximetry, possibly with monitoring of chest wall movements or the pulse transit time, may be sufficient to exclude OSA and to suggest whether or not there is a non-respiratory cause for excessive daytime sleepiness.

Intermediate and high clinical probability for OSA

Snoring with observed apnoeas and excessive daytime sleepiness is an example. Confirmation of apnoeas or paradoxical rib cage and abdominal movements, or desaturations, is required. Oximetry, ideally with a chest wall movement detector and airflow sensor, provides this information. The frequency of arousals can be assessed either from heart rate or from pulse transit time variations.

Complex clinical presentation

Excessive daytime sleepiness with snoring plus symptoms of the restless legs syndrome is an example. Polysomnography is advisable to evaluate the relative contributions of each of the possible causes.

Failure to respond to CPAP treatment

If compliance with CPAP is satisfactory and an adequate pressure is provided, there is a high probability that an undiagnosed and probably non-respiratory factor is responsible for the persisting symptoms. Polysomnography is the investigation of choice.

Treatment

The aims of treatment of OSA are:
1 Relief of symptoms and improvement in the quality of life.
2 Reduction of the risk of accidents.
3 Prevention of medical complications such as hypertension, myocardial infarction, strokes and premature death.

The treatments used to achieve these aims fall into several groups.

Established first-line treatments

These can be initiated in general practice, often without the need for a sleep study, and are aimed at relieving the factors which contribute to upper airway obstruction.

Weight loss

Weight loss should be attempted in patients who are obese, particularly if weight gain has coincided with an increase in neck size indicated by a change in shirt collar requirements and a worsening of symptoms or of sleep study findings. It is of help in around 50% of obese subjects with OSA, but weight is frequently regained.

Hypnotics

Benzodiazepines and other hypnotics should be avoided.

Alcohol intake

The intake of alcohol should be reduced.

Smoking cessation

Stopping smoking may help, but often leads to weight gain which worsens the OSA.

Improvement in nasal airway

This may be achieved with treatment for, for instance, rhinitis with inhaled steroids or with external or internal mechanical nasal dilators (page 249) or surgery (page 250).

Sleeping on the side rather than in the supine position

'Postural' or 'positional' treatment is difficult to maintain [34]. This type of treatment is said to lead to a conditioned reflex whereby the lateral position is maintained, but there is little evidence for this. Sleeping with a pillow wedged under the shoulders to prevent returning to the supine position is preferable to fixing a ball, foam or similar object into the back of the nightclothes since this causes arousals from sleep each time the supine position occurs [35]. Equipment which delivers an electric shock when it detects a snoring sound works on similar principles and has similar disadvantages.

Sleeping with the neck slightly extended may help prevent OSA by increasing the pharyngeal diameter.

Avoidance of sleep deprivation

Sleep deprivation reduces the respiratory drive to both hypoxia and hypercapnia, increases the threshold for arousal, alters sleep architecture and may impair upper airway muscle function.

Drug treatment of cause

Obstructive sleep apnoeas due to endocrine abnormalities such as hypothyroidism or acromegaly may be effectively treated by drug or other therapy of the underlying condition. Appetite suppressants, such as sibutramine, and drugs that prevent fat absorption, such as orlistat, may also be effective in the obese.

Non-established treatments

Oxygen

This abolishes the desaturations detected in sleep studies, but apnoeas may be more prolonged because it removes the hypoxic drive to breathe and to arousal. There is also a risk of nocturnal hypercapnia in severe OSA. Little change of sleep quality or daytime symptoms has been reported.

Surface active and muscle activating agents

Application of preparations containing chemicals that alter the surface properties of the upper airway or increase the muscle tone has been used, but there is little evidence regarding their effectiveness.

Muscle training

Attempts have been made to train the pharyngeal muscles by vocal exercises and singing so that they are more active during sleep, but these are ineffective.

Electrical stimulation of upper airway muscles

Implantation of electrical stimulation devices triggered by changes in rib cage movements, to 'pace' the pharyngeal dilator muscles in time with inspiration, have been developed. Direct stimulation of the hypoglossal (12th cranial) nerve, with hook electrodes, and of the genioglossus muscle has been employed. It is important that the site of obstruction is localized to the base of the tongue before these are attempted.

Ventilatory stimulant drugs

Progesterone is ineffective in relieving OSA and while theophyllines may have a slight effect they have the disadvantage of reducing the total sleep time. Almitrine, acetazolamide and doxapram are also ineffective.

Modification of upper airway muscle control and function

5HT agonists can increase genioglossal activity in animals, but have not been shown to be effective in humans, probably because of the complex effects of 5HT receptors and the range of other neurotransmitters that control upper airway function.

REM sleep suppressant drugs

Both tricyclic antidepressants and selective serotonin re-uptake inhibitors (SSRIs) reduce the duration of REM sleep and are effective if OSA are confined or almost confined to REM sleep. Protriptyline 5–20 mg nocte has been most widely used, but has been withdrawn in the UK. It is non-sedating, but side-effects such as constipation and urinary retention are common with a dose of more than around 10 mg. Selective serotonin re-uptake inhibitor antidepressants, such as paroxetine, may also reduce the loss of upper airway muscle activity during NREM sleep. They reduce the frequency of OSA in NREM sleep slightly.

Second-line treatments

These are reserved for subjects who have frequent and severe OSA, who have daytime hypercapnia, or who are resistant to first-line measures, either because they are ineffective or because of poor compliance. Referral to a specialist centre is usually required for a sleep study and assessment for these treatments (Fig. 10.4). They fall into four groups.

Wakefulness promoting drugs

Modafinil has been shown to improve excessive daytime sleepiness in OSA when other treatments have failed or are contraindicated. It does not treat the

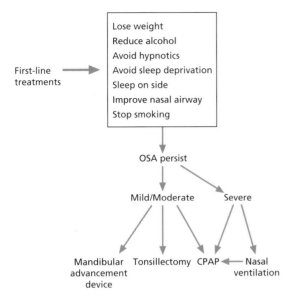

Fig. 10.4 Treatment of obstructive sleep apnoeas (OSA). CPAP, continuous positive airway pressure; REM, rapid eye movement.

physiological effects of OSA such as transient hypertension during apnoeas, and its effect on preventing long-term complications such as strokes or myocardial infarction is unknown. It should, however, be considered if excessive daytime sleepiness persists despite optimization of treatment, particularly nasal CPAP. Treatment with modafinil has not been shown to reduce compliance with nasal CPAP.

Mechanical devices

Nasal dilators
These reduce the nasal resistance to airflow and thereby cause the intrapharyngeal pressure to be less negative and reduce the likelihood that the airway will close. Internal nasal dilators have a spring which stretches the nares. They only dilate the anterior part of the airway, may be difficult to tolerate and often become displaced. External dilators are applied to the nose just anterior to the distal end of the nasal cartilage. They are better tolerated, rarely become displaced and are probably at least as effective as the internal dilators.

Soft palate supports
These devices keep the soft palate and uvula elevated, but are poorly tolerated and there is little evidence regarding their effectiveness.

Tongue retaining and protrusion devices
These prevent the tongue from falling back into the pharyngeal airway and in addition may cause mandibular advancement. They do not have any effect on dentition or the temporomandibular joints, but increase the production of saliva. A suction bulb is used to anchor the tip of the tongue to the teeth or lips and hold it forwards. This causes soreness of the tongue, with poor tolerance of the treatment, although it can be moderately effective.

Mandibular advancement or positioning devices
These hold the mandible and hyoid forwards during sleep and may also modify upper airway muscle activity [36]. The contraction of the genioglossus muscle is increased, possibly because it is stretched, and it becomes less compliant. The dimensions of the upper airway are increased, particularly at the level of the tongue base rather than at palatal level. The diameter increases especially anteroposteriorly, but also laterally, due to an effect on the anterior and posterior digastric muscles.

There are two main types of mandibular advance devices. First, soft thermoplastic one-piece devices, similar to a gum shield, which can be individually moulded by the subject to fit over the upper and lower teeth. Some of these have an orifice to enable mouth breathing to take place, but they are non-adjustable, bulky and only enable limited protrusion of the mandible. The two-piece devices, which are of harder material and usually individually made by a dental surgeon from a dental impression, have hooks and ridges which join the two parts. These can be adjusted to vary the degree of jaw protrusion for each individual, even during the night if necessary. They are lightweight and may be better tolerated than the one-piece designs.

Both types of device should allow some lateral as well as vertical jaw movement so that the patient can talk and yawn, and to reduce temporomandibular joint problems, but they should prevent any anteroposterior movement of the mandible. They should lead to only minimal (3 mm) vertical opening of the mouth, since this rotates the mandible and narrows the airway. The advancement of the mandible should be approximately 75% of the distance between the natural resting position and the most protruded position possible, as long as this is comfortable. An inability to protrude the mandible more than 0.6 cm makes it unlikely that a mandibular advancement device will be effective.

The indications for mandibular advancement devices are mild to moderate obstructive sleep apnoeas which are unresponsive to first-line treatments and in which surgery or CPAP either have failed or are contraindicated. The devices are most beneficial in the following situations.

1 If the apnoeas originate at the level of the base of the tongue, especially if there is retrognathia.
2 If the apnoeas are worse in the supine position [37].
3 If the apnoeas are mild or moderate.
4 In subjects who cannot tolerate alternative treatments such as CPAP.

The contraindications to mandibular advancement devices are as follows.

1 Temporomandibular joint dysfunction.
2 Insufficient or excessively mobile anterior teeth, dentures which are removed at night, extensive dental crown and bridge work, and periodontal disease.
3 Marked obesity, which mass-loads the airway whatever the body position.
4 Nasal obstruction with devices which impede oral breathing. Most newer single-piece devices and all two-piece devices allow oral breathing.
5 Poorly controlled epilepsy.

Mandibular advancement devices often cause discomfort, increased salivation, particularly in the first two weeks, a perception of an abnormal bite, dental hypersensitivity and gagging. They may become displaced, especially if the gums of the lower jaw are not covered with single-piece devices. There may be long-term effects on dental occlusion. Compliance is around 50% at 3 years.

These devices rarely completely abolish snoring, but may significantly improve mild to moderate obstructive sleep apnoeas. A reduction of the apnoea–hypopnoea index to less than 10 per hour is usually taken as a successful outcome. A reduction of around 50% of the number of sleep apnoeas is achievable in around 50% of those with sleep apnoeas. Improvements in daytime sleepiness, memory and ability to learn have been demonstrated with mandibular advancement devices. Localization techniques, such as sleep nasendoscopy, have been used as a predictor of response to this type of treatment, but there is little evidence regarding their value.

Surgery

Upper airway surgery has been proposed for OSA on the basis that it may widen the airway, cause scar tissue which reduces its compliance and alter upper airway reflexes beneficially [38]. It has the advantage of being a single procedure compared with most of the other treatments for OSA which require regular long-term application. The results of most surgical procedures, except adenotonsillectomy, have, however, been disappointing unless OSA is only mild. In general, upper airway surgery should be avoided in the obese, or if the airway obstructs at multiple sites or levels, since a localized surgical approach is unlikely to correct all of these.

The operations that have been proposed include the following.

Nasal surgery
This is rarely effective in OSA, although it may improve the sensation of nasal obstruction and occasionally enables a lower CPAP level to be effective.

Palatal surgery
This is rarely indicated in OSA, whether by a conventional surgical, laser or radio frequency technique. It is only effective in around 15% of those with significant OSA, and is hardly ever of value if OSA is severe. Palatal surgery may cause mouth leaks if CPAP is subsequently used with a nasal mask and an oronasal mask may be needed.

Tongue volume reduction surgery (linguoplasty)
Resection of the tongue base can be carried out surgically or with a laser or radio frequency technique. This may have a very limited application in OSA. The technique of suture suspension of the tongue base has been developed but its role in OSA is unknown.

Tonsillectomy and adenoidectomy
These are effective in around 90% of children. Tonsillectomy is also effective in adults if the tonsils are significantly enlarged.

Excision of obstructing mass
Excision of any mass which narrows the airway, such as an upper airway benign tumour, may improve OSA.

Laryngeal surgery
This may be of value if there are anatomical or neurological abnormalities affecting the larynx.

Orthognathic surgery
Orthognathic surgery primarily involves maxillary and mandibular advancement using osteotomy and rapid maxillary expansion techniques with screws to open the mid-palatal suture. These are particularly valuable

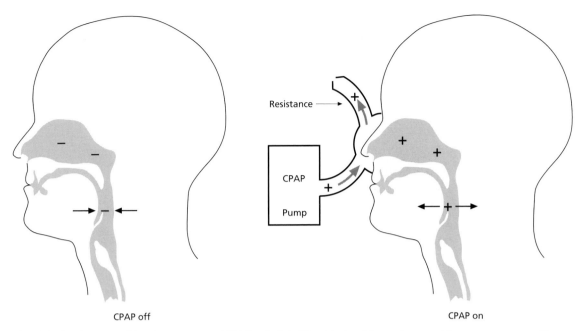

Fig. 10.5 Continuous positive airway pressure (CPAP) principle. The right-hand figure shows positive pressure generated by the CPAP pump being conducted to the upper airway and expanding it at pharyngeal level. The left-hand figure indicates spontaneous breathing without CPAP with negative pressure in the upper airway drawing the pharyngeal walls together.

for upper jaw abnormalities in children. These techniques advance the mid-face and jaw. Although around 10 mm bony advancement is usually sought, the soft tissues usually advance only 5–6 mm.

Orthognathic surgery is indicated in those with severe obstructive sleep apnoeas, usually with an apnoea–hypopnoea index of greater than 20 per hour, who have failed to improve or been intolerant of CPAP [39] and ideally have been shown to benefit from a mandibular advancement device, but could not tolerate it.

Assessment for orthognathic surgery is complex and involves detailed imaging of the upper airway. It should be carried out in specialist centres, but can be effective, especially if micrognathia or retrognathia is the cause of the OSA.

Initial complications of orthognathic surgery include damage to teeth, nerve injury, and infection. Late complications include dental malocclusion, temporomandibular joint discomfort and occasionally nasopharyngeal incompetence. Late skeletal relapse with narrowing of the airway is rare. There may also be cosmetic benefits in addition to improving sleep apnoeas.

Hyoid surgery
Hyoidoplasty involves moving the hyoid forward, or rotating it and fixing it to the anterior margin of the mandible or to the thyroid cartilage. It can be combined with mandibular advancement.

Tracheostomy
This was recommended frequently before nasal CPAP and other treatments were available. It bypasses the upper airway obstruction, but is now only required if OSA is life threatening and neither nasal CPAP nor intubation are available, or if CPAP cannot be tolerated or is ineffective, as occasionally occurs with laryngeal disorders. An alternative to a tracheostomy is insertion of a minitrach or transtracheal oxygen catheter.

Bariatic surgery
This does not have any direct effect on OSA, but by assisting weight loss it may indirectly improve it (page 14).

Nasal continuous positive airway pressure (CPAP) and bilevel pressure support
The principle of CPAP is that it increases the pressure within the upper airway during both inspiration and expiration (Fig. 10.5). It acts as a pneumatic splint, counteracting the forces that tend to close the airway. It may also have effects on upper airway reflexes

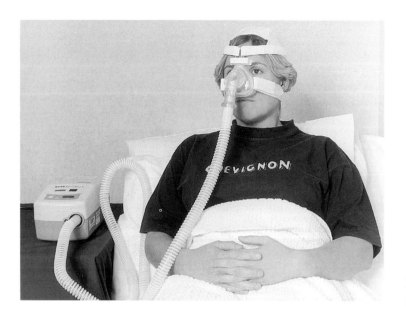

Fig. 10.6 Continuous positive airway pressure (CPAP) mask and pump.

which activate the upper airway dilator muscles. Continuous positive airway pressure also increases the functional residual capacity slightly. This increases the oxygen stores and therefore reduces the degree of oxygen desaturation during an apnoea. It also reflexly increases the upper airway diameter, reduces the left ventricular preload and reduces any pulmonary oedema.

Equipment
A CPAP system comprises the following.

Continuous positive airway pressure pump. This is a pump with a high flow capacity which delivers air at pressures which can be adjusted and then maintained almost constant during both inspiration and expiration (Fig. 10.6). The pressure can be kept at a fixed value throughout the night or varied or gradually reached over 20–30 min after the onset of sleep using a pressure 'ramp'. This is useful for patients who find it difficult to tolerate the required pressure while they are falling asleep.

Continuous positive airway pressure systems are powered either by mains electricity or by an external battery and most have a dual voltage or continually variable voltage facility. Their pressure range is around 4–20 cmH$_2$O, but the degree of pressure stability during each respiratory cycle varies between CPAP systems. The pressure tends to increase during expiration as air is added to the circuit from the patient, and to fall during inspiration according to the patient's

inspiratory flow rate. The CPAP level that is required is usually assessed by gradually increasing the pressure during the night of the study until indices of apnoeas, such as desaturations or evidence of airflow obstruction, are satisfactorily controlled. Use of predictive equations to assess the CPAP level is an unsatisfactory alternative, but methods such as the forced oscillation technique and variable pressure CPAP systems may be of value.

The noise of most CPAP systems is around 40 decibels. The air can be humidified with a heated water humidifier if necessary, usually because of nasal symptoms. Most CPAP systems have an electronic clock which measures either the duration for which the machine is switched on or the time for which a predetermined pressure is applied. The latter is of more value in assessing the patient's compliance since it measures the time that the CPAP is applied to the face rather than simply how long it has been switched on.

Continuous positive airway pressure circuit. This comprises the connecting tubing between the pump and the mask. An exhalation valve or leak is placed in the circuit close to the patient or in the mask in order to prevent rebreathing and carbon dioxide retention. The efficiency of these leaks or valves varies from system to system.

Mask and headgear. A nasal mask is usually sufficient, but occasionally a full face mask which includes the mouth as well is needed, either because of persistent mouth leaks or because the nasal airway is significantly blocked. The masks are made of silicon or similar inert flexible material and should be fitted individually to provide a comfortable seal around the nose, or nose and mouth. Nasal plugs or seals which fit into or around the nares are alternatives, particularly in patients who find masks claustrophobic. The mask, plugs or seals are held in place by headgear of a cap or strap design which fits around the skull.

Variable and fixed CPAP systems

Most CPAP systems are set to provide a fixed pressure during sleep, but variable pressure (intelligent, auto-continuous, auto-CPAP) machines alter the applied pressure according to algorithms designed to detect OSA. The CPAP level is adjusted on a breath by breath basis to prevent OSA [40], with the aim of abolishing microarousals and minimizing the applied pressure.

Some autotitrating CPAP systems sense vibrations similar to those which lead to snoring. Others detect airflow limitation from a flattening of the pressure profile, or using a forced oscillation technique in which small pressure oscillations are applied to the mouth and any increase in impedance indicates narrowing of the airway. All these techniques have limitations and may lead to inaccuracies associated with the subject being awake rather than asleep at night, mouth leaks, central sleep apnoeas or the presence of significant lung disease or cardiac failure.

Variable pressure CPAP systems have been used for the following purposes.

Diagnostic techniques. Their accuracy varies according to the methods used to adjust the pressure. None have been well evaluated. Errors particularly from mouth breathing and displacement of nasal pressure transducers may be significant, and none of the techniques assess whether the subject is asleep or awake.

Titration of CPAP level. The pressure which relieves 90 or 95% of obstructive episodes has been recommended, but artefacts and events during arousals often make interpretation difficult [41]. It is unknown exactly which obstructive events need to be eliminated, and if every episode of airflow limitation is to be responded to, the level of CPAP required will be significantly increased.

This technique does, however, have the advantage of reducing the costs associated with initially titrating CPAP since no supervision is needed. This loss of personal contact may reduce the patient's understanding and acceptance of the equipment and worsen long-term compliance.

Long-term treatment. Autotitrating CPAP systems usually have a slightly lower mean applied pressure than fixed pressure CPAP systems, but the peak pressure is higher and there is more pressure variation [42]. This may cause microarousals and sleep fragmentation. The pressure applied is usually greatest at sleep onset and in stages 1 and 2 NREM sleep, and lowest in stages 3 and 4 NREM sleep. There is also a danger that autotitrating systems may react inadequately and too slowly to hypoventilation during REM sleep and central sleep apnoeas.

Compliance has not been shown to be significantly improved with variable compared with fixed pressure systems [43]. Variable CPAP systems may be indicated in some groups of OSA patients, such as those in whom the required pressure differs substantially according to sleep stage and position, and who might require a significantly higher mean pressure with a fixed pressure system. Autotitrating CPAP systems are more expensive than fixed pressure systems.

Nasal bilevel pressure support ventilation

Nasal intermittent positive pressure ventilation (NIPPV) is occasionally required to treat OSA. The same system is used as for hypercapnic respiratory failure due to other conditions (page 272). A positive inspiratory pressure is combined with an expiratory pressure of approximately one-third of the inspiratory level. This combination both provides inspiratory support to increase the alveolar ventilation and also prevents the upper airway from closing during expiration.

Its indications are as follows.

Obesity hypoventilation syndrome. If the daytime P_{CO_2} is raised to more than about 7 kPa, nasal bilevel pressure support is usually preferable to nasal CPAP. Nasal positive pressure ventilation may only be required for a few days until sleep deprivation has been relieved and the P_{CO_2} has returned to normal. At that stage the transfer to nasal CPAP may be made, although NIPPV is occasionally required in the long term.

Poor compliance with CPAP because of a high pressure requirement. The high expiratory pressure may be difficult to tolerate, and use of a bilevel pressure system, in which the inspiratory pressure is usually around three times the expiratory pressure, is often of benefit, and reduces the severity of nasal side-effects.

Indications for CPAP

The indications for nasal CPAP treatment are as follows.

1 Troublesome symptoms from OSA, e.g. excessive daytime sleepiness or lifestyle complications, such as potential loss of employment as a professional driver.

2 Frequent obstructive sleep apnoeas (usually more than 15–20 per hour) which suggest that complications are likely unless treatment is provided [44]. The threshold for initiating CPAP should be lower in the presence of other cardiovascular risk factors or a history of angina, myocardial infarction or stroke.

3 Hypercapnia while awake. Treatment for the first few nights with nasal positive pressure ventilation may be needed before transferring to CPAP.

Side-effects of CPAP

Several problems may arise while CPAP is being used (Table 10.5). The most important are discussed below.

Air leaks. These may occur around the mask and although the CPAP pump can compensate for considerable leaks these should be minimized, particularly if the air is directed into or close to the eyes which can cause conjunctivitis. This can be prevented by a better fitting mask or headgear.

Table 10.5 CPAP complications and corrective measures.

Complication	Corrective measure
Air leak	Change mask or headgear Try chin strap or collar Alter head and neck position Consider face mask
Nasal symptoms	Inhaled steroid or ipratropium Minimize mouth leak Heated water humidification
Skin ulceration	Change mask or headgear Protect skin with, e.g., granuflex
Claustrophobia	Use smaller mask or nasal seals
Aerophagy	Reduce level of CPAP
Noise of CPAP	Reassure Ear plugs

CPAP, continuous positive airway pressure.

Air leaks through the mouth are common, and can be minimized by the use of a chin strap, collar and attention to the head and neck position, or if necessary the use of a face mask instead of a nasal mask.

Upper airway symptoms. The most common symptoms are a sensation of nasal blockage, nasal discharge or occasionally nose bleeds, dry mouth and throat. A blocked nose is often noticed within one or two nights of starting CPAP. Nasal symptoms may respond to inhaled nasal steroids, or if the nasal discharge is watery nasal ipratropium is of value. Correction of the unidirectional airflow by application of a chin strap or a full face mask often improves nasal symptoms, but if they persist, heated water humidification of the inspired air or the use of a face mask which includes the mouth as well as the nose are usually effective.

Skin problems. Soreness, redness and ulceration of the skin at the contact points with the mask are common. These can be prevented by attention to the mask selection and fitting, and to the headgear. Once an ulcer has formed a barrier such as granuflex is usually required to assist healing and this can also be used prophylactically. A *Staphylococcal* folliculitis occasionally occurs and responds to fucidic acid cream.

Claustrophobia. Some patients feel claustrophobic with a nasal or face mask, but may be able to tolerate nasal seals or plugs. Many subjects are able to overcome claustrophobia by gradually increasing the time they apply the nasal or oronasal mask.

Aerophagy. Air entering the pharynx under pressure may pass through the cricopharyngeal sphincter into the oesophagus instead of entering the trachea. Abdominal distension, belching and the passing of flatus rectally may result. Reduction in the CPAP level usually relieves these symptoms.

Noise. The noise of most CPAP systems is around 40 decibels, but the air leak from the mask or from the circuit close to the patient can also cause a disturbing noise. Ear plugs may be of help to either the patient or the partner.

Failure of continuous positive airway pressure

Continuous positive airway pressure treatment usually causes an improvement in symptoms and in sleep study findings even after a single night at an appropriate level. Failure to improve may, however, be due to one or more of the following.

Incorrect diagnosis. The apnoeas may be central rather than obstructive or the observed desaturations could be due to ventilation–perfusion mismatching rather than to apnoeas. OSA may not be the only diagnosis. Excessive daytime sleepiness may be mainly due to the restless legs syndrome or periodic limb movements, sleep restriction or shift work and OSA may be of secondary importance.

Insufficient CPAP level. The usual level of CPAP that is required is 5–15 cm or occasionally up to 20 cm of water. The pressure is usually adjusted so that oxygen desaturations and markers of autonomic arousal, such as heart rate changes, are abolished, but other criteria such as reduction in airflow limitation can be used. If the pressure is too low the apnoeas will only be partially relieved and symptoms may not disappear. A higher pressure is needed in the supine than in the lateral position and in REM than in stages 3 and 4 NREM sleep. The pressure that is required often falls slightly over the first few weeks after treatment is initiated, possibly because of relief of sleep fragmentation and of oedema of the upper airway. If the patient's weight changes the required CPAP level may alter again at a later stage.

Technical problems. Worsening leaks or nasal obstruction may prevent CPAP from being effective.

Poor compliance. Compliance with CPAP is often measured by the number of hours used per night, but a better measure is whether or not the CPAP use is sufficient to relieve symptoms. The time needed may be only around 4 h per night for many patients. Failure to achieve this may be due to inadequate education and explanation at the time of initiation of treatment, a pressure set too low, pressure-related side-effects, claustrophobia or rejection of the equipment psychologically by the patient or partner. Some patients take the CPAP mask off during their sleep, possibly during a confusional arousal, but use of a low-pressure alarm in the circuit which wakes the subject and alerts him or her to replace the mask is often effective.

Compliance is best if the patient has been well instructed and educated in the need for CPAP when it is initiated, if there is symptomatic improvement and if there are few initial side-effects [45]. Good compliance is associated with low anxiety, high self-esteem, an internal locus of control, and active coping strategies by the subject. Occasionally patients have difficulty in tolerating high CPAP levels, but this is not a factor for most subjects. It probably explains why the variable pressure CPAP systems have no compliance advantage over fixed pressure models.

Obese subjects under the age of 40 with worse symptoms and significant initial improvement have the best compliance rates. Regular follow-up with attention given to psychological aspects of accepting the equipment, relief of complications and modification of the CPAP level according to its effectiveness are all important in maintaining compliance. The compliance with nasal CPAP is greater than with most other treatments for long-term medical conditions such as hypertension or diabetes mellitus. The overall compliance rate varies between 45% and 90% in different centres, largely according to the selection of patients for CPAP, and the level of education and supervision that is provided.

Outcomes of CPAP treatment

Most of the effects of CPAP on OSA are apparent soon after starting effective treatment [46].

Symptoms. Symptoms both during the night and during the day improve within one or two nights and the improvement is virtually complete within around two weeks. Excessive daytime sleepiness improves both subjectively and objectively. The reduction in snoring and nocturnal restlessness often improves the partner's sleepiness as well. Mood changes, difficulty in concentrating and other cognitive problems usually resolve. The risk of road traffic accidents is reduced to the level of a normal subject with effective CPAP treatment [47], and the utilization of healthcare resources diminishes significantly. The overall quality of life improves.

A few patients, however, remain sleepy, despite regular use of CPAP. This may be due to either a pre-existing neurological abnormality or one that is induced by the apnoeas, possibly repeated brief episodes of hypoxia, which is irreversible.

Physiological changes. The obstructive apnoeas and desaturations are relieved by CPAP (Fig. 10.7). Sleep architecture usually returns to normal, but there is often REM sleep rebound during the first couple of nights after starting CPAP, particularly if OSA occur frequently during REM sleep and if there was sleep-onset REM before treatment was started.

The ventilatory response to carbon dioxide returns to normal and disturbed circadian rhythms, including

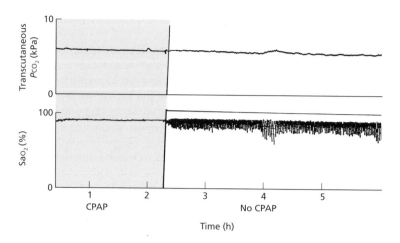

Fig. 10.7 Effects of continuous positive airway pressure (CPAP) on Sao_2 and transcutaneous Pco_2. Oximetry tracing in lower figure shows constant value of 95% using CPAP during the first third of the night, but without this there are frequent desaturations to a minimum of 66%. These are associated with transient rises in transcutaneous Pco_2 shown in the upper tracing indicating episodes of hypoventilation.

changes in the temperature cycle, are normalized. Most of the factors which increase the risk of cardiovascular disease, such as those affecting systemic inflammation and endothelial function, also improve, although long-term studies to assess whether this reduces the incidence of stroke and myocardial infarction have not been carried out. Fibrinogen levels and platelet activation and aggregation also return to normal with CPAP.

During the night the apnoeas and oxygen desaturations are relieved and rapid changes in blood pressure and heart rate during each apnoea disappear. Right ventricular function and pulmonary artery pressure during the day also normalize. CPAP reduces the upper airway resistance, increases functional residual capacity, reduces left ventricular afterload and sympathetic activity and the work of breathing. It may also reduce upper airway oedema by preventing repetitive vibration trauma.

Life expectancy. The effect of CPAP on life expectancy has not been established.

Discontinuation of CPAP treatment
Continuous positive airway pressure does not cure OSA but it is able to control or suppress the tendency to obstruct the upper airway. If CPAP is not used for any reason the OSA returns, although it may be several nights before its full intensity is seen because of factors, such as absence of sleep deprivation on the first night, which progress as the time without CPAP increases.

A trial without CPAP is justified if it is possible to treat or relieve the underlying cause of OSA. Loss of weight, treatment of, for instance, hypothyroidism or tonsillectomy may all enable CPAP to be withdrawn. If some OSA persists, an alternative treatment such as a mandibular advancement device can be tried.

Snoring

Overview
Simple snoring is a common problem in which noise is generated in the upper airway but is not associated with airflow limitation.

Prevalence
The prevalence of snoring is hard to assess because of the difficulty in quantifying it. It is usually complained of by the patient's partner who is only capable of reporting it if he or she is awake. It is said that around 35% of adults snore occasionally and 10% on most nights, and that it is approximately four times more common in men than in women. It is particularly common in children between the ages of 2 and 6, it becomes progressively less common through the teenage years after involution of the tonsils and adenoids, but becomes more frequent again in early middle age and increases in prevalence up to around the age of 75 years. Beyond this age it becomes less of a problem, because of the increase in prevalence of deafness among the partners.

Pathophysiology
Snoring is due to vibration of the tissues of the upper airway, usually during inspiration but occasionally during expiration or both. Unlike OSA there is no interruption of airflow into the lungs since the closure of the airway is at most only momentary and is not sustained throughout one or more inspirations. The

noise of snoring is generated by turbulent flow in the column of air in the upper airway.

Vibration of the upper airway can occur at any level down to the larynx but usually involves the soft palate, base of the tongue and posterior pharyngeal wall. There is no cortical or autonomic arousal from sleep during simple snoring since the work of the inspiratory muscles does not progressively increase as in OSA and the upper airway resistance syndrome.

Aetiology

The aetiology of simple snoring is similar to that of OSA.

Clinical features

The complaint of snoring almost invariably comes from a listener, usually the bed partner of the patient (Table 10.6). The complaint usually reflects the degree of sleep disruption or dissatisfaction of the partner and varies according to the partner's arousability from sleep by the noise and the presence of any insomnia. Snoring can lead to significant sleep disruption with excessive daytime sleepiness and frustration and anger in the partner. This may be expressed by repetitive physical attempts to wake the snorer who may then become secondarily sleep deprived and feel guilty about the sleep disruption that the snoring is causing to the partner. There is no evidence that snoring causes noise-induced deafness either in the patient or in the partner.

The volume of the snoring varies considerably between patients and during any one night. The pitch of snoring generated at different levels in the upper airway can be recognized by the experienced listener. A stridor-like sound usually arises from the larynx. Acoustic analysis has shown that the frequency of sound generated at palatal level is around 200 Hz with frequent harmonics and can be distinguished from tongue base (predominantly around 1000 Hz) and laryngeal snoring. Snoring may be continuous or intermittent and can build up to a crescendo, in which

Table 10.6 Clinical features of snoring.

Noise usually inspiratory
Snoring usually regular, if not suspect UARS or OSA
No EDS unless sleep disrupted by the partner, UARS or
    OSA
Partner's sleep disrupted

EDS, excessive daytime sleepiness; OSA, obstructive sleep apnoeas; UARS, upper airway resistance syndrome.

case the upper airway resistance syndrome or OSA should be suspected.

Snoring may remain constant or may fluctuate only slightly in severity and frequency over many years, but occasionally it evolves into the upper airway resistance syndrome or OSA, at which time the character of the snoring changes. Until that point other features of OSA are absent although epidemiological surveys have shown an increased prevalence of excessive daytime sleepiness and hypertension in snorers. This is probably because these populations included subjects with undiagnosed upper airway resistance syndrome and OSA.

Assessment

History

This is similar to that for obstructive sleep apnoeas (page 245).

Physical examination

Physical examination may reveal pathology within the upper airway, obesity or retrognathia, as with OSA. An attempt to simulate snoring may be helpful in indicating at which level it is arising, particularly if the noise is recognized by the partner as being identical to snoring during sleep.

Investigations

Referral for investigation is required if simple first-line measures are insufficient or if surgery is being considered.

The assessment of snoring is similar to that of OSA since it is important not only to assess the snoring itself, but also whether the subject has OSA, because the management of the two conditions often differs.

Investigation includes the following.

Assessment of excessive daytime sleepiness
In contrast to OSA and UARS, excessive daytime sleepiness is not a consequence of simple snoring unless the partner's response to the snoring causes sleep disruption.

Sleep studies
These are required to assess whether OSA are present or whether the problem is simple snoring.

Assessment of severity of snoring
The primary impact of snoring is on the listener rather than on the snorer. This is subjective and varies not

only according to the loudness, frequency and pattern of the snoring, but also with the partner's quality of sleep, sensitization to the snoring noise and their emotional response to the noise and to being woken during the night. A visual analogue score of the severity or frequency of the snoring completed by the partner may be of help in assessing its perceived severity.

Localization of source of snoring
Localization of the source of snoring may be important since some of the surgical procedures are site-specific treatment and are likely to be ineffective if snoring is occurring at a different level or several levels in the airway. Localization techniques are not often used in assessing whether or not a tonsillectomy should be performed, but could be of value.

The localization techniques include the following.

Acoustic analysis. Acoustic analysis with external microphones has indicated that snoring generated by palatal flutter has a low frequency, usually around 200 Hz with frequent harmonics. It can be distinguished from tongue base snoring which has a predominant frequency of around 1000 Hz in a more chaotic pattern.

There is considerable variation in the acoustic pattern during an individual night, which reduces its value as a predictor of which type of surgery is likely to be most effective. It has not been found to be of value in predicting whether OSA is present.

Imaging techniques. Several techniques have been developed to assess the size and shape of the upper airway and the level of its obstruction, but they have a limited application, largely because they are usually carried out while the subject is awake and upright. These methods include X-ray lateral cephalometry, which only gives two-dimensional images, acoustic reflection, computerized tomography (CT), and magnetic resonance imaging (MRI) scans, which have the best resolution. Dynamic cine X-ray and CT scans provide information about the changes in the airway during breathing and may be carried out during sleep if excessive daytime sleepiness is severe.

Endoscopy. Nasendoscopy during wakefulness may be combined with a Mueller manoeuvre (a forced inspiration with the mouth and nose occluded) in order to localize the site of obstruction or vibration of the upper airway. Upper airway endoscopy while awake can be useful in selected patients to examine organic lesions of the upper airway and movements of the vocal cords and pharynx. The patient can also be asked to generate a snoring sound and ideally this should be identified as such by the partner at the time of nasendoscopy to identify the site of vibration of the upper airway.

'Sleep' nasendoscopy has been developed, but is more accurately termed 'sedative' or 'anaesthetic' nasendoscopy since it is carried out under sedation with, for instance, intravenous midazolam or propofol. This technique is subjective and hard to quantify and the results depend on the exact head and neck position and degree of sedation. It simulates sleep and gives a dynamic view of upper airway vibration and obstruction. Mandibular advancement can be carried out during the procedure to attempt to predict the response to mandibular advancement devices or orthognathic surgery. Although this technique has not been validated, it can be useful in predicting whether or not palatal surgery will be successful.

Physiological techniques. Flow-volume loops may indicate the presence of major airway obstruction and show a sawtooth pattern of fluttering, particularly on the expiratory limb.

Treatment

The aim of treatment of snoring is to render the patient sufficiently quiet for the partner to sleep. Simple snoring does not have any known adverse effects on the snorer. Improvement in the partner's sleep can be achieved by the following.

Treatment of the partner

It is important that the partner is aware that the snorer is not generating the noise voluntarily and reassurance about the absence of health risks to the snorer may be of help. The partner may be able to sleep better if he or she falls asleep before the snorer, and protection in the form of ear plugs or similar equipment may be useful. If these measures are ineffective and the snoring cannot be treated, an alternative is for the snorer and partner to sleep in separate bedrooms. Hypnotic drugs are occasionally taken by the partner to minimize the sleep disruption caused by the snoring, but are inadvisable as long-term treatment.

Treatment of the patient

First-line treatments
These are similar to measures for treating OSA.

Second-line treatments

These are similar in principle to those for OSA, but upper airway surgery is usually more effective because the site of snoring is often more localized than the site of obstruction in OSA. Mandibular advancement devices may be useful, but nasal CPAP is less frequently required than in OSA and wakefulness promoting drugs are not indicated.

Upper airway surgery. It is essential that a sleep study is performed before surgery is contemplated to assess whether OSA are sufficiently frequent to be a contra-indication to surgery. Localization techniques may also be useful. Surgery should not be recommended unless first-line treatments, in particular weight loss, have been attempted and is only indicated if snoring is sufficiently troublesome to the listener or has the potential to be so for a future partner. The snorer should be aware that there will be no direct personal benefit from surgery and there are risks with all the procedures. These include:

1 *Nasal surgery.* This is often effective if nasal polyps are present, but usually has little effect in other situations.

2 *Palatal surgery.* Resection of part of the palate together with a uvulectomy has been practised for many years (uvulopalatopharyngoplasty, UVPPP, UPPP) and is often combined with a tonsillectomy [48]. UPPP may lead to nasopharyngeal stenosis, nasal regurgitation of fluids due to palatal incompetence (velopharyngeal insufficiency), voice change and loss of taste.

A similar effect can be obtained with a laser (laser assisted uvulopalatoplasty (LAUP)) or with radio frequency techniques. A carbon dioxide laser is usually used to resect part of the palate or to stiffen it by delivering a pattern of laser burns which heal by fibrosis. Laser palatoplasty may be carried out as a single- or multi-stage procedure and can cause intense pain postoperatively. It only occasionally leads to palatal incompetence.

Radio frequency energy applied through a needle causes intrapalatal changes in the deeper muscular tissues, but does not affect the mucosa or palatal sensation [49]. It leads to necrosis of tissue and sub-mucosal fibrosis within around 8 weeks with loss of volume of the palate and an increase in its stiffness. It is less painful than the other procedures, but often needs to be repeated.

Palatal surgery is initially effective in around 70% of non-obese subjects if snoring has been localized to palatal level, although the response rate is slightly less with laser techniques and only around 30–60% with radio frequency methods. There is a slightly higher relapse rate with both of these two latter techniques than with UPPP. In around 20% of subjects snoring recurs after a laser palatoplasty during the first 2 years. Complications are less frequent with laser and radio frequency techniques than with surgery.

3 *Tonsillectomy and adenoidectomy.* This is effective in relieving snoring particularly in children.

4 *Tongue volume reduction surgery (linguoplasty).* This can be carried out with radio frequency or laser resection of a wedge of tongue tissue or less commonly by surgical resection.

5 *Excision of obstructing mass.* Excision of any mass, such as an upper airway benign tumour, causing snoring is occasionally indicated.

6 *Orthognathic surgery.* This is not indicated for snoring, but only for OSA.

Mandibular advancement devices

These may be effective, particularly if the snoring is worse in the supine position.

Nasal continuous positive airway pressure (CPAP) treatment

This is effective in relieving snoring, although compliance may be poor unless the subject is highly motivated since there is no symptomatic benefit to the patient.

References

1 Stradling JR, Davies RJO. Sleep 1: Obstructive sleep apnoea/hypopnoea syndrome: definitions, epidemiology, and natural history. *Thorax* 2004; 59: 73–8.

2 Stradling JR, Crosby JH. Predictors and prevalence of obstructive sleep apnoea and snoring in 1001 middle aged men. *Thorax* 1991; 46: 85–90.

3 Redline S, Tishler PV. The genetics of sleep apnea. *Sleep Med Rev* 2000; 4(6): 583–602.

4 Guilleminault C, Kim YD, Chowdhur S, Horia M, Ohayon M, Kushida C. Sleep and daytime sleepiness in upper airway resistance syndrome compared to obstructive sleep apnoeas syndrome. *Eur Respir J* 2001; 17: 838–47.

5 Horner RL. Motor control of the pharyngeal musculature and implications for the pathogenesis of obstructive sleep apnea. *Sleep* 1996; 19(10): 827–53.

6 Ayappa I, Rapoport DM. The upper airway in sleep: physiology of the pharynx. *Sleep Med Rev* 2003; 7(1): 9–33.

7 Friberg D, Ansved T, Borg K, Carlsson-Nordlander B, Larsson H, Svanborg E. Histological indications of a progressive snorers disease in an upper airway muscle. *Am J Respir Crit Care Med* 1998; 157: 586–93.

8 Rosenow F, McCarthy V, Caruso AC. Sleep apnoea in endocrine diseases. *J Sleep Res* 1998; 7: 3–11.

9 Zwillich CW. Sleep apnoea and autonomic function. *Thorax* 1998; 53(3): S20–4.

10 Marrone O, Bonsignore MR. Pulmonary haemodynamics in obstructive sleep apnoea. *Sleep Med Rev* 2002; 6(3): 175–93.

11 Eisensehr I, Noachtar S. Haematological aspects of obstructive sleep apnoea. *Sleep Med Rev* 2001; 5(3): 207–21.

12 Imagawa S, Yamaguchi Y, Ogawa K, Obara N, Suzuki N, Yamamoto M, Nagasawa T. Interleukin-6 and sleep tumor necrosis factor-a in patients with obstructive apnoea–hypopnea syndrome. *Respiration* 2004; 71: 24–9.

13 Lavie L, Vishnevsky A, Lavie P. Evidence for lipid peroxidation in obstructive sleep apnoea. *Sleep* 2004; 27(1): 123–8.

14 Meston N, Davies RJO, Mullins R, Jenkinson C, Wass JAH. Endocrine effects of nasal continuous positive airway pressure in male patients with obstructive sleep apnoea. *J Int Med* 2003; 254: 447–54.

15 Ip MSM, Lam B, Ng MMT, Lam WK, Tsang KWT, Lam KSL. Obstructive sleep apnea is independently associated with insulin resistance. *Am J Respir Crit Care Med* 2002; 165: 670–6.

16 Vgontzas AN, Bixler EO, Chrousos GP. Metabolic disturbances in obesity versus sleep apnoea: the importance of visceral obesity and insulin resistance. *J Int Med* 2003; 254: 32–44.

17 Shimizu K, Chin K, Nakamura T, Mauzaki H, Ogawa Y, Hosokawa R, Niimi A, Hattori N, Nohara R, Sasayama S, Nakao K, Mishima M, Nakamura T, Ohi M. Plasma leptin levels and cardiac sympathetic function in patients with obstructive sleep apnoea–hypopnoea syndrome. *Thorax* 2002; 57: 429–34.

18 Weitzenblum E, Chaouat A, Kessler R, Oswald M, Apprill M, Krieger J. Daytime hypoventilation in obstructive sleep apnoea syndrome. *Sleep Med Rev* 1999; 3: 79–93.

19 Beelke M, Angeli S, Sette MD, Carli F de, Canovaro P, Nobili L, Ferrillo F. Obstructive sleep apnea can be provocative for right-to-left shunting through a patent foramen ovale. *Sleep* 2002; 25(8): 856–62.

20 Neau J-P, Paquereau J, Meurice J-C, Chavagnat J-J, Gil R. Stroke and sleep apnoea: cause or consequence? *Sleep Med Rev* 2002; 6(6): 457–69.

21 Blyton DM, Sullivan CE, Edwards N. Reduced nocturnal cardiac output associated with preeclampsia is minimized with the use of nocturnal nasal CPAP. *Sleep* 2004; 27(1): 79–84.

22 Engleman H, Joffe D. Neurophysiological function in obstructive sleep apnoea. *Sleep Med Rev* 1999; 3: 59–78.

23 Findley LJ, Unverzagt MR, Suratt PM. Automobile accidents involving patients with obstructive sleep apnea. *Am Rev Respir Dis* 1988; 138: 337–40.

24 Engleman H, Joffe D. Neuropsychological function in obstructive sleep apnoea. *Sleep Med Rev* 1999; 3(1): 59–78.

25 Beebe DW, Gozal D. Obstructive sleep apnea and the prefrontal cortex: towards a comprehensive model linking nocturnal upper airway obstruction to daytime cognitive and behavioral deficits. *J Sleep Res* 2002; 11: 1–16.

26 He J, Kryger MH, Zorick FJ, Conway W, Roth T. Mortality and apnea index in obstructive sleep apnea. Experience in 385 male patients. *Chest* 1988; 94(1): 9–14.

27 Faulx MD, Larkin EK, Hoit BD, Aylor JE, Wright AT, Redline S. Sex influences endothelial function in sleep-disordered breathing. *Sleep* 2004; 27: 1113–20.

28 Kapsimalis F, Kryger MH. Gender and obstructive sleep apnea syndrome, Part 2: Mechanisms. *Sleep* 2002; 25(5): 499–506.

29 Whittle AT, Marshall I, Mortimore IL, Wraith PK, Sellar RJ, Douglas NJ. Neck soft tissue and fat distribution: comparison between normal men and women by magnetic resonance imaging. *Thorax* 1999; 54: 323–8.

30 Gaultier C. Obstructive sleep apnoea syndrome in infants and children: established facts and unsettled issues. *Thorax* 1995; 50: 1204–10.

31 Marcus CL. Sleep-disordered breathing in children. *Am J Respir Crit Care Med* 2001; 164: 16–30.

32 Raymond B, Cayton RM, Chappell MJ. Combined index of heart rate variability and oximetry in screening for the sleep apnoea/hypopnoea syndrome. *J Sleep Res* 2003; 12: 53–61.

33 Flemons WW, Littner MR, Rowley JA, Gay P, Anderson WM, Hudget DW, McEvoy RD, Loube DI. Home diagnosis of sleep apnea: a systematic review of the literature. *Chest* 2003; 124: 1543–79.

34 Jokic R, Klimaszewski A, Crossley M, Sridhar G, Fitzpatrick MF. Positional treatment vs continuous positive airway pressure in patients with positional obstructive sleep apnea syndrome. *Chest* 1999; 115: 771–81.

35 De Backer W. Non-CPAP treatment of obstructive sleep apnoea. *Monaldi Arch Chest Dis* 1998; 53: 625–9.

36 Thorpy M, Chesson A, Derderian S, Kader G, Millman R, Potolicchio S, Rosen G, Strollo PJ Jr, Wooten V. Practice parameters for the treatment of snoring and obstructive sleep apnea with oral appliances. *Sleep* 1995; 18: 511–13.

37 Marklund M, Persson M, Franklin KA. Treatment success with a mandibular advancement device is related to supine-dependent sleep apnea. *Chest* 1998; 114: 1630–5.

38 Sher AE, Schechtman KB, Piccirillo JF. The efficacy of surgical modifications of the upper airway in adults with obstructive sleep apnea syndrome. *Sleep* 1996; 19: 156–77.

39 Pirelli P, Saponara M, Guilleminault C. Rapid maxillary expansion in children with obstructive sleep apnea syndrome. *Sleep* 2004; 27(4): 761–6.

40 Braghiroli A, Sacco C, Carli S, Rossi S, Donner CF. Autocontinuous positive airway pressure in the diagnosis and treatment of obstructive sleep apnoea. *Monaldi Arch Chest Dis* 1998; 53: 621–4.

41 Littner M, Hirshkowitz M, Davila D, Anderson WM, Kushida CA, Woodson BT, Johnson SF, Wise MS. Practice parameters for the use of auto-titrating continuous positive airway pressure devices for titrating pressures and treating adult patients with obstructive sleep apnea syndrome. *Sleep* 2002; 25(2): 143–73.

42 Ayas NT, Patel SR, Malhotra A, Schulzer M, Malhotra M, Jung D, Fleetham J, White DP. Auto-titrating versus standard continuous positive airway pressure for the treatment of obstructive sleep apnea: results of a meta-analysis. *Sleep* 2004; 27(2): 249–53.

43 Hukins C. Comparative study of auto-titrating and fixed-pressure CPAP in the home: a randomized, single-blind crossover trial. *Sleep* 2004; 27(8): 1512–17.

44 Loube DI, Gay PC, Strohl KP, Pack AI, White DP, Collop NA. Indications for positive airway pressure treatment of adult obstructive sleep apnea patients. *Chest* 1999; 115: 863–6.

45 Collard P, Pieters T, Aubert G, Delguste P, Rodenstein DO. Compliance with nasal CPAP in obstructive sleep apnea patients. *Sleep Med Rev* 1997; 1(1): 33–44.

46 Ballester E, Badia JR, Hernandez L, Carrasco E *et al.* Evidence of the effectiveness of continuous positive airway pressure in the treatment of sleep apnea/hypopnea syndrome. *Am J Respir Crit Care Med* 1999; 159: 495–501.

47 George CFP. Reduction in motor vehicle collisions following treatment of sleep apnoea with nasal CPAP. *Thorax* 2001; 56: 508–12.

48 Cahali MB, Formigoni GGS, Gebrim EMMS, Miziara ID. Lateral pharyngoplasty versus uvulopalatopharyngoplasty: a clinical, polysomnographic and computed tomography measurement comparison. *Sleep* 2004; 27(5): 942–50.

49 Stuck BA, Maurer JT, Hein G, Hormann K, Verse T. Radiofrequency surgery of the soft palate in the treatment of snoring: a review of the literature. *Sleep* 2004; 27(3): 551–5.

11 Central Sleep Apnoeas and Hypoventilation

Introduction

Respiration depends on the muscles of the respiratory pump being able to draw air in through the airways to the gas exchanging areas of the lungs. The respiratory pump comprises not only the respiratory muscles, but also the bones and other soft tissues of the rib cage and abdomen, the controlling mechanisms in the brain and spinal cord and the peripheral nerves. The control of both the respiratory pump and the upper airway during sleep is different from that during wakefulness.

In this chapter the effects of sleep on the respiratory pump and its disorders are examined. Lung disorders are discussed in Chapter 12 and disorders of the upper airway in Chapter 10.

Central sleep apnoeas without hypoventilation

Pathogenesis

These apnoeas may appear in sleep because of upper airway reflexes or because of variations in respiratory rate in REM sleep with intervals of greater than 10 s between breaths. Changes in the apnoeic threshold for carbon dioxide at the time of NREM sleep-stage transitions also cause central apnoeas. During the apnoea the P_{CO_2} gradually rises and when it reaches the apnoeic threshold a period of hyperventilation then begins to lower the P_{CO_2} again. When it falls below the apnoeic threshold, or if there is a sleep-stage shift so that the threshold itself rises, another central apnoea will start. The ventilatory response to changes in P_{CO_2} is also increased with this type of central sleep apnoea and it lowers the P_{CO_2} during both sleep and wakefulness.

Hypoxia also increases ventilation but in a non-linear way so that it tends to overshoot and lower the P_{CO_2} below the apnoeic threshold. During the resulting central sleep apnoea the P_{CO_2} rises again until respiration restarts. This sequence is particularly significant if the apnoeic threshold is raised or when the ventilatory response to oxygen is exaggerated.

Clinical features

Central sleep apnoeas associated with a normal or low P_{CO_2} are much commoner in males than in females, except in the polycystic ovary syndrome in which testosterone secretion is increased. This gender difference is probably due to the testosterone-dependent higher apnoeic threshold in males. Central sleep apnoeas may be asymptomatic, but can cause significant sleep fragmentation due to arousals from sleep. These arousals may cause a sensation of breathlessness or sudden awakenings for no apparent reason. The arousals are less frequent than in obstructive sleep apnoeas because of the absence of any increased inspiratory muscle effort as an arousal stimulus.

Observation during sleep reveals an absence of respiratory movements, which differentiates these apnoeas from obstructive sleep apnoeas. These observations can be confirmed by sleep studies in which abdominal and chest wall movement recordings are combined with airflow and oximetry.

Treatment

Treatment is not usually required for central sleep apnoeas with a normal or low P_{CO_2} unless they cause significant insomnia or excessive daytime sleepiness due to sleep fragmentation. In these situations the treatment options are as follows.

1 Modification of sleep pattern. Consolidation of NREM sleep with benzodiazepines and similar drugs minimizes the number of sleep-stage shifts. Reduction of the duration of REM sleep by antidepressants may be effective if REM sleep is when most of the apnoeas occur.

2 Modification of respiratory drive. Relief of hypoxia with supplemental oxygen usually given through nasal cannulae reduces the hypoxic drive. Theophyllines and acetazolamide lower the apnoeic threshold for carbon dioxide and may be of help.

3 Nasal continuous positive airway pressure (CPAP) treatment. This modifies upper airway reflexes, and increases the lung volume and the quantity of oxygen stored in the lungs. It may be effective by itself or in combination with nocturnal oxygen, and possibly 0.5–1% carbon dioxide [1].

Cheyne–Stokes respiration (CSR, periodic breathing)

Cheyne–Stokes respiration is closely related to central sleep apnoeas. It is characterized by a regular waxing and waning of tidal volume with little change in respiratory frequency during the phases when breathing is taking place. Between these cycles there may be a short or prolonged apnoea, which if it exceeds 10 s is classified as a central sleep apnoea using conventional criteria. Occasionally, however, the waxing and waning of tidal volume occurs without any cessation of breathing (Cheyne–Stokes variant).

Pathogenesis

The cyclical changes in respiration are due to an instability in the respiratory control system (Fig. 11.1). Within each stage of NREM sleep the respiratory drive remains constant, but it differs between stages. The frequent changes, at the onset of sleep and with arousal, lead to an unstable respiratory pattern. As the stage of sleep deepens, the arterial $P\text{CO}_2$ which is required to act as a respiratory stimulus (the apnoeic threshold) rises. This leads to a central apnoea until the carbon dioxide reaches the apnoeic threshold, at which time it stimulates the chemoreceptors, particularly in the carotid bodies, which initiate an episode of hyperventilation to reduce the $P\text{CO}_2$ below the apnoeic threshold again [2].

The ventilatory response to carbon dioxide is greater than normal in CSR. This magnifies the hyperventilation response to the rise in $P\text{CO}_2$ and also causes the arterial $P\text{CO}_2$ to be slightly low during wakefulness and the mean $P\text{CO}_2$ to be low during sleep [3]. The hyperventilation causes a rapid and deep fall in the arterial $P\text{CO}_2$, and in CSR there is usually a prolongation of the time for the arterial blood to reach the peripheral chemoreceptors in the carotid body and thereby to influence respiration. The degree of this delay determines the length of the hyperpnoeic phase of CSR and the crescendo–decrescendo pattern of the tidal volume. The length of the apnoeic phase is largely determined by the extent to which the $P\text{CO}_2$ falls below the apnoeic threshold and its rate of rise, which is related to the metabolic production of carbon dioxide.

In CSR, but not in central sleep apnoeas, there are usually other factors which increase the ventilatory response. These include the presence of hypoxaemia. The ventilatory response to hypoxia increases hyperbolically as the $P\text{O}_2$ falls and this gain in ventilatory response accentuates the episodes of hyperventilation. The cycle of CSR is shortest in individuals with the greatest hypoxic ventilatory drive. Pulmonary vagal afferent stimulation, which in heart failure, for instance, is associated with pulmonary venous distension and stimulation of pulmonary C-fibres, also increases the respiratory drive.

Causes

Cheyne–Stokes respiration is associated with several conditions; these are described below.

Hypoxia

This may be due to a low arterial $P\text{O}_2$, including situations when this is the result of breathing gas with a low inspired oxygen concentration or air at low pressure. The low $P\text{O}_2$ at altitude increases the hypoxic ventilatory response which destabilizes respiratory control and causes 'high-altitude periodic breathing'. This type of CSR occurs in NREM sleep which becomes fragmented because of frequent arousals. The duration of stages 3 and 4 NREM sleep is reduced.

Reduction in lung volumes

This reduces the body stores of oxygen and makes hypoxia more marked during any transient apnoea.

Cardiac dysfunction

This is associated with CSR for several reasons. First, the hypoxia and pulmonary venous distension increase respiratory drive. Secondly, the prolonged circulation

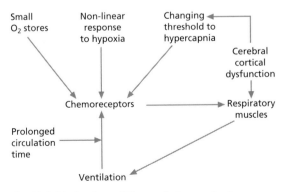

Fig. 11.1 Mechanisms of Cheyne–Stokes respiration.

time, which is often a feature of cardiac failure or low cardiac output states, leads to the CSR pattern. Lastly, cardiac disease is often associated with changes in the cerebral circulation so that its reactivity to changes in P_{CO_2} is lost and this alters the ventilatory response to P_{CO_2} [4].

Cheyne–Stokes respiration is associated with a poor prognosis if cardiac dysfunction is present. The 3-year survival is only around 50%. The high mortality may reflect the increased sympathetic activity during sleep which causes vasoconstriction leading to hypertension with a reduced cardiac output, dysrhythmias, a tachycardia with reduced stroke volume and an increase in the myocardial oxygen consumption.

Cerebral cortical dysfunction

Cheyne–Stokes respiration is common in disorders of the cerebral hemispheres which reduce the inhibition of the medullary respiratory centres so that reflex responses become accentuated. This probably contributes to the increased prevalence of CSR in the elderly.

Clinical features

Cheyne–Stokes respiration causes frequent arousals from sleep, especially in stages 1 and 2 NREM sleep. These may be detected as awakenings and insomnia, and if they are sufficiently frequent may result in excessive daytime sleepiness. The total sleep time and duration of stages 3 and 4 NREM and REM sleep are reduced if the CSR frequency is greater than around 20 episodes per hour. Occasionally the airway closes during the central apnoea and this combination of a central sleep apnoea and obstructive sleep apnoea is termed a mixed apnoea.

The CSR cycles are associated with an increase in sympathetic activity during the hyperpnoeic phase. At this time a tachycardia, an increase in cardiac output, a rise in blood pressure and an increase in the cerebral blood flow occur [5]. These effects are reversed during the apnoea. Cardiac dysrhythmias, such as atrial fibrillation, ventricular ectopics and atrioventricular block, may appear transiently during each CSR cycle.

Observation of the respiratory pattern is diagnostic and there may be snoring, usually because the upper airway closes towards the end of the apnoeic phase. During the apnoea neurological changes including eye closure, upward rotation of the eyes, conjugate gaze deviation, hyporeflexia, upgoing plantar reflexes, pupillary constriction and a reduction in tone of the limb muscles may be seen. These are all reversed during the hyperpnoeic phase.

Treatment

Treatment is often not required, but if CSR is symptomatic the following should be considered.

1 *Treatment of the underlying cause*, e.g. heart failure.

2 *Oxygen*. This stabilizes the respiratory control and is usually effective. Inspired 3% carbon dioxide also stabilizes the respiratory control, but leads to sympathetic hyperactivity and is impractical for long-term use.

3 *Respiratory stimulants*. These lower the threshold of the ventilatory response to P_{CO_2}. They include theophylline, but this also increases the gain of the respiratory control system by increasing the slope of the ventilatory response to carbon dioxide. Acetazolamide is effective through inducing a metabolic acidosis and has been used especially in high altitude periodic breathing [6].

4 *Sedative drugs*. Benzodiazepines consolidate sleep and reduce the number of sleep-stage changes.

5 *Nasal CPAP and nasal ventilation* (Fig. 11.2). These increase the mean intrathoracic pressure which

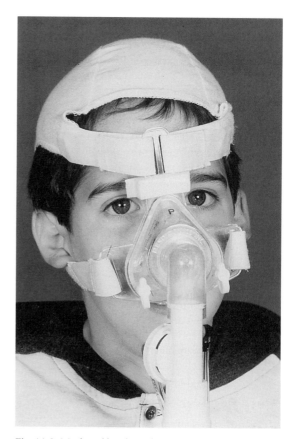

Fig. 11.2 Mask and headgear for nasal ventilation.

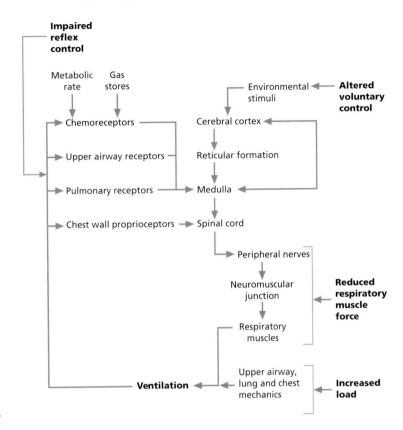

Fig. 11.3 Causes of ventilatory failure.

reduces pulmonary oedema and pulmonary venous congestion due to cardiac failure. The venous return to the right heart lessens, and the left ventricular end-diastolic volume, left ventricular transmural pressure-gradient and the left ventricular afterload are all reduced. Functional residual capacity rises which enlarges the oxygen stores and may reduce the work of breathing, thereby reducing oxygen consumption and carbon dioxide production. Upper airway reflexes may also be altered but occasionally the additional expiratory resistance due to the applied expiratory pressure causes the $P\text{CO}_2$ to rise and if it remains persistently above the apnoeic threshold the respiratory pattern stabilizes.

Nasal ventilation in particular reduces the respiratory muscle work and the oxygen consumption, and these various effects of CPAP and ventilation reduce the sympathetic drive and plasma noradrenaline levels [7].

Sleep hypoventilation

It is essential to distinguish 'central' apnoeas due to a loss of respiratory drive from those that are due to impaired respiratory mechanics or to widespread respiratory muscle weakness so that even a normal respiratory drive cannot be translated into detectable respiratory movements (Fig. 11.3). This latter group are better considered as 'pseudocentral' or 'peripheral' apnoeas, rather than due to any central abnormality [8]. They are characteristic of neuromuscular disorders that cause diaphragmatic weakness so that in REM sleep no functioning inspiratory chest wall muscles are left (Table 11.1). Impaired respiratory mechanics in, for instance, emphysema may also cause even a normal drive only to be able to develop a small tidal volume (hypopnoea) or even no detectable airflow.

Pathophysiology

Hypoventilation
The limitations of the respiratory pump in neuromuscular and skeletal disorders that affect the thoracic cage are apparent in sleep before they develop in wakefulness (Table 11.2). The ability to respond to the altered physiological environment during sleep is limited by the capacity of the respiratory drive,

High risk disorder, e.g. previous poliomyelitis, muscular dystrophy, thoracoplasty, scoliosis

Plus relevant symptoms, e.g.

Worsening breathlessness
Awakenings from sleep
Excessive daytime sleepiness
Early morning headaches
Swollen ankles

Plus vital capacity < 1.0–1.5 l

Table 11.1 When to suspect ventilatory failure.

Table 11.2 Neuromuscular and thoracic cage disorders causing respiratory failure during sleep.

Neurological
Carotid body disorders
Brainstem lesions
Central alveolar hyperventilation
Arnold–Chiari malformation
Cervical cordotomy
Spinal cord lesions
Motor neurone disease
Multiple system atrophy
Poliomyelitis
Spinal muscular atrophy

Disorders of peripheral nerves
Acute idiopathic polyneuropathy (Guillain–Barré syndrome)
Charcot–Marie–Tooth disease

Disorders of neuromuscular junction
Myasthenia gravis
Lambert–Eaton syndrome
Botulism

Disorders of respiratory muscles
Duchenne's muscular dystrophy
Myotonic dystrophy
Congenital myopathies
Acid maltase deficiency

Skeletal disorders
Scoliosis
Kyphosis
Thoracoplasty
Asphyxiating thoracic dystrophy (Jeune's disease)

respiratory muscle function and the mechanical properties of the respiratory system. In general, if the respiratory drive increases, the respiratory frequency rises, but the maximal tidal volume is less than in normal subjects. As a result, the physiological dead space is increased and alveolar ventilation falls with a reduction in Po_2 and a rise in Pco_2. As the respiratory frequency increases, the ratio of inspiratory to expiratory time rises so that the inspiratory muscles contract for longer with a risk of incipient respiratory muscle fatigue. This is usually avoided by the central respiratory control mechanisms adopting a strategy of either recruiting additional respiratory muscles such as the accessory muscles, alternating, for instance, diaphragmatic and intercostal muscle activity during each breath, or by inducing central sleep apnoeas. Each of these strategies reduces the work of the inspiratory muscles, but the alternative response is to cause an arousal from sleep.

If alveolar ventilation cannot be maintained, the respiratory control system sets the ventilation at a level which avoids muscle fatigue even though it leads to hypercapnia. Hypercapnia does enable more carbon dioxide to be excreted in a given volume of expired gas than with eucapnia for any level of respiratory muscle work. This adaptive mechanism tends to stabilize the arterial Pco_2. This is a respiratory stimulant acutely, but becomes progressively less so when it is prolonged. It also increases the cardiac output, and leads to a tachycardia, an increase in systolic blood pressure, and cerebral and cutaneous vasodilatation but visceral vasoconstriction. Its neurological effects include reduction in tendon reflexes, a flapping tremor of the hands, and frontal headaches which characteristically occur on awakening from sleep in the morning. It may also lead to confusion and even coma (carbon dioxide narcosis).

As the Pco_2 rises the arterial Po_2 falls and this may be accentuated, particularly in REM sleep, by a reduction in lung volume and a worsening of ventilation–perfusion matching and often a disproportionate fall in oxygen saturation according to its position on the oxyhaemoglobin dissociation curve. If hypoxia persists it may lead to polycythaemia in response to increased erythropoietin secretion by the kidneys. This increases the oxygen carrying capacity of the blood to maintain oxygen delivery to the tissues despite the low arterial Po_2. It also increases the blood viscosity, predisposing to venous and arterial thrombosis, and it increases both the pulmonary and systemic vascular resistance. This contributes to the risk of right and left ventricular hypertrophy and failure. Hypoxia also has a direct vasoconstrictor effect on the pulmonary arterioles and raises the pulmonary artery pressure.

The respiratory drive is intrinsically normal in most patients with neuromuscular and thoracic cage disorders, although it can be transiently impaired by, for instance, hypercapnia. Disorders which also affect the cerebral cortex, such as myotonic dystrophy, modify respiratory control, but through loss of the normal cortical inhibition of brainstem reflexes.

Respiration during REM sleep

The respiratory abnormalities are seen in REM before NREM sleep in all these disorders, apart for those, such as central alveolar hypoventilation and after cervical cordotomy, in which the medullary respiratory reflex control is directly affected [9]. REM sleep becomes fragmented and reduced in duration with frequent arousals, and only at a later stage is there loss of stages 3 and 4 NREM sleep. The main effects of REM sleep are as follows.

Increase in upper airway resistance

Weakness of the upper airway dilator muscles combines with the intense loss of muscle tone in REM sleep to predispose to upper airway obstruction. The risk of this is greater if the chest wall muscles are selectively spared and remain able to generate a sufficiently negative intra-airway pressure. Conversely, if the chest wall muscles, particularly the diaphragm, are involved then obstructive sleep apnoeas are less likely. The upper airway diameter is reduced through a reflex mechanism related to the loss of lung volume in REM sleep. The obstruction may occur at any level from the base of the tongue to the larynx, in which case stridor-like noises are often heard at night. If, however, the chest wall muscles are too weak to generate rapid airflow rates there may be little noise despite the upper airway obstruction (Table 11.3).

The high threshold for arousal during REM sleep prolongs the obstructive sleep apnoea and, together with the small oxygen stores in the lungs, tends to accentuate the oxygen desaturations. Resaturation after each apnoea is also slow because of the inability

Table 11.3 Neuromuscular causes of obstructive sleep apnoeas.

Multiple system atrophy
Syringobulbia
Posterior inferior cerebellar artery syndrome
Motor neurone disease
Arnold–Chiari malformation
Poliomyelitis
Muscular dystrophies, e.g. myotonic dystrophy, Duchenne's muscular dystrophy
Congenital myopathies

of the chest wall muscles to increase alveolar ventilation rapidly once arousal has occurred, either because of their weakness or, in thoracic cage deformities, because of the reduced chest wall compliance. With these neuromechanical defects hypercapnia between apnoeas is partly related to the inability to normalize the blood gases before the next apnoea begins. Secondary adaptive changes which maintain hypercapnia, as described above, develop, and even between apnoeas the weak muscles may be unable to compensate for the increase in the work of breathing through the narrowed upper airway. These effects are accentuated if the subject is obese, takes sedative drugs or alcohol or has any specific dysmorphic features which narrow the upper airway as in, for instance, nemaline myopathy.

Diaphragmatic dysfunction

The diaphragm is the only active inspiratory chest wall muscle in REM sleep, and hypoventilation may result if its function is impaired either due to intrinsic weakness or to derangement of chest wall mechanics which puts the diaphragm at a mechanical disadvantage, alters its length or reduces the chest wall compliance [10]. The most common causes are congenital myopathies such as acid maltase deficiency, muscular dystrophies such as Duchenne's muscular dystrophy or myotonic dystrophy, previous poliomyelitis and motor neurone disease, and chest wall disorders such as scoliosis, kyphosis or after a thoracoplasty.

Reduction in functional residual capacity

This reduces the upper airway diameter, and oxygen stores in the lungs, impairs ventilation–perfusion matching and reduces lung compliance, all of which may contribute to hypoxia, central sleep apnoeas or Cheyne–Stokes respiration and hypoventilation.

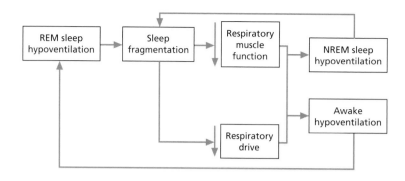

Fig. 11.4 Hypoventilation in sleep. NREM, non-rapid eye movement; REM, rapid eye movement.

Reduction in respiratory drive

This, as mentioned above, is rarely due to any intrinsic disorder related to the neurological condition but may be a consequence of sleep fragmentation or hypercapnia.

Respiration during NREM sleep

Reflex control of respiration is retained during NREM sleep and the main effects of this in neuromuscular and skeletal disorders are as follows.

Increase in upper airway resistance

This increases to a lesser extent than in REM sleep and obstructive sleep apnoeas are less common. They may, however, occur in degenerative disorders such as multiple system atrophy and motor neurone disease in which vocal cord adduction develops due to lesions in the nucleus ambiguus.

Cheyne–Stokes respiration

This arises with changes in sleep stage within NREM sleep and may lead to frequent arousals. The slow circulation time due to a cardiomyopathy in disorders such as Duchenne's muscular dystrophy and Friedreich's ataxia contributes to the central sleep apnoeas. Disorders affecting the cerebral cortex, with loss of its inhibitory effect on the medullary reflexes, also predispose to Cheyne–Stokes respiration together with any hypoxia that may be present.

Inactivation of chest wall muscles

There is a global reduction in chest wall muscle activity in NREM sleep in contrast to REM sleep. Neuromuscular disorders affecting these muscles accentuate this and predispose to hypoventilation. Disorders of the thoracic cage such as scoliosis which reduce its compliance may increase the work of breathing sufficiently for hypoventilation to occur even if the chest wall inspiratory muscles are intrinsically normal.

Arousals

Microarousals from sleep occur as a result of hypoxia and hypercapnia. The threshold for arousal is higher in REM than in NREM sleep and rises progressively from the lighter to the deeper stages of NREM sleep. Arousals are almost invariably seen initially in REM sleep, and the first abnormality of sleep architecture is fragmentation of REM sleep with REM sleep deprivation. If effective treatment is applied REM sleep rebound appears. Loss of stages 3 and 4 NREM sleep only occurs later if the respiratory abnormalities encroach into NREM sleep (Fig. 11.4).

The sleep fragmentation due to arousals reduces the ventilatory drive and probably both the strength and endurance of the respiratory muscles in the upper airway and chest wall. Hypoventilation worsens and hypoxia, which is initially a respiratory stimulus, can depress respiration if it becomes severe. Hypercapnia causes progressively less respiratory stimulation as the cerebrospinal fluid bicarbonate concentration rises and buffers the chemoreceptor response to $P\text{CO}_2$ changes. Hypoventilation tends to persist and once it appears in NREM as well as in REM sleep it soon appears during wakefulness. Loss of NREM sleep then leads to progressively worsening sleepiness during the day. The effects on respiratory drive are reversible and improve once sleep fragmentation is relieved, but are exacerbated by, for instance, sedative drugs and alcohol.

Sleep fragmentation affects particularly the function of the prefrontal cortex. Initially the ability to maintain attention and alertness during prolonged monotonous tasks is impaired, and this is followed by mood changes, loss of memory, poor concentration and impairment of motor performance. As sleep fragmentation becomes more severe, excessive sleepiness worsens and automatic behaviour and even hallucinations, which are probably due to intrusion of REM sleep into wakefulness, develop.

Causes

Respiratory drive disorders

Abnormalities of the respiratory drive may be readily reversible with appropriate treatment. Sleep deprivation and fragmentation reduce the respiratory drive and predispose to central sleep apnoeas. Drugs such as benzodiazepines and opiates and a metabolic alkalosis have a similar effect. Chronic hypercapnia increases the cerebrospinal fluid bicarbonate concentration, which increases its buffering capacity and thereby reduces the responsiveness to changes in $P\text{CO}_2$.

There are also several conditions in which abnormalities of respiratory control are permanent, or at least only partially reversible. These include the following.

Carotid body disorders

The carotid bodies increase ventilation in response to hypoxia during sleep and cause arousal if hypoxia becomes severe. Carotid body dysfunction may lead to failure to terminate either central or obstructive sleep apnoeas, and can lead to respiratory failure.

Central alveolar hypoventilation

This disorder occasionally occurs neonatally (congenital central hypoventilation syndrome), in which case it may be associated with other conditions such as Hirschsprung's disease, but more usually in early adult life. In this group it is usually idiopathic and presumably due to a functional defect in the medullary respiratory centres or their connections, but occasionally it is due to organic brainstem disease such as previous encephalitis, a stroke or a tumour.

The ventilatory response to hypoxia or hypercapnia or both is reduced. Central sleep apnoeas are seen initially most frequently in NREM sleep and are associated with hypercapnia which, when it becomes more severe, is present during wakefulness as well. It is more marked during intercurrent illnesses such as chest infections in which the work of breathing is increased beyond the capacity of the respiratory drive.

Polycythaemia and pulmonary hypertension may develop. Treatment with non-invasive ventilatory support, or occasionally by phrenic nerve stimulation, is effective in adults. Tracheostomy ventilation is required initially in children. If they fail to improve, phrenic nerve stimulation is preferable as a long-term treatment, but it is often possible to transfer to non-invasive ventilation. This may only be needed during sleep, or intermittently during the day as well.

Other medullary lesions

Any lesions in the medulla may disrupt respiratory control and lead to ventilatory failure during sleep. Tumours, haemorrhage, infarction, encephalitis, trauma, neurosurgery, irradiation, multiple sclerosis, syringobulbia and multiple system atrophy may all be responsible. These conditions usually cause a complex clinical picture because of the site of the lesion and this may make it difficult to assess the respiratory complications.

Arnold–Chiari malformation

This is due to herniation of the cerebellar tonsils through the foramen magnum and caudal displacement of part of the medulla. It can cause stretching or compression of the ninth and tenth cranial nerves and thereby leads to denervation of the carotid body, causing central apnoeas.

Cervical cordotomy

The main indication for this procedure is the relief of chronic pain, but if it is performed bilaterally the efferent pathways from the medullary respiratory centres can be severed so that the chest wall muscles are disconnected from reflex control. Central sleep apnoeas during NREM sleep arise and may be prolonged and cause fatal cardiac dysrhythmias, particularly during the first few nights after surgery. The degree of recovery varies.

Neuromuscular disorders

Generalized respiratory muscle weakness reduces the lung volumes, including the vital capacity. The maximal inspiratory and expiratory pressures are reduced and the respiratory frequency increases and tidal volume falls. Hypoventilation occurs in sleep when the vital capacity falls below around 30% predicted or to around 1–1.5 l. It is seen in REM sleep before NREM sleep [11].

Selective diaphragmatic weakness leads to paradoxical inward inspiratory abdominal movement in the supine position and the sensation of orthopnoea. This commonly causes severe sleep fragmentation with relative preservation of oxygenation and $P\text{CO}_2$ at night. Unilateral diaphragmatic weakness rarely causes sleep-related problems in adults, but can do so in infants who are more dependent on diaphragmatic function. The most important causes of selective diaphragmatic weakness are given in Table 11.4.

Table 11.4 Causes of bilateral diaphragm weakness.

| High cervical cord lesions |
| Motor neurone disease |
| Poliomyelitis |
| Acute idiopathic polyneuropathy |
| Myasthenia gravis |
| Systemic lupus erythematosis |
| Acid maltase deficiency |
| Muscular dystrophies |

Scoliosis

Scoliosis is due to rotation and lateral deviation of the spine. The inspiratory muscles are at a mechanical disadvantage due to distortion of the rib cage and diaphragmatic function is impeded. The chest wall compliance is reduced and there is ventilation–perfusion mismatching. The initial abnormality during sleep is hypoventilation during REM sleep [12].

Kyphosis

This is an anteroposterior deformity of the spine. It generally affects respiration if it is of early onset, usually before the age of 4 years, and if it is severe and in the mid or upper thoracic spine. It is usually due to tuberculous osteomyelitis of the spine and causes similar respiratory problems in sleep to scoliosis.

Disorders of the ribs

Congenital abnormalities rarely cause hypoventilation. Apart from a flail chest due to multiple traumatic rib fractures, the most important condition is that following a thoracoplasty. This was frequently performed for pulmonary tuberculosis before effective chemotherapy was introduced in the 1950s. Up to 11 ribs were resected, leading to a severe restrictive defect with paradoxical movement of the rib cage on the operated side. Diaphragmatic excursion is reduced and the combination of pleural thickening, loss of intercostal muscles and usually extensive pulmonary damage due to the tuberculous infection causes hypoventilation, initially during REM sleep and later in NREM sleep [13].

Disorders of the sternum

These rarely cause any respiratory disturbance during sleep, even if a depression deformity (pectus excavatum) or protrusion deformity (pectus carinatum) is severe.

Clinical features

Respiratory disturbances during sleep may be asymptomatic but as they worsen they cause arousals from sleep which may become sufficiently frequent to cause excessive daytime sleepiness and difficulty in maintaining sleep. Early morning headaches due to carbon dioxide retention may develop. The partner may be aware of snoring or stridor-like noises as well as an irregular respiratory pattern. Worsening breathlessness on exertion and ankle swelling are common and diaphragm weakness may cause orthopnoea so that sleep takes place in a chair instead of in bed.

Natural history

Age has an important influence on the clinical features. Below the age of around 3 years respiration is more dependent on the diaphragm than in later life and the rib cage is very compliant. Any weakness of the diaphragm predisposes to its fatigue and to respiratory failure, particularly since there is a greater proportion of REM sleep in children than in adults, and this is when respiration is particularly dependent on the diaphragm.

The rate at which the clinical features develop depends on how the balance between the capacity of the respiratory pump and its load changes. A transient intercurrent and often treatable illness such as a chest infection or asthma may precipitate nocturnal (and waking) respiratory failure. Age-related changes in respiratory drive, respiratory muscle strength and endurance and the compliance of the chest wall may switch the balance in favour of hypoventilation. The rate of progression of the underlying disorder is another important factor. Stable conditions such as childhood proximal spinal muscular atrophy hardly alter for many years, whereas some conditions are rapidly progressive such as motor neurone disease and multiple system atrophy, and in others, such as multiple sclerosis, the course fluctuates unpredictably. The sequence of progression of abnormalities is fairly predictable in some disorders, such as Duchenne's muscular dystrophy, and knowledge of this is important in managing the respiratory complications that appear during sleep. In other conditions, such as motor neurone disease, there may be any combination or sequence of weakness of upper airway and chest wall muscles together with bulbar weakness which can cause aspiration of saliva, food and drink into the tracheobronchial tree.

The respiratory effects of these conditions during sleep can also be influenced by unrelated disorders.

These include obesity which not only increases upper airway resistance but also mass-loads the chest wall muscles, impairs ventilation–perfusion matching and, if it is gross, can impair muscle contractility. Tobacco smoking can increase upper airway resistance as well as intrapulmonary airflow resistance, and if it causes emphysema the lung compliance increases leading to hyperinflation.

Assessment

History

A careful history is essential to accurately assess respiratory disorders during sleep (Chapter 3). The issues that should be considered are as follows.

1 How severe is the sleep disruption? How frequent are the arousals from sleep and what is their cause? Is the patient aware of any breathlessness or choking? Are there early morning headaches on awakening, suggesting carbon dioxide retention?

2 How severe is the excessive daytime sleepiness? This can be assessed using the techniques described in Chapter 3. Respiratory disorders and excessive daytime sleepiness may be due to sleep fragmentation caused by central or obstructive apnoeas, or to the sedative effect of hypercapnia (carbon dioxide narcosis).

3 Are there any features to indicate worsening of pulmonary or cardiovascular function, such as deteriorating breathlessness, ankle swelling or orthopnoea? This may be caused either by pulmonary oedema or by bilateral diaphragm weakness.

4 What is the cause? Is there a history of a previous relevant illness such as poliomyelitis or of a muscular dystrophy or other chronic neurological disorder? Is there a scoliosis or kyphosis or has the subject undergone a thoracoplasty? Are there features of chronic bronchitis, emphysema (chronic obstructive pulmonary disease, COPD) or asthma? Is there any inappropriate drug treatment which may be acting as a respiratory sedative, e.g. opiate analgesics or benzodiazepines?

Physical examination

Physical examination may reveal central cyanosis indicating hypoxia, or signs of hypercapnia such as a tachycardia with a large-volume pulse, warm hands and feet, a flapping tremor of the hands, reduction of tendon reflexes, small pupils and, occasionally, confusion and papilloedema. Neurological examination may show features of a neurological disorder including respiratory muscle weakness. Paradoxical inward inspiratory abdominal movement in the supine position indicates diaphragmatic weakness. There may be physical signs of a chest wall deformity and of airflow obstruction with hyperinflation, as well as right heart failure and pulmonary hypertension.

Investigations

Most patients with significant symptoms of a respiratory disorder during sleep, or abnormal physical signs, require referral to a specialist centre. Arterial blood gases while awake should be estimated. A sleep study with analysis of oxygen saturation, transcutaneous P_{CO_2} and, ideally, airflow, rib cage and abdominal movement is of value. Polysomnography is only needed if other causes of sleep disturbances, such as periodic limb movements in sleep, are being considered.

Lung function tests, including lung volumes, maximal inspiratory and expiratory mouth pressures, vital capacity in the lying and sitting position, and occasionally ventilatory responses to oxygen and carbon dioxide, may be needed. A chest X-ray, electrocardiogram and echocardiogram are usually indicated.

Treatment

A range of treatments is available and in general the simpler measures should be tried first.

Treat the underlying disorder

Very few of the neuromuscular and thoracic cage disorders are amenable to curative treatment but measures such as physiotherapy may be of help and prompt, energetic treatment of asthma and infective exacerbations is essential. Treatment of unrelated conditions which adversely affect respiratory function, such as obesity or tobacco smoking, may also be of value.

Oxygen

Supplemental oxygen can relieve hypoxia during sleep, but by removing the hypoxic ventilatory drive it may prolong both central sleep apnoeas and obstructive sleep apnoeas, worsen hypoventilation and lead to a rise in P_{CO_2}. If oxygen is administered the oxygen saturation and transcutaneous P_{CO_2} should be carefully monitored during sleep and the flow rate kept to the minimum that is required to raise the oxygen saturation to an acceptable level, such as 90%.

Discontinue sedatives

Any respiratory sedative medication such as opiate

analgesics, sedating antidepressants and benzodiazepines and related drugs should be discontinued if possible.

Respiratory stimulants

A variety of drugs, such as almitrine and progesterone, have been tried, but none of these is effective in improving ventilation during sleep. Methylxanthines can improve Cheyne–Stokes respiration, partly through an effect on cerebral blood flow and also by lowering the threshold for the ventilatory response to hypercapnia. Acetazolamide, which is a carbonic anhydrase inhibitor, causes a metabolic acidosis. It may relieve Cheyne–Stokes respiration particularly at altitude and reduces the arterial P_{CO_2} slightly in other disorders.

Inotropic drugs

These have been used in an attempt to improve respiratory muscle contractility, but the results have been disappointing.

REM sleep suppressants

Tricyclic antidepressants and selective serotonin re-uptake inhibitors reduce the duration of REM sleep-related abnormalities including upper airway obstruction. Protriptyline 5–20 mg nocte has been most widely used and is non-respiratory sedating, but has been withdrawn in the UK.

Phrenic nerve pacemaker (diaphragmatic stimulation, electrophrenic respiration)

This treatment is effective if the phrenic nerve, its nucleus in C3–C5 segments of the spinal cord and the diaphragm are intact. Its indication is in respiratory failure due to brainstem disorders that have disturbed the medullary respiratory control and high cervical tetraplegics, but not in patients with, for instance, phrenic nerve damage or muscular dystrophies in whom the contractility of the diaphragm is impaired.

Ventilatory support

Mechanical ventilatory support is an external source of energy which reduces the work of breathing and compensates for apnoeas, hypopnoeas and hypoventilation. It can be provided during wakefulness as well as during sleep.

Indications

In general, long-term ventilatory support is indicated if respiratory failure is causing troublesome symptoms, potentially serious complications such as polycythaemia

or pulmonary hypertension, or is likely to lead to these problems or to premature death.

It may also be indicated in asymptomatic high-risk patients, such as those with Duchenne's muscular dystrophy [14] or poliomyelitis, in order to delay or prevent complications from nocturnal respiratory failure. In neuromuscular conditions causing selective diaphragmatic weakness, such as motor neurone disease, assisted ventilation gives symptomatic relief to nocturnal breathlessness, even if there is no evidence for hypoventilation during sleep.

Ventilatory failure should be suspected when there are awakenings from sleep, early morning headaches, excessive daytime sleepiness, worsening breathlessness and ankle swelling, in a patient with a high-risk disorder, such as following a thoracoplasty or with a kyphosis or scoliosis, especially if the vital capacity is less than 1–1.5 l.

Techniques

Non-invasive techniques are preferred to tracheostomy ventilation unless there is upper airway obstruction which prevents them from being effective, or the airway has to be protected because of a risk of aspiration, or ventilatory support is needed almost continuously.

The methods of ventilatory support are as follows.
1 Positive pressure ventilation. This can be achieved during sleep by the following methods.

   (a) Tracheostomy ventilation. This invasive method of ventilation is surprisingly well tolerated but requires a higher level of care in the home than the non-invasive methods. Complications such as tube displacement, obstruction, impairment of swallowing and occasionally a tracheo-oesophageal fistula or tracheo-innominate artery fistula may develop.

   (b) Mask and mouthpiece ventilation. The nasal masks used for ventilatory support are similar to those used for nasal CPAP (Fig. 11.3), but oronasal masks are occasionally required. If neither can be tolerated a mouthpiece or nasal seals are alternatives. The mask connects to either a pressure or volume preset ventilator. The former is more frequently used, and in neuromuscular and skeletal disorders it is common for the peak inspiratory pressure to be 20–25 cmH$_2$O with a positive end expiratory pressure of 2–4 cmH$_2$O to prevent alveolar closure. The inspiratory time is 0.8–1.0 s with an expiratory time of around 2 s. A sensitive trigger and short response time are preferable in view of the rapid respiratory rate adopted by these patients.

These systems are usually well tolerated, but several difficulties are recognized. Ulceration of the skin of the bridge of the nose is a common problem. The mask may become displaced during sleep, air-leaks around the mask or through the mouth may develop and upper airway symptoms such as a dry or blocked nose may develop. Functional upper airway obstruction may be seen and, if air enters the oesophagus rather than the trachea, abdominal distension with frequent belching, nausea and the passing of flatus may arise.

These complications can usually be overcome by careful attention to the mask and ventilator settings, but occasionally ventilation through a mouthpiece is required. This may lead to dental complications, and air-leaks through the nose.

2 Negative pressure ventilation. With these techniques the chest and abdomen are enclosed in an airtight rigid chamber from which air is evacuated by a ventilator connected to it through wide-bore tubing. Air is drawn in through the mouth and nose. Three types of negative pressure ventilation are available.

(a) Tank ventilation (iron lung). The patient lies supine on a mattress within the chamber which encloses the whole body up to the neck. Access to the subject is limited and this equipment is large, heavy and expensive, but effective. It is rarely used for long-term nocturnal respiratory support, for which a cuirass or jacket is usually preferable.

(b) Jacket ventilation. A framework of metal or plastic provides the rigidity and this is covered by an airtight garment from which air is evacuated by a negative pressure ventilator.

(c) Cuirass ventilation. The properties of rigidity and impermeability to air are combined in a single structure, the cuirass shell, which is usually individually constructed to fit the patient so that it encloses the anterolateral aspects of the rib cage and abdomen (Fig. 11.5). A cuirass is light and durable and, unlike a mask, does not lead to claustrophobia, but it can induce upper airway obstruction due to loss of the normal sequence of activation of the upper airway muscles during inspiration.

Mechanisms of action

The mechanisms of action of non-invasive ventilation in sleep hypoventilation are still uncertain (Fig. 11.6). It consolidates stages 3 and 4 NREM sleep, which is particularly important in relieving symptoms such as excessive daytime sleepiness, and probably in improving the respiratory drive. It also reduces the arterial

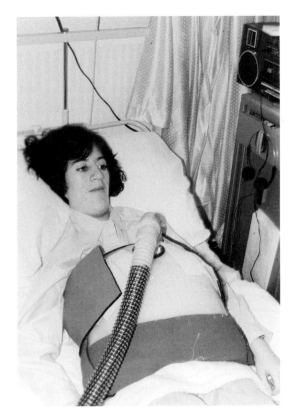

Fig. 11.5 Cuirass shell enclosing the patient's rib cage and abdomen with tubing connecting it to a negative presure ventilator.

P_{CO_2} while ventilation is applied, and this reduces the cerebrospinal fluid bicarbonate concentration and increases the ventilatory response to hypercapnia.

Non-invasive ventilation also improves the chest wall mechanics by increasing the respiratory excursion of the rib cage and the compliance of the soft tissues of the chest wall. It improves the metabolic environment in which the respiratory muscles function. Hypercapnia, acidosis, hypoxia and other endocrine and metabolic factors which impair contractility can be normalized. It also influences the cardiac output and blood supply to the diaphragm and other respiratory muscles, which is important since muscle fatigue is thought to be related to the balance between the metabolic activity and the quantity of blood flowing to the muscles.

Mechanical ventilation can also affect the intrinsic contractility of the respiratory muscles. Atrophy and functional impairment of respiratory muscles with myofibril damage can develop if these are completely unloaded and respiratory muscle activity abolished

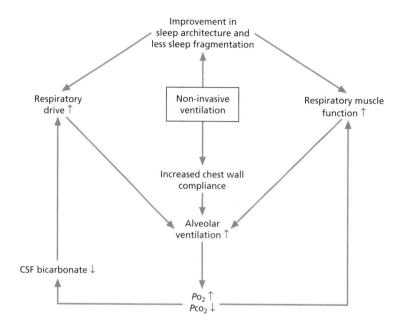

Fig. 11.6 Mechanisms of action of non-invasive ventilation.

[15]. Most non-invasive ventilatory systems, however, only provide partial respiratory support, which avoids this complication, and if the ventilator is appropriately adjusted it can even become a respiratory muscle training or conditioning device.

Outcomes of treatment
The main outcomes of ventilatory support are as follows.

Quality of life. Nocturnal non-invasive ventilation improves the symptoms of respiratory failure and quality of life. It relieves breathlessness on exertion, improves sleep quality and relieves daytime sleepiness and early morning headaches [16]. Everyday activities such as shopping and cleaning can be carried out more easily. It may be possible to return to work which was previously too physically or mentally demanding.

Physiological changes. Nocturnal ventilation not only improves arterial oxygen saturation and transcutaneous Pco_2 during sleep, but also normalizes the blood gases during wakefulness [17]. These improvements may be seen within 1–2 days of initiating treatment and the full effect is usually apparent within 1–4 weeks. Small improvements in vital capacity and maximal inspiratory and expiratory mouth pressures and respiratory drive may be seen.

Survival. There are no controlled studies of survival in chronic respiratory failure due to neuromuscular and skeletal disorders. In a stable condition such as scoliosis the 1-year survival is around 90% and 5-year survival around 80% [18]. Those with a thoracoplasty have a slightly worse outlook with survival at 3 years 75–85% and at 5 years over 65%, probably because of extensive pulmonary disease from the tuberculous infection [13].

Death may occur from a recurrence of chronic respiratory failure, despite ventilatory support, because of poor compliance, or due to an acute intercurrent illness, particularly a chest infection.

The prognosis is worse if the underlying neuromuscular disease is progressive, as in motor neurone disease and Duchenne's muscular dystrophy, or if there is bulbar muscle weakness with a risk of aspiration pneumonia [19].

References

1 Thomas RJ, Daly RW, Weiss JW. Low-concentration carbon dioxide is an effective adjunct to positive airway pressure in the treatment of refractory mixed central and obstructive sleep-disordered breathing. *Sleep* 2005; 28(1): 69–77.
2 Khoo MCK, Gottschalk A, Pack AI. Sleep-induced periodic breathing and apnea: a theoretical study. *J Appl Physiol* 1991; 70: 2014–24.

3 Fanfulla F, Mortara A, Maestri R *et al.* The development of hyperventilation in patients with chronic heart failure and Cheyne–Stokes respiration. A possible role of chronic hypoxia. *Chest* 1998; 114: 1083–90.

4 Naughton MT. Heart failure and central apnoea. *Sleep Med Rev* 1998; 2: 105–16.

5 Lorenzi-Filho G, Dajani HR, Leung RST, Floras JS, Bradley TD. Entrainment of blood pressure and heart rate oscillations by periodic breathing. *Am J Respir Crit Care Med* 1999; 159: 1147–54.

6 Swenson ER. Carbonic anhydrase inhibitors and ventilation: a complex interplay of stimulation and suppression. *Eur Respir J* 1998; 12: 1242–7.

7 Philip-Joet FF, Paganelli FF, Dutau HL, Saadjian AY. Hemodynamic effects of bilevel nasal positive airway pressure ventilation in patients with heart failure. *Respiration* 1999; 66: 136–43.

8 Shneerson J. Sleep in neuromuscular and thoracic cage disorders. *Eur Resp Mono* 1998; 3: 324–44.

9 Bye PTP, Ellis ER, Issa FG, Donnelly PM, Sullivan CE. Respiratory failure and sleep in neuromuscular disease. *Thorax* 1990; 45: 241–7.

10 White JES, Drinnan MJ, Smithson AJ, Griffiths CJ, Gibson GJ. Respiratory muscle activity and oxygenation during sleep in patients with muscle weakness. *Eur Respir J* 1995; 8: 807–14.

11 Bourke SC, Gibson GJ. Sleep and breathing in neuromuscular disease. *Eur Respir J* 2002; 19: 1194–201.

12 Midgren B, Petersson K, Hannsson L, Eriksson L, Airikkala P, Elmqvist D. Nocturnal hypoxaemia in severe scoliosis. *Br J Dis Chest* 1988; 82: 226–36.

13 Shneerson JM. Respiratory failure in tuberculosis: a modern perspective. *Clin Med* 2004; 4: 72–6.

14 Hukins CA, Hillman DR. Daytime predictors of sleep hypoventilation in Duchenne musclar dystrophy. *Am J Respir Crit Care Med* 2000; 161: 166–70.

15 Sassoon CSH, Caiozzo VJ, Manka A, Sieck GC. Altered diaphragm contractile properties with controlled mechanical ventilation. *J Appl Physiol* 2002; 92: 2585–95.

16 Hill NS, Eveloff SE, Carlisle CC, Goff SG. Efficacy of nocturnal nasal ventilation in patients with restrictive thoracic disease. *Am Rev Respir Dis* 1992; 145: 365–71.

17 Simonds AK, Elliott MW. Outcome of domiciliary nasal intermittent positive pressure ventilation in restrictive and obstructive disorders. *Thorax* 1995; 50: 604–9.

18 Leger P, Bedicam JM, Cornette A *et al.* Nasal intermittent positive pressure ventilation. Long term follow-up in patients with severe chronic respiratory insufficiency. *Chest* 1994; 105: 100–5.

19 Shneerson JM, Simonds AK. Noninvasive ventilation for chest wall and neuromuscular disorders. *Eur Respir J* 2002; 20: 480–7.

12 Medical Disorders

Introduction

Medical disorders often cause secondary insomnia and excessive daytime sleepiness and occasionally lead to abnormal sensory experiences and motor activity during sleep. These and abnormalities of upper airway function and respiratory pump disorders have been dealt with in previous chapters. This chapter discusses the wide range of other medical disorders which are associated with sleep. Many of these cause symptoms primarily related to the physiological system that is affected, and sleep-related aspects may be less conspicuous.

Assessment

History

A careful history is essential to accurately assess these medical disorders. The details of the symptoms at the moment of waking, the responses made to these, and any other observed activities are important. The time of the events during the night and the degree of recall may help to establish the nature of the events.

Physical examination

Physical examination may reveal abnormalities specific to the disorder, and investigations relevant to the system involved may be required.

Investigations

Polysomnography is only occasionally needed, for instance to distinguish gastro-oesophageal reflux from obstructive sleep apnoeas as a cause of nocturnal choking, through nocturnal pH monitoring.

Principles of treatment

The aims of treatment are as follows.
1 To explain the nature of the disorder to the subject and to reassure when appropriate.
2 To provide specific treatment for the disorder. This may be, for instance, drug treatment for asthma or nocturnal angina.
3 To modify sleep–wake patterns by:
  (a) sleep hygiene – the aim is to reinstate the normal sleep–wake pattern and prevent these episodes;
  (b) behavioural therapy, e.g. in nocturnal enuresis.

Neurological conditions

Neurodevelopmental disorders

Many of these disorders have abnormalities of sleep, such as an absence of sleep spindles or a reduction in REM sleep duration. In autism and Asperger's syndrome there is an increased number of REM sleep episodes, but they are briefer than normal. There is also an increased prevalence of sleep terrors and an awareness of poor sleep at night.

Primary sleep disorders such as the restless legs syndrome and obstructive sleep apnoeas may exacerbate developmental problems and cause excessive daytime sleepiness, manifested as hyperactivity, aggression and poor cognitive development. Around 20% of those with attention deficit hyperactivity disorder are said to have the restless legs syndrome. In Down's syndrome and cerebral palsy there is a predisposition to sleep apnoeas.

Sleep disorders may also be the result of the care and care environment. Children with developmental disorders often live in residential and nursing homes and are inactive for much of the day with little exposure to bright light. Improvement in these aspects of sleep hygiene and altering the timing of sleep onset and ensuring a regular wake-up time in the morning are important. Behavioural techniques such as instituting a regular wind-down routine in the evenings to build associations with sleep may be helpful. Failure of the parents and carers to set limits at bedtime should be corrected, and rewarding of good behaviour and scheduled wakenings just before an anticipated difficulty in sleep should be considered. Hypnotics are of little help in long-term management, but wakefulness promoting drugs, such as modafinil, may improve alertness during the day.

Nocturnal and early morning headaches

There are several causes for nocturnal and early morning headaches [1].

Tension headaches

These may result from any condition that causes sleep fragmentation, such as obstructive sleep apnoeas or insomnia, particularly when this is associated with the chronic fatigue syndrome or fibromyalgia. Polysomnography usually shows a reduction in total sleep time, sleep efficiency and duration of stages 3 and 4 NREM sleep. The headaches usually improve if the underlying sleep disorder can be treated.

Sinus headaches

These are due to changes in pressure within the sinuses and often occur at a regular time soon after waking.

Bruxism

This may cause facial pain referred from the temporomandibular joints.

Migraine

Migraines have a complex relationship to sleep. They are often relieved during the day by sleep but, conversely, may develop after waking from sleep, particularly REM sleep, at night. Migraines are commoner when the subject is tired, and possibly after oversleeping, and they are often followed by sleepiness. They are commoner in sleep walkers and narcolepsy than in normal subjects, and changes in 5HT neurotransmission may be responsible. The link between migraine and sleep may reflect alterations in autonomic function, possibly related to changes in 5HT transmission, between sleep and wake states.

Cluster headaches (migrainous neuralgia)

These are often intense, occur unilaterally around the eye, and are associated with lachrymation, nasal discharge and facial vasodilatation. They are 10 times more common in males than in females, occur particularly between the ages of 40 and 60 years and last for 30–180 min. They are most frequent in spring and autumn when the change in the length of exposure to light is greatest, and are also associated with low plasma peak melatonin and cortisol concentrations.

Seventy-five per cent of cluster headaches occur during sleep and they often appear at the same time each night for several weeks before going into remission. They are most common in REM sleep, and at the transition between REM and NREM sleep. Metabolic activity is increased during these episodes in the cingulate gyrus and hypothalamus close to the suprachiasmatic nuclei. This probably alters the balance between parasympathetic and sympathetic systems to cause the unilateral vascular and secretory changes which underlie the clinical features. The headaches may worsen during REM sleep rebound when REM sleep suppressant drugs such as tricyclic antidepressants are discontinued, and may be exacerbated by obstructive sleep apnoeas.

Chronic paroxysmal hemicrania

This is probably a variant of cluster headaches and is associated with vasomotor symptoms. The episodes are brief and more frequent with up to 10–20 attacks occurring each 24 h. They occur at a regular time each night and are closely related to REM sleep, which they often cause to become fragmented.

Hypnic headache

This unusual condition has been described in the elderly. The headaches occur only during sleep, are diffuse usually bilateral and frontal and may be associated with dreaming. They occur at a consistent time each night for each individual usually between 1.00 and 3.00 AM and last for 30–60 min. They are said to be related to REM sleep but no cause has been established. They may respond to caffeine, indomethacin or lithium.

Intracranial hypertension

The intracranial pressure normally rises during REM sleep, possibly because of changes in the cerebral blood flow. Distortion of the dura mater or vasodilatation itself, possibly related to the action of nitric oxide, stimulates pain receptors in the intracranial vessels.

Raised intracranial pressure causes headaches which are usually bifrontal, and may be associated with nausea and vomiting. They usually clear within 20–60 min after waking in the morning. They are associated with space-occupying intracranial lesions, severe hypertension, hypercapnia, particularly in REM sleep, causing cerebral vasodilatation, cerebral oedema following a hypoglycaemic episode, and benign intracranial hypertension.

Respiratory conditions

The changes in respiration which affect the respiratory pump are described in Chapter 11 and upper airway disorders are discussed in Chapter 10. This section covers only those conditions in which the changes in lung function itself are predominant.

Asthma

Asthma is characterized by a widespread but variable increase in airflow resistance together with hyper-inflation of the lungs. It has a circadian rhythm irrespective of the many environmental factors that affect its severity (Fig. 12.1) [2]. Nocturnal asthma may cause frequent arousals from sleep, particularly after the first cycle of NREM and REM sleep, and it may lead to excessive daytime sleepiness. The arousals are partly due to the increased work of breathing, but

also to frequent coughing, and they improve once the asthma is controlled.

The lowest peak flow rates in asthmatics are recorded at around 4.00 AM. There is a normal cir-cadian fluctuation in peak flow rates of less than 10–15%, with the highest values at around 4.00 PM, but this is exaggerated in asthmatics, perhaps with a slight shift in the time of the lowest peak flow rates as well.

The cause of the increase in amplitude of the changes in airflow obstruction is uncertain (Fig. 12.2). It is probably not primarily related to the onset of sleep itself since the peak flow rates fall even if the subject remains awake at night, although the fall is greater during sleep. The changes are not related to any par-ticular sleep stage, but a major factor appears to be the reduction in lung volume. This is probably due to the generalized inhibition of motor activity during

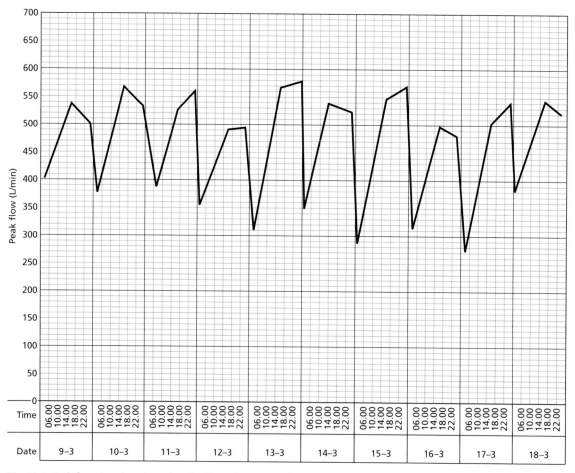

Fig. 12.1 Peak flow chart in asthma showing diurnal pattern with early morning dips.

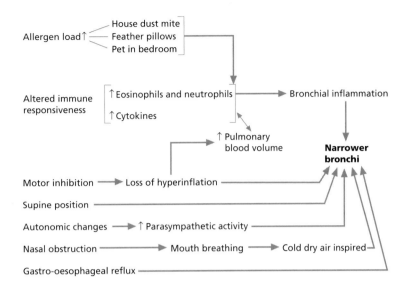

Fig. 12.2 Causes of nocturnal asthma.

sleep, particularly REM sleep. This leads to relaxation of the chest wall muscles with abolition of any reflex hyperinflation in response to airflow obstruction and a failure to respond to any intrapulmonary reflexes during sleep which would increase the lung volume. As the lung volume falls the diameter of the airways decreases and, if they are already narrowed, the increase in airflow resistance may be considerable. The reduction in lung volume is greater in the supine position, but posture by itself is not the only factor since there is still a circadian fluctuation in airflow obstruction even if the subjects lie in bed continuously throughout the 24 h.

During sleep the intrapulmonary blood volume increases. This reduces the volume of air within the lungs slightly, but more importantly increases the number of inflammatory cells and the quantity of mediators within the lung. This raises the potential for any bronchial inflammation. Broncho-alveolar lavage has shown more eosinophils and neutrophils in the aspirate at 4.00 AM than at 4.00 PM, and the quantity of cytokines, for instance IL-1β, is also increased. Transbronchial biopsies have shown an increase in the eosinophilic alveolar infiltrate at night in proportion to the severity of nocturnal asthma. The increase in lung inflammation is not related to nocturnal changes in cortisol levels, or to serum IgE which peaks at midday.

There are several other factors which could affect airway function at night in asthma. First, the increase in parasympathetic activity causes bronchoconstriction and the importance of this is indicated by the

degree of improvement which can be obtained with atropinic drugs at night. The lower blood levels of adrenaline at night compared to during the daytime are probably not significant, but the increased nasal resistance associated with the alternating changes in the patency of the right and left nasal airway (nasal cycle) may cause mouth breathing which leads to cool, dry air entering the lungs, which can induce asthma. Gastro-oesophageal reflux is also common during sleep and this can cause reflex bronchoconstriction. Temperature changes in the bedroom and exposure to allergens, such as house dust mites, feathers in pillows and the hair or fur of pets who may have slept in the bedroom, may also exacerbate the nocturnal tendency of asthma to worsen.

Respiratory failure due to asthma usually occurs at night partly because asthma is more severe during sleep, but also because of abnormalities of respiratory control. Asthmatics at risk of developing respiratory failure often have a reduced hypoxic and hypercapnic ventilatory response to bronchoconstriction, and some also increase their inspiratory time which reduces the time available for expiration and so predisposes to air trapping.

The differential diagnosis of nocturnal asthma includes left ventricular failure, obstructive sleep apnoea, choking during sleep due to, for instance, gastro-oesophageal reflux, and nocturnal angina (Table 12.1). Nocturnal cough due to asthma should be distinguished from a postnasal drip.

It is not only important to avoid any factors that may precipitate nocturnal asthma, but also to use

Table 12.1 Sleep-related causes of some common symptoms.

Headaches	Cluster headache, raised intracranial pressure, e.g. hypercapnia, hypnic headache
Chest pain	Angina, myocardial infarction, gastro-oesophageal reflux, oesophageal spasm, peptic ulcer
Breathlessness	Asthma, left ventricular failure, bilateral diaphragmatic paralysis, CSR, CSA, OSA
Cough	Asthma, post nasal drip, gastro-oesophageal reflux
Choking	OSA, pharyngeal pooling of saliva, gastro-oesophageal reflux, vocal cord adduction asthma, left ventricular failure
Nocturia	OSA, prostatic hypertrophy, renal disease, diabetes mellitus or insipidus

CSA, central sleep apnoeas; CSR, Cheyne–Stokes respiration; OSA, obstructive sleep apnoeas.

long-acting drug treatments which lasts throughout the night. Care should be taken with theophyllines, leukotriene receptor antagonists and systemic glucocorticoids which, although they are often effective in relieving nocturnal asthma, can also cause insomnia.

Chronic bronchitis and emphysema (chronic obstructive pulmonary disease, COPD)

In chronic bronchitis and emphysema the arterial Po_2 falls during sleep, partly due to hypoventilation which leads to a rise in the arterial Pco_2 and partly to worsening of ventilation and perfusion matching within the lungs. The cardiac output is maintained, but the pulmonary artery pressure rises because of hypoxic vasoconstriction. REM sleep is initially fragmented and later there is loss of stages 3 and 4 NREM sleep. The oxygen saturation dips, particularly during REM sleep. Chronic hypoxia may lead to polycythaemia, hypercapnia during wakefulness and other physiological changes described in Chapter 11. Excessive daytime sleepiness, shortness of breath at night with frequent awakenings, ankle swelling and cognitive impairments, particularly of memory, are common.

The essential physiological feature of chronic bronchitis and emphysema is expiratory air flow limitation [3]. The expiratory phase is prolonged and, if it cannot be completed before the onset of the next inspiration, air trapping with intrinsic positive end

expiratory pressure (PEEP) develops. The impaired ventilation–perfusion matching requires an increase in the ventilation to normalize the arterial Po_2, but the pattern of respiratory rate and tidal volume adopted by the patient fluctuates continuously. The reduced lung compliance and hyperinflation increase the work of breathing and reduce the length of the inspiratory muscles, particularly the diaphragm, and thereby impair their effectiveness.

During sleep the upper airway narrows, particularly in REM rather than NREM sleep, increasing the airflow resistance. This prolongs the inspiratory time, reduces the expiratory time, and increases the risk of air trapping and intrinsic PEEP. The alternative strategies of reducing the tidal volume (hypopnoea) or of slowing the respiratory rate both lead to alveolar hypoventilation.

The combination of upper airway obstruction with chronic airflow limitation has been termed the 'overlap syndrome', although this term is of little value. The combination of these two conditions predisposes to hypercapnia, both during sleep and during wakefulness. This is partly because the airflow obstruction prevents the respiratory muscles from normalizing the blood gases rapidly enough after arousal and before the next apnoea, and also because, once hypercapnia is established during the night, it leads to hypercapnia while awake as well. This sequence of

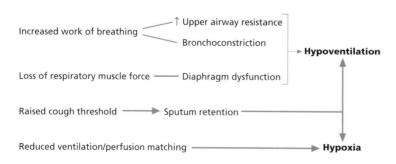

Fig. 12.3 Effects of sleep on chronic obstructive pulmonary disease (COPD).

events can be suspected if daytime hypercapnia occurs when the forced expiratory volume in 1 s (FEV1) is greater than about 1.0–1.5 l.

Diaphragmatic dysfunction during sleep is related to hyperinflation, in which the diaphragm shortens and alters its configuration so that it contracts horizontally and draws the lateral rib cage inwards instead of expanding it. These ineffective contractions are particularly important in REM sleep when the diaphragm is the only active inspiratory chest wall muscle. Prolonged and deep oxygen desaturations associated with hypercapnia may result.

A third factor is the fall in lung volume during REM sleep which increases airflow resistance, reduces ventilation–perfusion matching and leads to an increase in the work of breathing and a fall in the Po_2. The higher cough threshold during REM sleep and in the deeper stages of NREM sleep predisposes to retention of secretions in the airways which increases the airflow resistance and the work of breathing.

These changes are superimposed on a fluctuating chemoreceptor drive in response to rapid micro-oscillations in the arterial Pco_2 and Po_2 and changes in the activation of mechanoreceptors according to the tidal volume, respiratory rate and airflow during each breath. The Po_2 is often located near the inflection point of the oxyhaemoglobin dissociation curve so that any slight fall causes a disproportionately large oxygen desaturation compared to normal.

The central and obstructive sleep apnoeas that result from these abnormalities cause repeated arousals and fragmentation of sleep. REM sleep is particularly shortened and fragmented, and later in the natural history stages 3 and 4 NREM sleep are similarly affected. Hypercapnia occurs particularly in REM sleep, and later in NREM sleep as well. Arousals may be associated with a sensation of breathlessness on waking, and lead to excessive daytime sleepiness. Early morning headaches due to carbon dioxide retention may appear. Most patients prefer to sit upright rather than lie flat, in order to optimize diaphragmatic function.

The approach to treatment is similar to that described in Chapter 11 for nocturnal respiratory complications due to neuromuscular and skeletal disorders. Long-term oxygen treatment is advisable if the Po_2 remains persistently below around 7.3 kPa during the day with an oxygen saturation of less than 85–90% at night, but if this is associated with significant daytime hypercapnia (Pco_2 greater than about 8 kPa) non-invasive ventilatory support with or without supple-mental oxygen is preferable. Improvement in survival, in symptoms and in the physiological abnormalities has been demonstrated. The ventilator should be set with a slow respiratory rate, short inspiratory time, high inspiratory flow-rate, small tidal volume, long expiratory time and PEEP, together with a sensitive triggering system in order to coordinate the patient's respiratory activity with the ventilator and to minimize the risk of air trapping.

Cystic fibrosis

The respiratory changes in cystic fibrosis during sleep are similar to those in chronic bronchitis and emphysema, but sleep fragmentation may be exacerbated by frequent coughing and deterioration in airflow obstruction by retention of tracheobronchial secretions [3, 4]. The oxygen saturation falls, particularly if the subject is hypoxic during wakefulness, and it is lowest during REM sleep. Pulmonary hypertension, right heart failure and hypercapnia during wakefulness as well as sleep may eventually result, as in chronic bronchitis and emphysema.

Parenchymal disorders

The effects of these on sleep have been very little studied, but interstitial lung diseases can cause frequent arousals from sleep. The respiratory frequency, which is rapid during wakefulness, hardly changes during NREM sleep. In REM sleep an unstable respiratory pattern appears and leads to oxygen desaturations which are often considerable because of the low initial Po_2 which is close to the inflection point of the oxy-haemoglobin dissociation curve. These desaturations are, however, usually less marked in sleep than during exercise. They may be relieved either by treatment of the lung disease itself or by supplemental oxygen at night. This is often needed during the day as well. Ventilatory support is rarely required.

Sudden infant death syndrome (SIDS)

Sudden infant death syndrome is a heterogeneous disorder that affects children usually between the ages of 2 and 4 months. It is thought to occur only during sleep and is commonest in premature infants and in the winter. It usually follows or is associated with an upper respiratory infection.

'Apparent life threatening events' (ALTEs) are episodes which are frightening to the observer and characterized by a cessation of breathing, colour change, loss of muscle tone, choking or gagging. These episodes, unlike SIDS, occur during wakefulness. Their cause is uncertain, but in some patients gastro-oesophageal reflux, epilepsy, cardiac dysrhythmias and obstructive sleep apnoeas are present. The child recovers fully from these episodes, unlike SIDS, and the risk of death is low.

The cause of SIDS has not been satisfactorily explained despite intense investigation. It is probably multifactorial and the relative contributions of each component are likely to differ in each child.

A common feature is a failure of arousal from sleep in the presence of a difficulty with respiration [5]. The failure to arouse may be due to a neurological developmental abnormality, possibly determined prenatally. Abnormalities of cardiac autonomic control probably contribute. The respiratory stimulus may be a chest infection or possibly an allergic reaction within the lungs [6], but may often be obstructive sleep apnoeas.

Apnoeas of prematurity are more common if the birthweight is low, but are less frequent at postconception ages of greater than 40 weeks, which is when SIDS usually occurs. Congenital malformations of the mandible may cause obstructive sleep apnoeas and while defects in the medullary respiratory centres could lead to central apnoeas, the link between these and SIDS has never been firmly demonstrated.

Cardiovascular conditions

The metabolic rate and cardiac output fall during NREM sleep and the loss of sympathetic vasoconstriction reduces the systemic vascular resistance so that the blood pressure falls. NREM sleep is cardioprotective despite the drop in perfusion pressure. In contrast, in REM sleep autonomic control is unstable. Fluctuations in heart rate and blood pressure are common and the cerebral blood flow increases. These changes protect against some cardiovascular problems during sleep, but predispose to others.

Cardiac dysrhythmias

The increased parasympathetic activity in sleep reduces the heart rate and atrioventricular node conduction, and increases the threshold for ventricular fibrillation. The heart rate accelerates, however, at the moment of an arousal because of an increase in sympathetic activity.

NREM sleep tends to prevent supraventricular tachycardias, paroxysmal atrial fibrillation and ventricular dysrhythmias, especially in stages 3 and 4 NREM sleep. Sinus bradycardia and atrioventricular node conduction defects may appear. Occasionally

the fall in perfusion pressure in NREM sleep can trigger dysrhythmias, particularly if there is coronary artery disease.

Prolonged sinus arrests may be seen in REM sleep, particularly in young males. Asystole for up to 2.5 s is conventionally regarded as normal, but this may become as long as 9 s in sleep in otherwise healthy subjects, probably because of an increase in parasympathetic activity. This is probably a normal variant, although it has been termed the 'REM sleep-related sinus arrest' syndrome. Sinus dysrhythmia is also prominent in young males, particularly during phasic REM sleep, and occasionally even Mobitz Type 1 second-degree atrioventricular block may occur.

Waking in the morning leads to an increase in myocardial oxygen requirements, blood pressure and heart rate, probably because of a change from the supine to the standing position and increased catecholamine secretion and sympathetic activity in response to environmental stimuli. The fibrinogen level and platelet aggregation also increase. Ventricular ectopics frequently occur at this time, but can be prevented by beta blockers. Sudden death presumed to be cardiac in origin is most common between 7.00 AM and 11.00 AM, probably due to ventricular tachycardia and fibrillation.

Cardiac dysrhythmias during and immediately after sleep may present with arousals and awareness of palpitations, breathlessness or angina, but they are often asymptomatic. Continuous 24-h electrocardiogram recording is required to establish the diagnosis. Polysomnography is rarely needed. Drug or ablation treatment may be required.

Hypertension

The blood pressure normally falls by 5–15% during NREM sleep, but to a lesser extent and in a much more variable fashion during REM sleep, in which both the cardiac output and peripheral vascular resistance fluctuate considerably. The dip in blood pressure during sleep is often absent when hypertension is present during wakefulness, possibly because of persistence of sympathetic vasoconstrictor over-activity.

The blood pressure rises rapidly on waking, whether this is a brief arousal from sleep or at the end of the nocturnal sleep episode. This and blood pressure fluctuations during sleep may contribute to an increased risk of stroke. This risk is greatest in obstructive sleep apnoeas where the rapidly alternating parasympathetic and sympathetic activity leads to transient rises in blood pressure of up to 50%. Strokes are most frequent between 6.00 and 9.00 AM and the increase in circulating catecholamines and in platelet aggregation on waking may contribute to this.

Angina and myocardial infarction

Cardiac ischaemia is common in sleep, particularly during the second half of the night [7]. It is more often silent (asymptomatic) in sleep than during exercise. During sleep, cardiac output falls as a result of a slower heart rate rather than any change in stroke volume. In NREM sleep, blood pressure also falls and the drop in perfusing pressure reduces the coronary artery blood flow. An exaggeration of this hypotension (over-dipping), especially in stages 3 and 4 NREM sleep, may cause clinically significant cardiac ischaemia, especially in the presence of coronary artery disease. The peak time for myocardial infarction during NREM sleep is between 12.00 and 2.00 AM when stages 3 and 4 are most likely. Despite this, NREM sleep is largely cardioprotective because of the low metabolic rate and the constant, but low, cardiac output.

In REM sleep, however, the major change is that the myocardial oxygen requirements increase. Sympathetic activity is enhanced, although erratically, and there is vasoconstriction within the skeletal muscles. The heart rate, blood pressure and peripheral vascular resistance all rise, but are unstable. Depression of ST segments of the electrocardiogram by more than 1 mm is frequent and angina is also more common in REM than in NREM sleep. REM sleep is also associated with the Prinzmetal variant angina in which coronary artery spasm, presumably due to a shift towards sympathetic dominance, leads to ST segment elevation. This is commonest between 4.00 and 8.00 AM.

The process of awakening is probably even more of a risk for cardiac ischaemia than REM sleep. The chance of a myocardial infarction rises between 4.00 and 9.00 AM and is three times more common at this time than in the evening (Fig. 12.4). Unstable angina

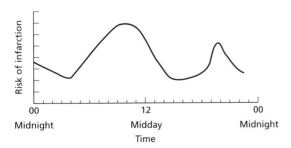

Fig. 12.4 Timing of myocardial infarction.

and sudden cardiac death both show a similar pattern. This is probably due to increased sympathetic activity, increased platelet activation and aggregability, an increase in the fibrinogen level and a reduction in fibrinolysis, together with the onset of physical exertion which raises the blood pressure and heart rate. The coronary artery vasoconstriction, together with an in-crease in heart rate and blood pressure, probably leads to plaque rupture which triggers the thrombotic process.

Obstructive sleep apnoeas can also induce cardiac ischaemia, especially in REM sleep. This is partly due to hypoxia, but also to shift of the interventricular septum to the left as the right ventricle dilates. This reduces the volume of the left ventricle during systole, reduces the left ventricular compliance and increases its work. Increase in sympathetic activity also contributes to ischaemia by causing coronary artery vasoconstriction. Angina occurs occasionally, but cardiac dysrhythmias are more common.

Coronary artery bypass grafting is usually followed by insomnia which gradually improves over several weeks or months and occasionally for up to 2 years. The total sleep time is reduced together with a reduction in the duration of stages 3 and 4 NREM sleep [8]. These changes may be partly due to postoperative anxiety and pain, and poor sleep hygiene, due, for instance, to noise in the hospital ward, but also to cerebral dysfunction due to the general anaesthetic and extracorporeal circulation.

Heart failure

Approximately 1% of adults have heart failure of New York Health Association (NYHA) grade 3 or 4. While diastolic heart failure affects particularly women and the elderly, systolic heart failure is much commoner.

Cardiac effects

The raised filling pressure is associated with venoconstriction, and cardiac dilatation with a reduced ejection fraction. Cardiac function is often further impaired by remodelling or fibrosis, and intermittent dysrhythmias. The cardiac oxygen demands increase because of the increased left ventricular afterload due to hypertension from the systemic vasoconstriction resulting from increased sympathetic activity.

Circulatory effects

The renin–angiotensin–aldosterone axis is stimulated and antidiuretic hormone (ADH) is secreted with the result that sodium and water are retained. Sympathetic

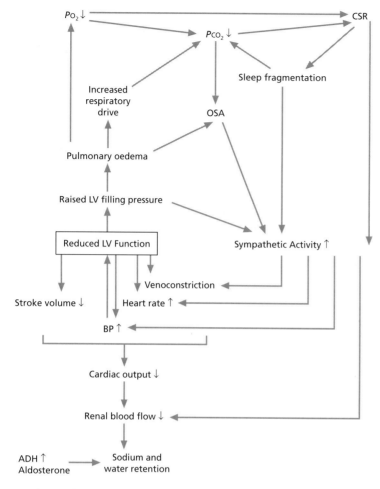

Fig. 12.5 Physiological responses to heart failure.

LV = Left ventricle
BP= Blood pressure
ADH = Antidiuretic hormone
CSR = Cheyne Stokes respiration
OSA = Obstructive sleep apnoea

activity increases and raises the heart rate, causes venoconstriction and increases cardiac contractility. The baroreceptors in the heart and major arteries have a reduced sensitivity.

Atrial and brain natriuretic peptides are secreted and cytokines, such as IL-6 and TNF alpha, are produced. These impair endothelial function and may also lead to skeletal muscle wasting. Metabolic influences such as insulin resistance also contribute to skeletal muscle wasting.

Respiratory effects

Cardiac failure has several important sleep-related respiratory effects. It may cause breathlessness at night,

particularly when lying flat, with frequent awakenings, daytime sleepiness and cognitive changes. Physical fatigue, due both to cardiac failure and to drug treatment, particularly beta blockers, may be present.

Left ventricular failure increases the ventilatory response to carbon dioxide. This is partly due to stimulation of J receptors by pulmonary oedema and also because of an increase in the gain of the central nervous system control system. In addition, hypoxia due to ventilation–perfusion mismatching in the lung increases the response to carbon dioxide and is itself a respiratory stimulant.

As a result the arterial $P\text{CO}_2$ falls during wakefulness and remains low during sleep. The normal rise in arterial P_{CO_2} of 2–3 mmHg at sleep onset does not occur. The P_{CO_2} during sleep is therefore close to the apnoeic threshold and if ventilation increases slightly, for instance with an arousal at the end of an apnoea, the arterial P_{CO_2} may fall below the apnoeic threshold and lead to a central sleep apnoea. The reduced oxygen stores in the lungs as a result of the reduced lung volume accentuate the oscillations in P_{O_2}, which further destabilize respiration [9].

Approximately 40% of patients with cardiac failure have central apnoeas and 10% have obstructive apnoeas [10]. These cause repeated arousals from sleep leading to excessive daytime sleepiness. The increased sympathetic activity due to the arousals increases the systemic vasoconstriction and the left ventricular afterload. Central apnoeas are therefore not only a marker of cardiac failure, but also worsen it.

Obstructive sleep apnoeas and cardiac failure are related particularly to obesity in males and age in females. Their cause is uncertain, but mixed apnoeas commonly develop when the airway closes during a primarily central apnoea. In addition, a low arterial P_{CO_2} is associated with narrowing of the glottis and possibly of the rest of the upper airway as well, and the reduction in lung volumes due to pulmonary oedema causes a reflex reduction in pharyngeal diameter. Upper airway oedema also narrows its lumen and contributes to obstructive sleep apnoeas.

The effects of obstructive sleep apnoeas on cardiac function are described on page 237. They can lead to left ventricular hypertrophy with a reduction in stroke volume. Arousals at the end of each apnoea increase the sympathetic activity and the heart rate and blood pressure. These changes may be sustained during the day as well as occurring during the night.

Cheyne–Stokes respiration appears if the circulation time is slow and if there is a high chemoreceptor gain due, for instance, to an increased ventilatory response to P_{CO_2}, particularly in the presence of hypoxia (page 263). Cheyne–Stokes respiration in sleep due to heart failure is associated with a poorer survival compared to patients with a similar ejection fraction, but no Cheyne–Stokes respiration.

Treatment of respiratory effects

Acute cardiac failure

In acute left ventricular failure there is oedema of the small airways which increases the airway resistance, and ventilation–perfusion mismatching which causes hypoxia. Pulmonary oedema reduces the lung compliance and lung volumes, and increases the work of breathing. The myocardial oxygen supply falls, due to hypoxia, and there may also be a metabolic acidosis. The sympathetic activity increases the heart rate and blood pressure.

Treatment with diuretics, nitrates and opiates reduces sympathetic activity and leads to vasodilatation. Nevertheless intubation and ventilation may still be required, although the intubation rate can be reduced by around 30% by the application of continuous positive airway pressure. This reduces ventilation–perfusion mismatching, offsets intrinsic PEEP, reduces the work of breathing, and reduces the left ventricular afterload and preload. Continuous positive airway pressure is safe if the left ventricular end-diastolic pressure is greater than 12 cmH$_2$O, but if it is less than this it may cause hypotension and possibly myocardial infarction. Bilevel pressure support ventilation may be better tolerated with a lower expiratory pressure, but is more likely to reduce the arterial P_{CO_2}.

Chronic cardiac failure

Drug therapy. Standard drug therapy, apart from beta blockers, has little effect on the arousal index, sleep quality or ventricular dysrhythmias. Respiratory stimulants, such as theophyllines and acetazolamide, may have some benefit.

Oxygen. This reduces the hypoxic drive to breathe and thereby may increase the arterial P_{CO_2} and reduce the frequency of central apnoeas as well as the afterload due to peripheral vasoconstriction.

Continuous positive airway pressure (CPAP) treatment.
1 Central sleep apnoeas. A level of at least 10 cmH$_2$O is required to have a significant effect on preload. CPAP is in effect a left ventricular assist device, which reduces the cardiac diameter and thereby by Laplace's law reduces the wall tension. It reduces sympathetic activity which leads to a fall in heart rate and blood pressure, with less peripheral vasoconstriction, and this reduces the left ventricular afterload. The left ventricular ejection fraction may increase and, if this reduces the circulation time, Cheyne–Stokes respiration will be less evident. Any reduction in pulmonary oedema also reduces ventilation–perfusion mismatching, reduces the respiratory drive, increases arterial P_{CO_2} and tends to relieve any central apnoeas and Cheyne–Stokes respiration.

Central apnoeas may not be abolished immediately and CPAP should be reassessed after around 1 month with a repeat sleep study. Abolition of central apnoeas may not be sufficient to have the desired effect on preload, which makes it difficult to assess the optimum level of CPAP.

2 Obstructive sleep apnoeas. CPAP acutely relieves upper airway obstruction, reduces sympathetic drive and thereby reduces blood pressure. This reduction in left ventricular afterload increases the ejection fraction, reduces pulmonary oedema, and increases the arterial Po_2. In the long term the left ventricular ejection fraction increases and the left ventricle becomes smaller.

Non-invasive ventilation. Conventional pressure or volume present nasal ventilation increases the functional residual capacity and lung compliance by recruitment of alveoli through relief of pulmonary oedema. It also reduces ventilation–perfusion mismatching, but impairs venous return. It reduces the work of breathing and the metabolic rate so that there is less oxygen requirement and carbon dioxide elimination.

Nasal ventilation should not be used if there is unstable cardiac ischaemia or low blood pressure. If there is a low filling pressure its main effect is to reduce cardiac output by impairing venous return. Nasal pressure support ventilation is indicated if the arterial Pco_2 is raised, if CPAP is poorly tolerated, or if the breathlessness persists despite CPAP. Inspiratory pressures of 10–15 cmH_2O and 5 cmH_2O expiratory pressure are usually effective.

Adaptive servoventilation has been proposed as a method of providing sufficient pressure to have the benefits of CPAP without leading to overventilation and a lowering of the Pco_2. This type of ventilator adjusts the applied pressure frequently during sleep, with the aim of stabilizing the respiratory pattern. It reduces brain natriuretic peptide and urinary catecholamine excretion and improves daytime sleepiness.

Cardiac pacing. Cardiac resynchronization therapy may be indicated in heart failure with left bundle branch block. This delays left ventricular contraction and leads to desynchronization of the two ventricles, and a reduction in cardiac output. Insertion of a pacemaker resynchronizes ventricular function and can be combined with an implanted defibrillator. It increases the cardiac output, improves left ventricular failure and central sleep apnoeas and Cheyne–Stokes respiration in sleep.

Primary pulmonary hypertension

The raised pulmonary artery pressure causes right ventricular hypertrophy and a reduction in cardiac output with a slow circulation time. This predisposes to central sleep apnoeas [11], but oxygen desaturations at night are common even without any apnoeas, presumably due to impaired ventilation–perfusion matching. The hypoxia is associated with a low arterial Pco_2, both during wakefulness and during sleep, and it may fall below the apnoeic threshold with subsequent central sleep apnoeas. Cheyne–Stokes respiration is common, but may resolve with supplemental oxygen at night.

Gastro-intestinal conditions

Swallowing disorders

The flow of saliva almost ceases during sleep, and the frequency of swallowing falls, particularly in stages 3 and 4 NREM sleep.

Waking with a sensation of choking due to pooling of saliva in the pharynx occasionally occurs in otherwise normal elderly subjects. It appears to be unrelated to gastro-oesophageal reflux, but is precipitated by hypnotic and other central nervous system depressant drugs. It probably reflects a deterioration in the swallowing mechanism with age, which is amplified by sleep. This condition has been termed the 'sleep-related abnormal swallowing syndrome'.

Choking during sleep has several other causes. The most common is vocal cord adduction triggered by gastro-oesophageal reflux. Waking feeling unable to breathe in or out or to speak is often terrifying. The sensation of choking is located in the throat and may last for a few seconds or up to a minute. There is often a need to get out of bed and drink a glass of water and occasionally consciousness may be lost. The attacks may recur several times over a few weeks, before going into remission. They can be relieved by antiacid secretion preparations, e.g. high-dose proton pump inhibitors. These episodes may be confused with the sensation of choking with obstructive sleep apnoeas, although this is briefer, nocturnal asthma, and vocal cord adduction due to, for instance, motor neurone disease. The 'sleep choking syndrome' probably does not exist as a discrete entity.

Gastro-oesophageal reflux

This is more common during sleep than during wakefulness. The lower oesophageal sphincter tone is reduced during sleep, and gastric fluid can reflux

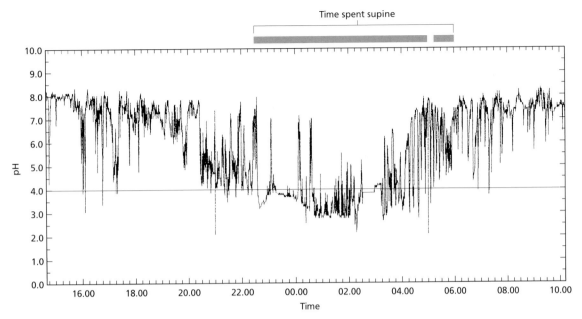

Fig. 12.6 Oesophageal pH recording showing acid reflux in sleep. The oesophageal pH frequently falls below 4 at night, whereas it rarely does so during the day.

into the oesophagus, particularly in the supine position. The tone of the upper oesophageal sphincter (cricopharyngeus) may also fall during sleep, allowing oesophagopharyngeal reflux.

The refluxed gastric acid may stay in contact with the oesophageal and pharyngeal mucosa for prolonged periods because of the infrequency of swallowing and reduced peristalsis after swallowing. This slow clearance of acid contributes to oesophagitis. Gastro-oesophageal reflux is common in obstructive sleep apnoeas, partly because of the association with obesity, but also because of the fluctuations in intrathoracic pressure during the apnoeas. If swallowing does occur more readily it may lead to sufficiently frequent arousals to cause excessive daytime sleepiness. Reflux can be diagnosed by continuous oesophageal pH recordings which show the duration as well as the extent of the fall in pH (Fig. 12.6). The frequency of episodes of reflux is usually taken as the number in which the pH remains less than 4 for at least 12 s.

Nocturnal gastro-oesophageal reflux may cause the following.

1 *Arousals during sleep without any heartburn.* This can lead to considerable sleep fragmentation and excessive daytime sleepiness [12].

2 *Sudden awakening due to retrosternal pain as a result of oesophagitis.*

3 *Chest pain, due to diffuse oesophageal spasm.* This is more common during sleep than during wakefulness.

4 *Choking caused by vocal cord adduction.*

5 *Nocturnal cough and wheeze.* These symptoms are due to reflex-induced asthma, due to reflux of acid into the lower oesophagus and, less commonly, to a direct effect of the refluxed fluid on the airways.

6 *Sleep bruxism.* This may be associated with sleep-related gastro-oesophageal reflux.

Peptic ulceration

Gastric acid secretion is partly under parasympathetic control. Basal secretion reaches a peak between 9.00 PM and 2.00 AM and is not closely related to NREM or REM sleep. In patients with duodenal ulcers the secretion of gastric acid increases both during the day and at night compared to normal subjects. This can be abolished by a vagotomy, indicating that autonomic changes both during wakefulness and during sleep contribute to these abnormalities.

Epigastric pain may cause awakening which usually occurs 1–4 h after the onset of sleep, and may be relieved by food. The differential diagnosis includes nocturnal angina. Upper gastro-intestinal endoscopy may be required to establish the diagnosis.

Intestinal motility disorders

The contractions of the stomach are less frequent in sleep and gastric emptying is slower than during wakefulness. This probably also applies to the small and large intestines. The changes in motility may underlie the worsening of abdominal pain at night in the irritable bowel syndrome, which can cause insomnia [13]. Colonic motility is particularly reduced in stages 3 and 4 NREM sleep and its reduction during sleep is associated with the infrequent need to defaecate and the common requirement for this soon after wakening, particularly after food. Nocturnal diarrhoea is a feature of extensive inflammation in, for instance, ulcerative colitis, and of diabetes when this causes an autonomic neuropathy. This may modify the control of bowel motility or secretion of bile salts during sleep.

Genitourinary tract disorders

Renal disorders

The normal diurnal rhythm of urinary output is abolished or even reversed in chronic renal disease, adrenal gland insufficiency and in the presence of oedema. This leads to nocturia which may also occur if there is bladder outflow obstruction, due, for instance, to prostatic hypertrophy, or with diuretic treatment.

The diurnal fluctuation in renal function may also be related to the tendency for episodes of gout to arise during sleep. Most of the uric acid which is produced by purine metabolism is excreted through the kidneys and a reduction in urate clearance at night may be responsible for hyperuricaemia.

Renal failure

Sleep disturbances are common in renal failure, particularly in the elderly. Around 80% of patients complain of difficulty in initiating sleep (page 183) and it is also common for excessive daytime sleepiness to be a problem [14]. Polysomnography shows a reduction in total sleep time with increased sleep fragmentation and duration of stages 1 and 2 NREM sleep, and with reduction of stages 3 and 4 NREM sleep and REM sleep.

A 'subclinical' uraemic encephalopathy, and antihypertensive and antidepressant drugs may contribute to daytime sleepiness. Anxiety and depression from the stress of the illness and its treatment are common. Bone pain associated with dialysis may lead to insomnia. Dialysis also increases cytokine production, alters body temperature control and influences melatonin secretion.

In addition to these problems renal failure is associated with the following.

Sleep apnoeas

Central apnoeas are due to hypocapnia associated with a metabolic acidosis and an unstable respiratory pattern. Obstructive apnoeas are more common than in normal subjects and may be at least partly due to 'toxins' which alter central nervous system respiratory control. The association with obesity is less marked than in normal subjects, but the apnoeas appear to increase the risk of cardiovascular complications and may contribute to hypertension. They respond to nasal continuous positive airway pressure.

Restless legs and periodic limb movements in sleep

These are present in up to 70% of those on dialysis, both peritoneal and haemodialysis. The cause is probably multifactorial, but includes iron deficiency due to dietary restriction and blood loss, changes in dopamine and possibly opioid availability in the brain, and a peripheral neuropathy due to the renal failure. The frequency of periodic limb movements has been shown to predict mortality in renal failure, but periodic limb movements and the restless legs syndrome improve with renal transplantation. They also respond to conventional drug treatment for restless legs and periodic limb movements in sleep, including dopaminergic agents and gabapentin.

Nocturnal enuresis (bed wetting, enuresis nocturna)

Overview

Nocturnal enuresis is the persistent involuntary incontinence of urine during sleep after the age of 5 years. It usually represents a transient phase of inadequate neurological control over the detrusor muscle of the bladder.

Occurrence

It is slightly more frequent in males than in females. It is more common in monozygotic twins and is often familial. It affects 15% of children at the age of 5 years, 10% at 6 years and 5% at 10 years, but is rare in adults unless there is an organic cause.

Pathogenesis

Nocturnal enuresis is probably due to the following.

1 Immaturity of the central nervous system which fails to inhibit contraction of the detrusor muscle. Once this generates a sufficiently high pressure within the bladder, involuntary relaxation of the bladder neck occurs and this is followed by micturition. The failure to inhibit the detrusor may be familial or provoked by stress or other psychological problems. Some subjects may also have a small or non-compliant bladder which contributes to nocturnal urinary frequency.

2 Failure to arouse from stages 3 and 4 NREM sleep, which is more prolonged and consolidated in children than in adults, predisposes to enuresis.

Clinical features

Nocturnal enuresis is normal up to the age of around 5 years, but not after this age if it is persistent and frequent or if control of micturition has been acquired during wakefulness. It is often exacerbated by family stresses or over-attentiveness to the problem of bed wetting. Sedative drugs may exacerbate it by impairing neurological control of the bladder during sleep.

The child may awaken unaware of having wet the bed and dreams relating to bed wetting may follow rather than cause the event. In children enuresis tends to occur during the first third of the night, and may be associated with other conditions such as obstructive sleep apnoeas and constipation and respond to treatment of these.

Investigations

Polysomnography is not required to make the diagnosis, but often reveals partial or complete arousals, usually from stages 3 and 4 NREM, occasionally from stages 1 and 2 NREM, and least commonly from REM sleep. Sleep cystometry shows an increase in bladder reactivity to external stimuli and an increase in detrusor muscle contraction prior to micturition. The pressure within the bladder rises to a level which would be sufficient to trigger involuntary micturition during wakefulness and therefore probably during sleep as well.

Differential diagnosis

1 Anatomical abnormalities, e.g. bladder neck obstruction, ureteric stenosis. These often cause daytime enuresis or sleep enuresis after a period of continence has been established (secondary enuresis).

2 Vesico-ureteric reflux. This is often associated with detrusor instability and detrusor–sphincter incoordination which leads to enuresis.

3 Central nervous system abnormalities, e.g. lumbar spinal cord disorders.

4 Acquired disorders, e.g. recurrent urinary tract infections.

5 Disorders causing increased volume of urine, e.g. diabetes mellitus, diabetes insipidus, obstructive sleep apnoeas.

6 Nocturnal epilepsy causing urinary incontinence.

Problems

1 Embarrassment, particularly for older children.

2 Secondary psychological reactions.

Treatment

1 Treat any contributory factor, e.g. obstructive sleep apnoeas.

2 Discontinue hypnotic drugs.

3 Reduce oral fluid intake in the evenings and avoid any diuretics, such as caffeine, in drinks.

4 Family support.

5 Training methods:

(a) Bladder training exercises during wakefulness, such as delaying micturition during the day to increase the functional bladder capacity.

(b) Sphincter training exercises involving repeatedly interrupting the urinary stream while micturating.

(c) Conditioning methods involving, for instance, enuresis alarms, which are triggered by urination, which wake the child. This leads to an increase in the awareness of incontinence and earlier sensing of detrusor muscle activity, but may take several months to be effective.

(d) Arousal techniques involving setting an alarm at regular intervals during the night before bed wetting occurs so that the child can urinate before the bladder fills.

6 Drug treatment. Cholinergic drugs such as oxybutynin can be used to stabilize the detrusor muscle and increase the functional capacity of the bladder. Tricyclic antidepressants, such as imipramine, have anticholinergic and antidiuretic effects, but may cause drowsiness and gastro-intestinal side-effects. Either nasal or oral desmopressin, a synthetic analogue of vasopressin (antidiuretic hormone, ADH), reduces the volume of urine at night even in the absence of diabetes insipidus.

There is a rapid response to desmopressin treatment which makes it suitable for short-term use, for instance if the child is away from home. None of these drugs, however, should be used in children under the age of around 7 years. They may be combined with training methods and ideally should not be used for longer than 3 months.

Impaired sleep-related penile erections

Penile erections occur predominantly during REM sleep, although they may persist into NREM sleep and after awakening. In adults their absence indicates either an alteration in sleep architecture with reduction or fragmentation of REM sleep, as in severe obstructive sleep apnoeas, or an organic cause for impotence. This may be diabetes mellitus or drugs, including selective serotonin re-uptake inhibitors and tricyclic antidepressants, and beta blockers and REM-suppressant drugs, including amphetamines and related drugs. Erections during sleep and on waking are retained with most psychogenic causes of impotence.

Painful penile erections

In this rare condition erections during sleep cause a deep penile pain, whereas those during wakefulness, such as during intercourse, are painless [15]. The pain is most intense and prolonged during the second half of the night when REM sleep is most prominent, although the erections are often more prolonged than normal and less closely linked to REM sleep so that they extend into NREM sleep. They may cause frequent nocturnal awakenings with fragmentation particularly of REM sleep. They appear to be triggered by anxiety, particularly regarding sexual relationships, and fluctuate in severity, often remitting spontaneously.

They are not associated with Peyronie's disease, which causes penile pain during erections in wakefulness as well as in sleep, and in which the pain is related to local anatomical abnormalities. Benzodiazepines and beta blockers may be of help, possibly through relieving anxiety, but there is usually only a temporary response to antidepressants.

Rheumatological disorders

Rheumatoid arthritis

This is characterized by early morning stiffness and pain, although the precise cause of this remains uncertain. Sleep is unrefreshing and there is a reduced duration of stages 3 and 4 NREM sleep and REM sleep. REM sleep deprivation also lowers the pain threshold. Polysomnography shows alpha intrusion into stages 3 and 4 NREM sleep as well as a reduced sleep efficiency.

Obstructive sleep apnoeas in rheumatoid arthritis are often due to crico-arytenoid arthritis which may respond initially to systemic steroid treatment. Surgery is occasionally required, but nasal continuous positive airway pressure is usually effective. The restless legs syndrome and periodic limb movements in sleep are also common in rheumatoid arthritis, probably because of iron deficiency associated with gastrointestinal blood loss.

Cutaneous disorders

Night sweats (sleep hyperhidrosis)

There are two to four million cutaneous eccrine sweat glands which are innervated by the sympathetic nervous system with acetylcholine as the neurotransmitter. The volume and tonicity of the sweat are controlled largely by the preoptic nucleus in the hypothalamus in order to regulate the body temperature.

Night sweats may be a physiological response to a rise in temperature, but many normal subjects complain of excess sweating at night without any demonstrable fever. This is probably due to an increased sympathetic stimulation of sweat glands and is often related to anxiety or stress, or is a response to sleep disorders such as obstructive sleep apnoeas. Menopausal night sweats are related to fluctuations in blood oestrogen levels. Night sweats also occur in thyrotoxicosis, with infections such as pulmonary tuberculosis, in lymphomas, particularly Hodgkin's disease, and occasionally in hypothalamic lesions.

Sweating at night can lead to frequent awakenings from sleep. Treatment is unsatisfactory, except for the sweats related to the menopause which respond to oestrogen replacement treatment. If night sweats are drenching and require frequent changes of nightclothes, either extensive tuberculosis or a lymphoma, such as Hodgkin's disease, should be suspected.

Nocturnal pruritus (itch)

Pruritus during sleep may be due to an identifiable skin disorder, but often occurs in the absence of this. It is most common in stages 1 and 2 NREM sleep and is probably secondary to cutaneous vasodilatation. It may also occur during REM sleep, but is least frequent in stages 3 and 4 NREM sleep. Sedating antihistamines, such as chlorpheniramine, are usually effective.

Immunological disorders and infections

Fever and infections

Fever in response to an infection is due to pyrogens, such as IL-1, some of which are also sleep factors. Both Gram positive and negative bacteria and, to a lesser extent, viral infections cause an initial increase in sleepiness and in the duration of NREM sleep with inhibition of REM sleep and later an inhibition of stages 3 and 4 NREM sleep. The induction of the fever and of NREM sleep are independent effects of cytokines. Prolongation of sleep is associated with a better survival in severe infections. The altered sleep pattern modifies the profile of melatonin secretion and this also affects the immune response to the infection.

Systemic mastocytosis

This rare disorder is associated with profound lethargy, possibly due to liberation of sleep-promoting mediators such as PGD2 from mast cells.

Paroxysmal nocturnal haemoglobinuria

In this uncommon condition, lysis of red blood cells intravascularly during sleep leads to nocturnal haemoglobinuria. It usually presents with the passing of red or brown urine after waking or with symptoms of anaemia. The condition is equally common in males and females and occurs usually between the ages of 20 and 40 years. The red cells are deficient in CD59 and HRF proteins which inhibit the C9 fraction of complement from binding to the cell membrane. C5 convertase complexes, produced by the alternative pathway of complement activation, bind to the cells. The lack of CD59 and HRF leaves the cells vulnerable to insertion of terminal complement components, especially C9, into the membrane and this leads to cell lysis. It is uncertain how sleep influences these events.

Acute severe illness and surgery

The same changes in NREM and REM sleep are seen as a response to a variety of intense physical stresses, such as myocardial infarction, stroke, acute heart failure, trauma in intensive care unit patients and after surgical procedures. Initially stages 3 and 4 NREM and REM sleep are shortened, but after a few days they increase (sleep rebound) [16]. These changes are seen, for instance, after a cholecystectomy performed by a laparotomy, but not after a laparoscopic cholecystectomy in which the surgical trauma is minimized.

General anaesthesia has little effect on subsequent sleep, and regional anaesthetics, such as an epidural, do not influence sleep. Pain is often severe enough to reduce stages 3 and 4 NREM sleep and REM sleep for 2–4 days after surgery, and the increase in catabolic hormone production, such as noradrenaline and ACTH, after trauma or surgery may modify sleep.

Coronary artery bypass grafting is followed by a prolonged reduction in total sleep time and in the duration of stages 3 and 4 NREM sleep and is associated with daytime naps. These changes last for several months, and may be the result of altered cerebral function due to the anaesthesia and surgical procedure.

Cancer

Some of the impact of cancer on sleep is specific to individual types of malignancy [17]. Cerebral metastases, for instance, can occasionally disrupt circadian rhythms or cause other specific effects on sleep–wake control. Most of the problems, however, may arise irrespective of the nature of the tumour. Sleep hygiene is often disturbed because of progressively less exercise and lack of exposure to bright light during the day, increasingly frequent naps and the use of the bedroom as a living room as well as place to sleep. Episodes of hospitalization expose the subject to increased sensory stimulation, particularly noise and light, throughout the day and often at night.

Insomnia is often due to anxiety and depression about the illness and its outcomes. Pain may disturb sleep and symptoms due to cancer therapy such as nausea and vomiting following chemotherapy, and insomnia with glucocorticoid drugs, and nocturia following diuretic treatment are common.

Excessive daytime sleepiness may be due to sleep fragmentation brought on by the factors leading to sleeplessness at night. Sedative medication, such as antidepressants and anticonvulsants, may contribute. Excessive sleepiness may also be due to neurological involvement by the tumour or to cerebral irradiation.

Sleep disorders due to cancer and its treatment are under-recognized and the initial step is to identify the problem and analyse its causes. Advice about reducing the frequency of naps, increasing exercise if possible, improving the sleep environment and maintaining regular sleep–wake routines may help. Changes in drug treatment and its timing may promote sleep at night and wakefulness during the day. Provision of specific treatment for drug-induced problems such as the restless legs syndrome due to antidepressants, or for obstructive sleep apnoeas induced by weight gain following glucocorticoid treatment, should be considered. Cognitive behavioural therapy to modify beliefs about cancer may be of help. Negative attitudes such as believing that the cancer will return if the subject does not sleep need to be addressed.

References

1 Jennum P, Jensen R. Sleep and headache. *Sleep Med Rev* 2002; 6(6): 471–9.

2 Martin RJ, Banks-Schlegel S. Chronobiology of asthma. *Am J Respir Crit Care Med* 1998; 158: 1002–7.

3 Bradley S, Solin P, Wilson J, Johns D, Walters EH, Naughton MT. Hypoxemia and hypercapnia during exercise and sleep in patients with cystic fibrosis. *Chest* 1999; 116: 647–54.

4 Schulz R, Baseler G, Ghofrani HA, Grimminger F, Olschewski H, Seeger W. Nocturnal periodic breathing in primary pulmonary hypertension. *Eur Respir J* 2002; 19: 658–63.

5 Simpson JM. Infant stress and sleep deprivation as an aetiological basis for the sudden infant death syndrome. *Early Hum Dev* 2001; 61: 1–43.

6 Coombs RRA, Holgate ST. Allergy and cot death: with special focus on allergic sensitivity to cows' milk and anaphylaxis. *Clin Exp Allergy* 1990; 20: 359–66.

7 Bonsignore MR, Smirne S, Marrone O, Insalaco G, Salvaggio A, Bonsignore G. Myocardial ischemia during sleep. *Sleep Med Rev* 1999; 3(3): 241–55.

8 Edéll-Gustafsson UM, Hetta JE, Arén CB, Hamrin EKF. Measurement of sleep and quality of life before and after coronary artery bypass grafting: a pilot study. *Int J Nurs Prac* 1997; 3: 239–46.

9 Naughton MT. Heart failure and central apnoea. *Sleep Med Rev* 1998; 2(2): 105–16.

10 Javaheri S, Parker TJ, Liming JD, Corbett WS, Nishiyama H, Wexler L, Roselle GA. Sleep apnea in 81 ambulatory male patients with stable heart failure. Types and their prevalences, consequences and presentations. *Circulation* 1998; 97: 2154–9.

11 Schulz R, Baseler G, Ghofrani HA, Grimminger F, Olschewski H, Seeger W. Nocturnal periodic breathing in primary pulmonary hypertension. *Eur Respir J* 2002; 19: 658–63.

12 Penzel T, Becker HF, Brandenburg U, Labunski T, Pankow W, Peter JH. Arousal in patients with gastro-oesophageal reflux and sleep apnoea. *Eur Respir J* 1999; 14: 1266–70.

13 Moldofsky H. Sleep and pain. *Sleep Med Rev* 2001; 5(5): 387–98.

14 Parker KP. Sleep disturbances in dialysis patients. *Sleep Med Rev* 2003; 7(2): 131–43.

15 Calvet U. Painful nocturnal erection. *Sleep Med Rev* 1999; 3: 47–57.

16 Rosenberg J. Sleep disturbances after non-cardiac surgery. *Sleep Med Rev* 2001; 5(2): 129–37.

17 Lee K, Cho M, Miaskowski C, Dodd M. Impaired sleep and rhythms in persons with cancer. *Sleep Med Rev* 2004; 8: 199–212.

Further Reading

1 Aldrich MS. *Sleep Medicine*. New York: Oxford University Press, 1999.
2 Bazil CW, Malow BA, Sammaritano MR. *Sleep and Epilepsy: The Clinical Spectrum*. Amsterdam: Elsevier, 2002.
3 Billiard M, ed. *Sleep. Physiology, Investigations and Medicine*. New York: Kluwer Academic, 2003.
4 Chokroverty S, ed. *Sleep Disorders Medicine*, 2nd edn. Boston: Butterworth, 1999.
5 Chokroverty S, Hening WA, Walters AS. *Sleep and Movement Disorders*. Philadelphia: Butterworth–Heinemann, 2003.
6 Culebras A. *Clinical Handbook of Sleep Disorders*. Boston: Butterworth–Heinemann, 1996.
7 Culebras A. *Sleep Disorders and Neurological Disease*. New York: Marcel Dekker, 2000.
8 Dement WC, Vaughan C. *The Promise of Sleep*. New York: Delacorte Press, 1999.
9 Kryger MH, Roth T, Dement WC. *Principles and Practice of Sleep Medicine*, 4th edn. Philadelphia: Elsevier. Saunders, 2005.
10 Lee-Chiong TL Jr, Satera MJ, Carskadon MA. *Sleep Medicine*. Philadelphia: Hanley and Belfus, 2002.
11 McNicholas WT, Phillipson EA. *Breathing Disorders in Sleep*. London: W.B. Saunders, 2002.
12 Mindell JA, Owen JA. *A Clinical Guide to Pediatric Sleep: Diagnosis and Management of Sleep Problems*. Philadelphia: Lippincott, Williams and Wilkins, 2003.
13 Poceta JS, Mitler MM, eds. *Sleep Disorders, Diagnosis and Treatment*. New Jersey: Humana Press, 1998.
14 Silber MH, Krahn LE, Morgenthaler TI. *Sleep Medicine in Clinical Practice*. London: Taylor and Francis, 2004.
15 Stores G, Wiggs L, ed. *Sleep Disturbance in Children and Adolescents with Disorders of Development: Its Significance and Management*. Cambridge: Cambridge University Press, 2001.
16 Stradling JR. *Handbook of Sleep-Related Breathing Disorders*. Oxford: Oxford University Press, 1993.
17 Thorpy MJ. *Handbook of Sleep Disorders*. New York: Marcel Dekker, 2000.
18 Thorpy MJ, Yager J. *The Encyclopedia of Sleep and Sleep Disorders*. New York: Facts on File, 1991.

Appendix 1

Horne Ostberg: Questionnaire to Determine Morningness and Eveningness in Human Circadian Rhythms

Instructions

1. Please read each question very carefully before answering
2. Answer ALL questions
3. Answer questions in numerical order
4. Each question should be answered independently of others. Do NOT go back and check your answers
5. All questions have a selection of answers. For each question place a cross alongside ONE answer only. Some questions have a scale instead of a selection of answers. Place a cross at the appropriate point along the scale
6. Please answer each question as honestly as possible. Both your answers and the results will be kept in strict confidence
7. Please feel free to make any comments in the section provided below each question

The Questionnaire

1. Considering only your own 'feeling best' rhythm, at what time would you get up if you were entirely free to plan your day?

AM 5   6   7   8   9   10   11   12

2. Considering only your own 'feeling best' rhythm, at what time would you go to bed if you were entirely free to plan your evening?

PM 8   9   10   11   12 AM   1   2   3

3. If there is a specific time at which you have to get up in the morning, to what extent are you dependent on being woken up by an alarm clock?

Not at all dependent . . . . ☐
Slightly dependent . . . . ☐
Fairly dependent . . . . ☐
Very dependent . . . . ☐

4. Assuming adequate environment conditions, how easy do you find getting up in the mornings?

Not at all easy . . . . ☐
Not very easy . . . . ☐
Fairly easy . . . . ☐
Very easy . . . . ☐

5. How alert do you feel during the first half hour after having woken in the morning?

Not at all alert . . . . ☐
Slightly alert. . . . . ☐
Fairly alert . . . . ☐
Very alert . . . . ☐

6. How is your appetite during the first half hour after having woken in the morning?

Very poor . . . . ☐
Fairly poor . . . . ☐
Fairly good. . . . . ☐
Very good. . . . . ☐

7. During the first half hour after having woken in the morning, how tired do you feel?

Very tired . . . . ☐
Fairly tired . . . . ☐
Fairly refreshed . . . . ☐
Very refreshed . . . . ☐

8. When you have no commitments the next day, at what time do you go to bed compared to your usual bedtime?

Seldom or never later . . . . ☐
Less than one hour later. . . . . ☐
1–2 hours later . . . . ☐
More than two hours later . . . . ☐

9. You have decided to engage in some physical exercise. A friend suggests that you do this one hour twice a week and the best time for him is between 7 AM and 8 AM. Bearing in mind nothing else but your own 'feeling best' rhythm, how do you think you would perform?

Would be on good form. . . . . ☐
Would be on reasonable form. . . . . . ☐
Would find it difficult. . . . . ☐
Would find it very difficult . . . . ☐

10. At what time in the evening do you feel tired and as a result in need of sleep?

PM 8 | 9 | 10 | 11 | 12 AM | 1 | 2 | 3

11. You wish to be at your peak performance for a test, which you know is going to be mentally exhausting and lasting for two hours. You are entirely free to plan your day. Considering you own 'feeling best' rhythm which one of the 4 testing times would you choose?

08:00 AM – 10:00 AM . . . . ☐
11:00 AM – 01:00 PM . . . . ☐
03:00 PM – 05:00 PM . . . . ☐
07:00 PM – 09:00 PM . . . . ☐

12. If you went to bed at 11:00 PM at what level of tiredness would you be?

Not at all tired . . . . ☐
A little tired . . . . ☐
Fairly tired . . . . ☐
Very tired . . . . ☐

13. For some reason you have gone to bed several hours later than usual, but there is no need to get up at any particular time the next morning. Which ONE of the following events are you most likely to experience?

Will wake up at usual time and will NOT fall asleep .... ☐
Will wake up at usual time and will doze thereafter .... ☐
Will wake up at usual time but will fall asleep again .... ☐
Will NOT wake up until later than usual .... ☐

14. One night you have to remain awake between 4.00 AM and 6.00 AM in order to carry out a night watch. You have no commitments the next day. Which ONE of the following alternatives will suit you best?

Would NOT go to bed until watch was over .... ☐
Would take a nap before and sleep after .... ☐
Would take a good sleep before and nap after .... ☐
Would take ALL sleep before watch .... ☐

15. You have to do two hours of hard physical work. You are entirely free to plan your day. Considering only your own 'feeling best' rhythm which ONE of the following times would you choose?

08:00 AM – 10:00 AM .... ☐
11:00 AM – 01:00 PM .... ☐
03:00 PM – 05:00 PM .... ☐
07:00 PM – 09:00 PM .... ☐

16. You have decided to engage in hard physical exercise. A friend suggests that you do this for one hour twice a week and the best time for him is between 10:00 PM and 11:00 PM. Bearing in mind nothing else but your own 'feeling best' rhythm how well do you think you would perform.

Would be on good form.......... ☐
Would be on reasonable form..... ☐
Would find it difficult........... ☐
Would find it very difficult .... ☐

17. Suppose that you could choose your own work hours. Assume that you worked a FIVE hour day (including breaks) and that your job was interesting and paid by results. Which FIVE CONSECUTIVE HOURS would you select?

12	1	2	3	4	5	6	7	8	9	10	11	12	1	2	3	4	5	6	7	8	9	10	11	12

Midnight   Noon   Midnight

18. At what time of the day do you think that you reach your 'feeling best' peak?

12	1	2	3	4	5	6	7	8	9	10	11	12	1	2	3	4	5	6	7	8	9	10	11	12

Midnight   Noon   Midnight

19. One hears about 'morning' and 'evening' types of people. Which ONE of these types do you consider yourself to be?

Definitely a morning type .... ☐
Rather more a morning type than an evening type .... ☐
Rather more an evening type than a morning type .... ☐
Definitely an evening type .... ☐

Appendix 2

Pittsburgh Sleep Quality Index (PSQI)

Instructions: The following questions relate to your usual sleep habits during the past month only. Your answers should indicate the most accurate reply for the majority of days and nights in the past month. Please answer all questions.

1. *During the past month, when have you usually gone to bed at night?*
   USUAL BED TIME:_____

2. *During the past month, how long has it usually taken you to fall asleep each night?*
   NUMBER OF MINUTES:_____

3. *During the past month, when have you usually gotten up in the morning?*
   USUAL GETTING UP TIME:_____

4. *During the past month, how many hours of actual sleep did you get at night?*
   (This may be different than the number of hours you spend in bed.)
   HOURS OF SLEEP PER NIGHT:_____

For each of the remaining questions, check the one best response. Please answer all questions.

5. *During the past month, how often have you had trouble sleeping because you . . .*
   (a) *Cannot get to sleep within 30 minutes*

| Not during the past month __ | Less than once a week __ | Once or twice a week __ | Three or more times a week __ |

   (b) *Wake up in the middle of the night or early morning*

| Not during the past month __ | Less than once a week __ | Once or twice a week __ | Three or more times a week __ |

   (c) *Have to get up to use the bathroom*

| Not during the past month __ | Less than once a week __ | Once or twice a week __ | Three or more times a week __ |

   (d) *Cannot breathe comfortably*

| Not during the past month __ | Less than once a week __ | Once or twice a week __ | Three or more times a week __ |

   (e) *Cough or snore loudly*

| Not during the past month __ | Less than once a week __ | Once or twice a week __ | Three or more times a week __ |

   (f) *Feel too cold*

| Not during the past month __ | Less than once a week __ | Once or twice a week __ | Three or more times a week __ |

   (g) *Feel too hot*

| Not during the past month __ | Less than once a week __ | Once or twice a week __ | Three or more times a week __ |

(h) *Had bad dreams*

| Not during the past month __ | Less than once a week __ | Once or twice a week __ | Three or more times a week __ |

(i) *Have pain*

| Not during the past month __ | Less than once a week __ | Once or twice a week __ | Three or more times a week __ |

(j) Other reason(s), please describe: _____

_____

How often during the past month have you had trouble sleeping because of this?

| Not during the past month __ | Less than once a week __ | Once or twice a week __ | Three or more times a week __ |

6. *During the past month, how would you rate your sleep quality overall?*

Very good: _____
Fairly good: _____
Fairly bad: _____
Very bad: _____

7. *During the past month, how often have you taken medicine (prescribed or 'over the counter') to help you sleep?*

| Not during the past month __ | Less than once a week __ | Once or twice a week __ | Three or more times a week __ |

8. *During the past month, how often have you had trouble staying awake while driving, eating meals, or engaging in social activity?*

| Not during the past month __ | Less than once a week __ | Once or twice a week __ | Three or more times a week __ |

9. *During the past month, how much of a problem has it been for you to keep up enough enthusiasm to get things done?*

No problem at all _____
Only a very slight problem _____
Somewhat of a problem _____
A very big problem _____

10. *Do you have a bed partner or roommate?*

No bed partner or roommate _____
Partner/roommate in other room _____
Partner in same room, but not same bed _____
Partner in same bed _____

If you have a roommate or bed partner, ask him/her how often in the past month you have had . . .

(a) *Loud snoring*

| Not during the past month __ | Less than once a week __ | Once or twice a week __ | Three or more times a week __ |

(b) *Long pauses between breaths while asleep*

| Not during the past month __ | Less than once a week __ | Once or twice a week __ | Three or more times a week __ |

(c) *Legs twitching or jerking while you sleep*

| Not during the past month __ | Less than once a week __ | Once or twice a week __ | Three or more times a week __ |

(d) *Episodes of disorientation or confusion during sleep*

| Not during the past month __ | Less than once a week __ | Once or twice a week __ | Three or more times a week __ |

(e) *Other restlessness while you sleep, please describe* _____

_____

| Not during the past month __ | Less than once a week __ | Once or twice a week __ | Three or more times a week __ |

Appendix 3

Shortform-36 Health Survey

INSTRUCTIONS: This survey asks for your views about your health. This information will help keep track of how you feel and how well you are able to do your usual activities.

Answer every question by marking the answer as indicated. If you are unsure about how to answer a question, please give the best answer you can.

1. In general, would you say your health is:

(circle one)

Excellent..1
Very good...2
Good..3
Fair 4
Poor..5

2. *Compared to one year ago*, how would you rate your health in general *now*?

(circle one)

Much better now than one year ago 1
Somewhat better now than one year ago 2
About the same as one year ago 3
Somewhat worse now than one year ago 4
Much worse now than one year ago 5

3. The following questions are about activities you might do during a typical day. Does *your health now limit you* in these activities? If so, how much?

(circle one number on each line)

ACTIVITIES	Yes, Limited A Lot	Yes, Limited A Little	No, Not Limited At All
a. **Vigorous activities,** such as running, lifting heavy objects, participating in strenuous sports	1	2	3
b. **Moderate activities,** such as moving a table, pushing a vacuum cleaner, bowling, or playing golf	1	2	3
c. Lifting or carrying groceries	1	2	3
d. Climbing **several** flights of stairs	1	2	3
e. Climbing **one** flight of stairs	1	2	3
f. Bending, kneeling, or stooping	1	2	3
g. Walking **more than a mile**	1	2	3
h. Walking **half a mile**	1	2	3
i. Walking **one hundred yards**	1	2	3
j. Bathing or dressing yourself	1	2	3

4. During the *past 4 weeks*, have you had any of the following problems with your work or other regular daily activities *as a result of your physical health*?

(circle one number on each line)

	YES	NO
a. Cut down on the **amount of time** you spent on work or other activities	1	2
b. **Accomplished less** than you would like	1	2
c. Were limited in the **kind** of work or other activities	1	2
d. Had **difficulty** performing the work or other activities (for example, it took extra effort)	1	2

5. During the *past 4 weeks*, have you had any of the following problems with your work or other regular daily activities *as a result of any emotional problems* (such as feeling depressed or anxious)?

(circle one number on each line)

	YES	NO
a. Cut down on the **amount of time** you spent on work or other activities	1	2
b. **Accomplished less** than you would like	1	2
c. Didn't do work or other activities as **carefully** as usual	1	2

6. During the *past 4 weeks*, to what extent has your physical health or emotional problems interfered with your normal social activities with family, friends, neighbours, or groups?

(circle one)

Not at all 1
Slightly 2
Moderately 3
Quite a bit 4
Extremely 5

7. How much *bodily* pain have you had during the *past 4 weeks*?

(circle one)

None 1
Very mild 2
Mild 3
Moderate 4
Severe 5
Very severe 6

8. During the *past 4 weeks*, how much did *pain* interfere with your normal work (including both work outside the home and housework)?

(circle one)

Not at all 1
A little bit 2
Moderately 3
Quite a bit 4
Extremely 5

9. These questions are about how you feel and how things have been with you *during the past 4 weeks*. For each question, please give the one answer that comes closest to the way you have been feeling. How much of the time during the *past 4 weeks* –

(circle one number on each line)

	All of the Time	Most of the Time	A Good Bit of the Time	Some of the Time	A Little of the Time	None of the Time
a. Did you feel full of life?	1	2	3	4	5	6
b. Have you been a very nervous person?	1	2	3	4	5	6
c. Have you felt so down in the dumps that nothing could cheer you up?	1	2	3	4	5	6
d. Have you felt calm and peaceful?	1	2	3	4	5	6
e. Did you have a lot of energy?	1	2	3	4	5	6
f. Have you felt downhearted and low?	1	2	3	4	5	6
g. Did you feel worn out?	1	2	3	4	5	6
h. Have you been a happy person?	1	2	3	4	5	6
i. Did you feel tired?	1	2	3	4	5	6

10. During the *past 4 weeks*, how much of the time has your *physical health or emotional problems* interfered with your social activities (like visiting with friends, relatives, etc.)?

(circle one)

All of the time 1
Most of the time 2
Some of the time 3
A little of the time 4
None of the time 5

11. How TRUE or FALSE is *each* of the following statements for you?

(circle one number on each line)

	Definitely True	Mostly True	Don't Know	Mostly False	Definitely False
a. I seem to get ill more easily than other people	1	2	3	4	5
b. I am as healthy as anybody I know	1	2	3	4	5
c. I expect my health to get worse	1	2	3	4	5
d. My health is excellent	1	2	3	4	5

Appendix 4

Functional Outcomes of Sleep Questionnaire

Some people have difficulty performing everyday activities when they feel tired or sleepy. The purpose of this questionnaire is to find out if you generally have difficulty carrying out certain activities because you are too sleepy or tired. In this questionnaire, when the words 'sleep' or 'tired' are used, it means the feeling that you can't keep your eyes open, your head is droopy, that you want to 'nod off', or that you feel the urge to take a nap. These words do *not* refer to the tired or fatigued feeling you may have after you have exercised.

DIRECTIONS: Please put a (Y) in the box for your answer to each question. Select only *one* answer for each question. Please try to be as accurate as possible. All information will be kept confidential.

	(0) I don't do this activity for other reasons	(4) No difficulty	(3) Yes, a little difficulty	(2) Yes, moderate difficulty	(1) Yes, extreme difficulty
1 Do you have difficulty concentrating on things you do because you are sleepy or tired?		☐	☐	☐	☐
2 Do you generally have difficulty remembering things because you are sleepy or tired?		☐	☐	☐	☐
3 Do you have difficulty finishing a meal because you become sleepy or tired?		☐	☐	☐	☐
4 Do you have difficulty working on a hobby (for example, sewing, collecting, gardening) because you are sleepy or tired?	☐	☐	☐	☐	☐
5 Do you have difficulty doing work around the house (for example, cleaning house, doing laundry, taking out the trash, repair work) because you are sleepy or tired?	☐	☐	☐	☐	☐
6 Do you have difficulty operating a motor vehicle for *short* distances (less than 100 miles) because you become sleepy or tired?	☐	☐	☐	☐	☐

	(0) I don't do this activity for other reasons	(4) No difficulty	(3) Yes, a little difficulty	(2) Yes, moderate difficulty	(1) Yes, extreme difficulty
7 Do you have difficulty operating a motor vehicle for *long* distances (greater than 100 miles) because you become sleepy or tired?	☐	☐	☐	☐	☐
8 Do you have difficulty getting things done because you are too sleepy or tired to drive or take public transportation?	☐	☐	☐	☐	☐
9 Do you have difficulty taking care of financial affairs and doing paperwork (for example, writing checks, paying bills, keeping financial records, filling out tax forms, etc.) because you are sleepy or tired?	☐	☐	☐	☐	☐
10 Do you have difficulty performing employed or volunteer work because you are sleepy or tired?	☐	☐	☐	☐	☐
11 Do you have difficulty maintaining a telephone conversation because you become sleepy or tired?	☐	☐	☐	☐	☐
12 Do you have difficulty visiting with your family or friends in *your* home because you become sleepy or tired?	☐	☐	☐	☐	☐
13 Do you have difficulty visiting your family or friends in *their* home because you come sleepy or tired?	☐	☐	☐	☐	☐
14 Do you have difficulty doing things for your family or friends because you are too sleepy or tired?	☐	☐	☐	☐	☐
15 Has your relationship with family, friends or work colleagues been affected because you are sleepy or tired?	☐	☐	☐	☐	☐
16 Do you have difficulty exercising or participating in a sporting activity because you are too sleepy or tired?	☐	☐	☐	☐	☐

	(0) I don't do this activity for other reasons	(4) No difficulty	(3) Yes, a little difficulty	(2) Yes, moderate difficulty	(1) Yes, extreme difficulty
17 Do you have difficulty watching a movie or videotape because you become sleepy or tired?	☐	☐	☐	☐	☐
18 Do you have difficulty enjoying the theatre or a lecture because you become sleepy or tired?	☐	☐	☐	☐	☐
19 Do you have difficulty enjoying a concert because you become sleepy or tired?	☐	☐	☐	☐	☐
20 Do you have difficulty watching TV because you are sleepy or tired?	☐	☐	☐	☐	☐
21 Do you have difficulty participating in religious services, meetings or a group or club because you are sleepy or tired?	☐	☐	☐	☐	☐
22 Do you have difficulty being as active as you want to be in the *evening* because you are sleepy or tired?	☐	☐	☐	☐	☐
23 Do you have difficulty being as active as you want to be in the *morning* because you are sleepy or tired?	☐	☐	☐	☐	☐
24 Do you have difficulty being as active as you want to be in the *afternoon* because you are sleepy or tired?	☐	☐	☐	☐	☐
25 Do you have difficulty keeping pace with others your own age because you are sleepy or tired?	☐	☐	☐	☐	☐

	(1) Very low	(2) Low	(3) Medium	(4) High
26 How would you rate your general level of activity?	☐	☐	☐	☐

(0) No intimate or sexual relationship	(4) No	(3) Yes, a little	(2) Yes, moderately	(1) Yes, extremely
☐	☐	☐	☐	☐

27　Has your intimate or sexual relationship been affected because you are sleepy or tired?

(0) I don't engage in sexual activity for other reasons	(4) No	(3) Yes, a little	(2) Yes, moderately	(1) Yes, extremely
☐	☐	☐	☐	☐
☐	☐	☐	☐	☐
☐	☐	☐	☐	☐

28　Has your desire for intimacy or sex been affected because you are sleepy or tired?

29　Has your ability to become sexually aroused been affected because you are sleepy or tired?

30　Has your ability to 'come' (have an orgasm) been affected because you are sleepy or tired?

Appendix 5

Medical Outcome Study Sleep Scale

YOUR SLEEP

1. How long did it usually take you to *go to sleep* during the *past 4 weeks*?

(Circle one of the numbers 1 to 5)

0–15 minutes	1
16–30 minutes	2
31–45 minutes	3
46–60 minutes	4
More than 60 minutes	5

2. On average, how many hours did you sleep *each night* during the *past 4 weeks*?

Write in the number of hours per night: ☐☐

How often during the *past 4 weeks* did you . . .

(Circle one number for each question)

	All of the time	Most of the time	A good bit of the time	Some of the time	A little of the time	None of the time
3. feel that your sleep was not peaceful (moving restlessly, feeling tense, speaking, etc., while sleeping)?	1	2	3	4	5	6
4. get enough sleep to feel rested when waking up in the morning?	1	2	3	4	5	6
5. wake up short of breath or with a headache?	1	2	3	4	5	6
6. feel drowsy or sleepy during the day?	1	2	3	4	5	6
7. have trouble going to sleep?	1	2	3	4	5	6

How often during the *past 4 weeks* did you . . .

(Circle one number for each question)

	All of the time	Most of the time	A good bit of the time	Some of the time	A little of the time	None of the time
8. wake up during your sleep and have trouble going back to sleep again?	1	2	3	4	5	6
9. have trouble staying awake during the day?	1	2	3	4	5	6
10. snore during your sleep?	1	2	3	4	5	6
11. take naps (5 minutes or longer) during the day?	1	2	3	4	5	6
12. get the amount of sleep you needed?	1	2	3	4	5	6

Appendix 6

Stanford Sleepiness Scale

1. Alert. Wide awake. Energetic.
2. Functioning at a high level, but not at peak. Able to concentrate.
3. Awake, but not fully alert.
4. A little foggy, let down.
5. Foggy. Beginning to lose interest in remaining awake. Slowed down.
6. Sleepy. Prefer to be lying down. Woozy.
7. Cannot stay awake. Sleep onset soon.
X. Asleep.

Appendix 7

Epworth Sleepiness Scale

How likely are you to doze off or fall asleep in the following situations, in contrast to just feeling tired? This refers to your usual way of life in the last few weeks. Even if you have not done some of these things recently, try to work out how they would have affected you. Use the following scale to choose the most appropriate number for each situation. Please tick one box on each line.

0 = Would never doze
1 = Slight chance of dozing
2 = Moderate chance of dozing
3 = High chance of dozing

Situation	0	1	2	3
Sitting and reading				
Watching television				
Sitting inactive in a public place (e.g. a theatre or a meeting)				
As a passenger in a car for an hour without a break				
Lying down in the afternoon, when circumstances permit				
Sitting and talking to someone				
Sitting quietly after lunch without alcohol				
In a car, while stopped for a few minutes in the traffic				

Appendix 8

Ullanlinna Narcolepsy Scale

1. *When laughing, becoming glad or angry or in an exciting situation, have the following symptoms suddenly occurred?*

Manifestation	Never	1–5 times during lifetime	Monthly	Weekly	Daily or almost daily
Knees unlocking	_____	_____	_____	_____	_____
Mouth opening	_____	_____	_____	_____	_____
Head nodding	_____	_____	_____	_____	_____
Falling down	_____	_____	_____	_____	_____

2. *How fast do you usually fall asleep in the evening?*

> 40 min	31–40 min	21–30 min	10–20 min	< 10 min
_____	_____	_____	_____	_____

3. *Do you sleep during the day (take naps)?*

No need	I wanted but cannot sleep	Twice weekly or less	On 3–5 days weekly	Daily or almost daily
_____	_____	_____	_____	_____

4. *Do you fall asleep unintentionally during the day?*

Situation	Never	Monthly or less	Weekly	Daily	Several times daily
Reading	_____	_____	_____	_____	_____
Travelling	_____	_____	_____	_____	_____
Standing	_____	_____	_____	_____	_____
Eating	_____	_____	_____	_____	_____
Other unusual	_____	_____	_____	_____	_____

Appendix 9

Restless Legs Syndrome Rating Scale

Have the patient rate his/her symptoms for the following ten questions. The patient and not the examiner should make the ratings, but the examiner should be available to clarify any misunderstandings the patient may have about the questions. The examiner should mark the patient's answers on the form.

In the past week . . .

(1) *Overall*, how would you rate the *RLS discomfort in your legs or arms?*

☐   Very severe
☐   Severe
☐   Moderate
☐   Mild
☐   None

(2) *Overall*, how would you rate the *need to move* around because of your RLS symptoms?

☐   Very severe
☐   Severe
☐   Moderate
☐   Mild
☐   None

(3) *Overall*, how much *relief* of your RLS arm or leg discomfort did you get from moving around?

☐   No relief
☐   Mild relief
☐   Moderate relief
☐   Either complete or almost complete relief
☐   No RLS symptoms to be relieved

(4) How severe was your *sleep disturbance* due to your RLS symptoms?

☐   Very severe
☐   Severe
☐   Moderate
☐   Mild
☐   None

(5) How severe was your *tiredness* or *sleepiness during the day due* to your RLS symptoms?

☐   Very severe
☐   Severe

In the past week . . .

- ☐ Moderate
- ☐ Mild
- ☐ None

(6) How severe was your *RLS as a whole*?

- ☐ Very severe
- ☐ Severe
- ☐ Moderate
- ☐ Mild
- ☐ None

(7) How *often* did you get RLS symptoms?

- ☐ Very severe (This means 6 to 7 days a week)
- ☐ Severe (This means 4 to 5 days a week)
- ☐ Moderate (This means 2 to 3 days a week)
- ☐ Mild (This means 1 day a week)
- ☐ None (This means less than one day a week)

(8) When you had RLS symptoms, how severe were they on average?

- ☐ Very severe (This means 8 hours or more per 24 hour per day)
- ☐ Severe (This means 3 to 8 hours per 24 hour day)
- ☐ Moderate (This means 1 to 3 hours per day 24 hour day)
- ☐ Mild (This means less than 1 hour per 24 hour day)
- ☐ None

(9) *Overall*, how severe was the impact of your RLS symptoms on your ability to carry out your *daily affairs*, for example carrying out a satisfactory family, home, social school or work life?

- ☐ Very severe
- ☐ Severe
- ☐ Moderate
- ☐ Mild
- ☐ None

(10) How severe was your *mood disturbance* due to your RLS symptoms – for example angry, depressed, sad, anxious or irritable?

- ☐ Very severe
- ☐ Severe
- ☐ Moderate
- ☐ Mild
- ☐ None

Appendix 10

Restless Legs Syndrome Quality of Life Questionnaire

The following are some questions on how your Restless Legs Syndrome might affect your quality of life. Answer each of the items below in relation to your life experience in the past 4 weeks. Please mark only one answer for each question.

In the past four weeks:

1. How distressing to you were your restless legs?

☐ Not at all ☐ A little ☐ Some ☐ Quite a bit ☐ A lot

2. How often in the past 4 weeks did your restless legs disrupt your routine evening activities?

☐ Never ☐ A few times ☐ Sometimes ☐ Most of the time
☐ All the time

3. How often in the past 4 weeks did restless legs keep you from attending your evening social activities?

☐ Never ☐ A few times ☐ Sometimes ☐ Most of the time
☐ All the time

4. In the past 4 weeks how much trouble did you have getting up in the morning due to restless legs?

☐ Not at all ☐ A little ☐ Some ☐ Quite a bit ☐ A lot

5. In the past 4 weeks how often were you late for work or your first appointments of the day due to restless legs?

☐ Never ☐ A few times ☐ Sometimes ☐ Most of the time
☐ All the time

6. How many days in the past 4 weeks were you late for work or your first appointments of the day due to restless legs?

Write in number of days ☐☐

7. How often in the past 4 weeks did you have trouble concentrating in the afternoon?

☐ Never ☐ A few times ☐ Sometimes ☐ Most of the time
☐ All the time

8. How often in the past 4 weeks did you have trouble concentrating in the evening?

☐ Never ☐ A few times ☐ Sometimes ☐ Most of the time
☐ All the time

In the past four weeks:

9. In the past 4 weeks how much was your ability to make good decisions affected by sleep problems?

☐ Not at all ☐ A little ☐ Some ☐ Quite a bit ☐ A lot

10. How often in the past 4 weeks would you have avoided travelling when the trip would have lasted more than two hours?

☐ Never ☐ A few times ☐ Sometimes ☐ Most of the time
☐ All the time

11. In the past 4 weeks how much interest did you have in sexual activity?

☐ Not at all ☐ A little ☐ Some ☐ Quite a bit ☐ A lot
☐ Prefer not to answer

12. How much did restless legs disturb or reduce your sexual activities?

☐ Not at all ☐ A little ☐ Some ☐ Quite a bit ☐ A lot
☐ Prefer not to answer

13. In the past 4 weeks how much did your restless legs disturb your ability to carry out your daily activities, for example carrying out a satisfactory family, home, social, school or work life?

☐ Not at all ☐ A little ☐ Some ☐ Quite a bit ☐ A lot

14. Do you currently work full or part time (paid work, unpaid or volunteer)?
(mark one box)

☐ YES If Yes please answer questions #15 through #18
☐ NO, because of my RLS – Thank you, you have now completed the questionnaire
☐ NO, due to other reasons – Thank you, you have now completed the questionnaire

15. How often did restless legs make it difficulty for you to work a full day in the past 4 weeks?

☐ Never ☐ A few times ☐ Sometimes ☐ Most of the time
☐ All the time

16. How many days in the past 4 weeks did you work less than you would like due to restless legs?

Write in number of days ☐☐

17. On the average, how many hours did you work in the past 4 weeks?

Write in number of hours ☐☐

18. On the days you worked less than you would like, on average about how many hours less did you work due to your restless legs.

Write in number of hours per day ☐☐

Index